The Case Against Conversion "Therapy"

The Case Against Conversion "Therapy"

Evidence, Ethics, and Alternatives

Edited by
Douglas C. Haldeman

 AMERICAN PSYCHOLOGICAL ASSOCIATION

Published by
American Psychological Association
750 First Street, NE
Washington, DC 20002
https://www.apa.org

Order Department
https://www.apa.org/pubs/books
order@apa.org

In the U.K., Europe, Africa, and the Middle East, copies may be ordered from Eurospan
https://www.eurospanbookstore.com/apa
info@eurospangroup.com

Typeset in Charter and Interstate by Circle Graphics, Inc., Reisterstown, MD

Printer: Gasch Printing, Odenton, MD
Cover Designer: Gwen J. Grafft, Minneapolis, MN

Library of Congress Cataloging-in-Publication Data

Names: Haldeman, Douglas C., editor.
Title: The case against conversion "therapy" : evidence, ethics, and alternatives / edited by Douglas C. Haldeman.
Description: Washington, DC : American Psychological Association, [2022] | Includes bibliographical references and index.
Identifiers: LCCN 2021022248 (print) | LCCN 2021022249 (ebook) | ISBN 9781433837111 (paperback) | ISBN 9781433837128 (ebook)
Subjects: LCSH: Homosexuality—Treatment—Moral and ethical aspects. | Sexual reorientation programs. | Sexual orientation. | Gays—Mental health.
Classification: LCC RC558 .C326 2022 (print) | LCC RC558 (ebook) | DDC 616.85/83—dc23
LC record available at https://lccn.loc.gov/2021022248
LC ebook record available at https://lccn.loc.gov/2021022249

https://doi.org/10.1037/0000266-000

Printed in the United States of America

10 9 8 7 6 5 4 3 2 1

Contents

Contributors

Sam Brinton, The Trevor Project

Linda F. Campbell, PhD, University of Georgia, Athens, GA, United States, and the Center for Counseling and Personal Evaluation

Raven K. Cokley, NCC, PhD, University of Georgia, Athens, GA, United States

Jack Drescher, MD, Columbia University, New York, NY, United States; New York University, New York, NY, United States; and Distinguished Life Fellow of the American Psychiatric Association

Judith M. Glassgold, PsyD, Rutgers University, Piscataway, NJ, United States

Frank B. Gorritz, APC, NCC, University of Georgia, Athens, GA, United States

Melissa J. Grey, PhD, Monroe County Community College, Monroe, MI, United States

Douglas C. Haldeman, PhD, John F. Kennedy University, Pleasant Hill, CA, United States, and Past President, California Psychological Association

Kristin A. Hancock, PhD, John F. Kennedy University, Pleasant Hill, CA, United States

Michael L. Hendricks, PhD, ABPP, Washington Psychological Center, PC, Washington, DC, United States

Sharon G. Horne, PhD, University of Massachusetts Boston, Boston, MA, United States

Mallaigh McGinley, Doctoral Student in Counseling Psychology at the University of Massachusetts Boston, Boston, MA, United States

Seth T. Pardo, PhD, San Francisco Department of Public Health, San Francisco, CA, United States

Thomas G. Plante, PhD, ABPP, Santa Clara University, Santa Clara, CA, United States, and Stanford University School of Medicine, Stanford, CA, United States

David P. Rivera, PhD, Queens College–City University of New York, Queens, NY, United States

Caitlin Ryan, PhD, ACSW, Family Acceptance Project, San Francisco State University, San Francisco, CA, United States

Anneliese A. Singh, PhD, LPC, Tulane University, New Orleans, LA, United States

Foreword

This is a timely book. At the time of its publication, the world is experiencing a growing regulation of conversion therapy (Drescher et al., 2016). In the United States, 20 states, the District of Columbia, and the Commonwealth of Puerto Rico ban licensed professionals from trying to change a person's sexual orientation or gender identity. Similar bans have been introduced in many other state legislatures. In U.S. states without bans, local municipalities have issued their own. Three Canadian provinces (Ontario, Manitoba, and Nova Scotia) also have bans, and in provinces without them, local, municipal bans exist. Additionally, bans are increasingly passed internationally.

How did we get here? Once upon a time, it was possible to walk into a mental health professional's office and ask for assistance in changing one's sexual orientation or gender identity. The opportunity to provide such a service was even offered to Sigmund Freud a century ago. In 1920, he published his thoughts about his clinical encounter with a teenage girl whose parents engaged him to change her behavior and sexual orientation. Freud (1955/1920) wryly noted,

> Parents expect one to cure their nervous and unruly child. By a healthy child they mean one who never causes his parents trouble, and gives them nothing but pleasure. The physician may succeed in curing the child, but after that it goes its own way all the more decidedly, and the parents are now far more dissatisfied than before. (p. 150)

Despite such misgivings, Freud took on the case, expressing pessimism to his readers (although he did not record what he said to the parents) about the prospects of effecting change:

> Such an achievement—the removal of genital inversion or homosexuality—is in my experience never an easy matter. . . . In general, to undertake to convert a fully developed homosexual into a heterosexual does not offer much more prospect of success than the reverse, except that for good practical reasons the latter is never attempted. (Freud, 1955/1920, p. 151)

The generation of psychoanalysts who came after Freud, unfortunately, approached the possibility of sexual orientation change with greater enthusiasm. While claiming direct lineage with Freud's ideas, they tinkered with his theories in ways that fit their own therapeutic agendas (Drescher, 1998). For example, Freud (1953/1905) said all humans were bisexual, but Sandor Rado (1940), whose work informed many psychoanalytic conversion therapy theorists, said they were not. Freud (1955/1920) said homosexuality was not an illness, by which he meant it was not a neurotic conflict, and Charles Socarides (1968) later asserted that it was.

The history of long, expensive, and ultimately ineffective psychoanalytic conversion talk therapies is troubling enough. Also disquieting were those offered by behaviorists of the mid-20th century: pain-inducing, aversive conditioning using electric shock; deprivation of food and liquids; smelling salts; and chemically induced nausea. These conversion therapy practitioners also experimented with biofeedback, hypnosis, masturbation reconditioning, cognitive behavior therapy, systematic desensitization, and combinations of these approaches (American Psychological Association, Task Force on the Appropriate Therapeutic Response to Sexual Orientation, 2009).

No matter that even to this day no one has yet established—scientifically, that is—the "causes" of a homosexual or heterosexual orientation or of a transgender or cisgender identity. After all, what need for true scientific knowledge when one had a working theory and desperate patients and families willing to pay to test one's theories?

The conversion therapy landscape would change dramatically after 1973, when the Board of Trustees (BOT) of the American Psychiatric Association voted to remove homosexuality from its list of mental disorders, the second edition of the *Diagnostic and Statistical Manual* (*DSM-II*, American Psychiatric Association, 1968). Detailed accounts of that history can be found elsewhere (Bayer, 1981; Drescher, 2015; Drescher & Merlino, 2007). In brief: Gay activists disrupted the 1970 annual meeting of the American Psychiatric Association in San Francisco. Those events catalyzed an internal process within the organization of committee meetings, hearings, interviews, scientific symposia, and journal publications (i.e., Green, 1972; Stoller et al., 1973). All this led to a closer scrutiny of the historic reasoning—that is, since the 19th century—for psychopathologizing homosexuality. Following a lengthy deliberative process by many of its committees, the American Psychiatric Association's BOT voted to remove homosexuality from the *DSM-II*.[1]

Following the 1973 change, the mental health landscape changed radically. National mental health organizations issued position statements in support of lesbian, gay, bisexual, and transgender civil rights. Mental health training programs eventually stopped teaching trainees how to try to change anyone's sexual orientation or gender identity. Today, one would be hard-pressed to find a psychiatric residency or clinical psychology program, a social work or nursing school, or a physician's assistant or counseling program that teaches any form of what has come to be known as sexual orientation conversion efforts (known as SOCE) or conversion therapy.

The American Psychiatric Association's 1973 decision did not lead to the immediate demise of conversion therapy practices within the mainstream. That change took time. Even up until the 1990s, the mental health mainstream took no positions on the issue. Consequently, one could reasonably interpret the professional mainstream's viewpoint as "There is no harm in trying."[2] Only after pioneers—such as this volume's editor, Douglas Haldeman (1991, 1994)—began writing about the troubling implications of allowing such practices did the mental health mainstream begin to take notice and speak up and speak out against them.

Once the mental health mainstream began speaking out against conversion therapy practices, legislatures started paying attention. However, banning licensed professionals from converting minors constitutes a large metaphorical hammer for a very small nail, as conversion therapy practitioners are usually unlicensed and most of their clients are not minors. Nevertheless, these bans serve the purpose of protecting the most vulnerable members of the public, underscore a change in social acceptance of lesbian, gay, bisexual, and transgender people, and send a message regarding the social unacceptability of conversion therapy efforts.

---

[1]This process, it should be noted, ultimately led American psychiatry to reformulate its entire diagnostic system and a significant transformation of psychiatric nosology in *DSM-III* (American Psychiatric Association, 1980).

[2]I attended a New York City conference on homosexuality in the 1980s where a prominent figure in the psychiatry world, who had been instrumental in removing homosexuality from the *DSM*, expressed such an opinion.

What should the next step be? Consumer protection laws. If conversion therapies were treated as the consumer fraud they are, both licensed and unlicensed practitioners would be subject to penalties for engaging in such practices. Such laws would also protect adults as well as children.

Which brings us to the necessity for this volume. Why is it relevant? Because conversion therapies are still being practiced. Often individuals ask, "Is that still going on?" Sadly, the answer is "Yes." People are being harmed, sometimes by well-meaning but misguided individuals and at other times by quacks and charlatans. We hope that this volume will spur the kind of social change needed to protect individuals of all ages from further harm.

—*Jack Drescher, MD*
Clinical Professor of Psychiatry, Columbia University
Adjunct Professor, New York University
New York, New York

REFERENCES

American Psychiatric Association. (1968). *Diagnostic and statistical manual of mental disorders* (2nd ed.). American Psychiatric Press.

American Psychiatric Association. (1980). *Diagnostic and statistical manual of mental disorders* (3rd ed.). American Psychiatric Press.

American Psychological Association, Task Force on the Appropriate Therapeutic Response to Sexual Orientation. (2009). *Report of the Task Force on the Appropriate Therapeutic Response to Sexual Orientation.*

Bayer, R. (1981). *Homosexuality and American psychiatry: The politics of diagnosis.* Basic Books.

Drescher, J. (1998). I'm your handyman: A history of reparative therapies. *Journal of Homosexuality, 36*(1), 19–42. https://doi.org/10.1300/J082v36n01_02

Drescher, J. (2015). Out of *DSM:* Depathologizing homosexuality. *Behavioral Sciences, 5*(4), 565–575. https://doi.org/10.3390/bs5040565

Drescher, J., & Merlino, J. P. (Eds.). (2007). *American psychiatry and homosexuality: An oral history.* Routledge.

Drescher, J., Schwartz, A., Casoy, F., McIntosh, C. A., Hurley, B., Ashley, K., Barber, M., Goldenberg, D., Herbert, S. E., Lothwell, L. E., Mattson, M. R., McAfee, S. G., Pula, J., Rosario, V., & Tompkins, D. A. (2016). The growing regulation of conversion therapy. *Journal of Medical Regulation, 102*(2), 7–12. https://doi.org/10.30770/2572-1852-102.2.7

Freud, S. (1953). A case of hysteria: Three essays on sexuality and other works. In S. Freud, *The standard edition of the complete psychological works of Sigmund Freud: Volume VII (1901–1905)* (pp. 123–246). Hogarth Press. (Original work published 1905)

Freud, S. (1955). The psychogenesis of a case of homosexuality in a woman. In S. Freud, *The standard edition of the complete psychological works of Sigmund Freud: Volume XVIII* (pp. 145–172). Hogarth Press. (Original work published 1920)

Green, R. (1972). Homosexuality as a mental illness. *International Journal of Psychiatry, 10*(1), 77–98.

Haldeman, D. C. (1991). Sexual orientation conversion therapy for gay men and lesbians: A scientific examination. In J. C. Gonsiorek & J. D. Weinrich (Eds.), *Homosexuality: Research implications for public policy* (pp. 149–160). Sage Publications. https://doi.org/10.4135/9781483325422.n10

Haldeman, D. C. (1994). The practice and ethics of sexual orientation conversion therapy. *Journal of Consulting and Clinical Psychology, 62*(2), 221–227. https://doi.org/10.1037/0022-006X.62.2.221

Rado, S. (1940). A critical examination of the concept of bisexuality. *Psychosomatic Medicine, 2*(4), 459–467. https://doi.org/10.1097/00006842-194010000-00007

Socarides, C. W. (1968). *The overt homosexual.* Grune & Stratton.

Stoller, R. J., Marmor, J., Bieber, I., Gold, R., Socarides, C. W., Green, R., & Spitzer, R. L. (1973). A symposium: Should homosexuality be in the APA nomenclature? *The American Journal of Psychiatry, 130*(11), 1207–1216. https://doi.org/10.1176/ajp.130.11.1207

The Case Against Conversion "Therapy"

INTRODUCTION

A History of Conversion Therapy, From Accepted Practice to Condemnation

DOUGLAS C. HALDEMAN

The patient was 25 years old, an aspiring actor working as a waiter. Gay-identified and cisgender, he had attended a university affiliated with his church. He was strikingly handsome. After his second serious suicide attempt, he had been referred for evaluation by a local hospital's emergency department. He explained that he had been seeing a psychologist at his university's counseling center. When Mark disclosed that he had been having same-sex fantasies for years and thought that he might be gay, the psychologist referred him to another therapist for "specialized treatment."

The "specialized treatment" was actually aversive conditioning in which Mark was asked to find homoerotic pictorial material that he found arousing. This material was made into slides, which were then presented to Mark at the same time that an electric shock was delivered to his hands, testicles, and penis. At the cessation of the shock, the slide image changed to that of a nude female in a seductive pose. In this method of "treating" unwanted same-sex attraction, widely known as "Playboy therapy," the patient's innate same-sex orientation was to be disrupted with aversive stimuli. The relief associated with the cessation of the shock was intended to augment opposite-sex responsiveness.

https://doi.org/10.1037/0000266-001
The Case Against Conversion "Therapy": Evidence, Ethics, and Alternatives,
D. C. Haldeman (Editor)

This method of treating same-sex attraction was notoriously ineffective and cruel; in fact, it was subsequently denounced by every major health care organization, as well as the creator of the method himself (Davison, 1976). It demonstrates the degree to which people have been willing to subject themselves to discomfort and even torture in order to expunge their shame and stay in the good graces of their families, social environments, and religious institutions. When I asked Mark why he had submitted to these monstrous interventions, he simply said, "I did what I thought I needed to do to live."

The year was 1983, and it marked the beginning of my interest in what was once known as "conversion therapy" or "reparative therapy." I should note from the outset that in the mental health literature these terms are being replaced by the less familiar but more accurate acronym sexual orientation change efforts (SOCE) because these methods do not constitute a legitimate, accepted form of therapy. There is no empirical basis for the theories of SOCE and no evidence of its success. To the contrary, there is ample evidence that SOCE can significantly harm people. No training protocols for SOCE exist, and nearly every major health care organization in the United States opposes SOCE. Therefore, to refer to these methods as therapy in any form elevates them to a status of which they are undeserving.

In recent years, as the transgender community has gained more visibility, methods similar to SOCE have been used on gender nonconforming individuals—primarily children—to try to make them identify with their sex assigned at birth. As with SOCE, these methods are neither empirically substantiated nor demonstrated to be effective. In fact, they may be very dangerous, as they are implicated in the disproportionate rate of serious mental health concerns and number of suicide attempts by transgender individuals (see Rivera & Pardo, Chapter 2; Glassgold & Ryan, Chapter 4, this volume). Given the nontherapeutic effects of so-called "conversion therapy" on transgender individuals, such efforts are now referred to as gender identity change efforts (GICE).

It is important to clarify that GICE are *not* intended to help trans people with gender transition. In other words, the "gender identity change" that is the goal of GICE is a change from a gender identity that *differs* from one's sex assigned at birth to a gender identity that is *consistent* with one's sex assigned at birth. Changing gender identity (the goal of GICE) is not the same as changing gender expression (the goal of gender transition). GICE are harmful, whereas gender transition to make one's outward expression of gender match their inner experience of gender has proven beneficial, sometimes even lifesaving.

SOCE and GICE, then, are the primary foci of this book, which explains their roots in sociocultural heterosexism and cisgenderism, their effects on the people who receive them, and implications for public policy and international issues. Before going further, however, additional terminology used throughout the book should be clarified. *Sexual orientation* refers to the internal experience of sexual and romantic attraction and arousal, which may or may not be consistent with an individual's sexual expression or behavior. *Gender identity* refers to one's internal concept of self as male, female, gender fluid, or other; this identity may or may not be consistent with the sex assigned at birth. *Gender expression* refers to the external appearance of one's gender identity, as indicated through behavior, clothing, haircut, and/or voice. A person's gender expression may or may not conform to socially defined behaviors and characteristics typically associated with being either masculine or feminine. Table 1 summarizes these and other terms for the reader.

Historically, both SOCE and GICE were uncritically assumed to be the treatments of choice for same-sex attraction and gender nonconformity, as both of these "conditions" were viewed as pathological by the psychomedico establishment. Same-sex attraction and behavior were excoriated in the medical literature as early as the 19th century by Austrian psychiatrist Richard Von Kraft-Ebbing, who ironically was a notorious cross-dresser. In *Psychopathia Sexualis*, Kraft-Ebbing (1892) denounced homosexuality along with "masturbation, sadism, masochism, and analingus" as evidence of serious psychopathology on the grounds that they do not lead to procreation and therefore serve no legitimate purpose. In Kraft-Ebbing's case, we may speculate that this position was due to a reaction formation seen many times since: Those most internally conflicted about their own same-sex desires are the most likely to vociferously demonize them publicly. Regardless, Kraft-Ebbing's views went largely unchallenged for decades—and are still viewed as legitimate by some, including many of the (mostly) conservative religious proponents of SOCE and GICE.

WHY THIS BOOK IS NEEDED

When I wrote my first chapter on SOCE in 1991, I never dreamed that we would still be talking about it 30 years later. After all, each of the major mental health organizations had discarded "homosexuality" as a form of psychopathology nearly 20 years earlier. The era of "gay liberation" had brought visibility to lesbian, gay, bisexual, transgender, and questioning or

TABLE 1. Defining Terms

Term	Definition
Sexual orientation	"A multidimensional aspect of human experience, comprised of gendered patterns in attraction and behavior, identity related to these patterns, and associated experiences, such as fantasy" (Rosario & Scrimshaw, 2014, pp. 555–596; as cited in APA, 2021c, p. 1).
Sexual orientation change efforts	"A range of techniques used by a variety of mental health professionals and non-professionals with the goal of changing sexual orientation" (APA, 2021c, p. 1). The term is gradually replacing *conversion therapy* in the professional literature because efforts to change someone's sexual orientation do not qualify as therapy.
Gender identity	"A person's deep felt, inherent sense of being a girl, woman, or female; a boy, a man, or male; a blend of male or female; [or another] gender" (APA, 2015, p. 862).
Gender expression	"The presentation of an individual including physical appearance, clothing choice and accessories, and behaviors that express aspects of gender identity" (APA, 2015, p. 861).
Cisgender person	"A person whose gender identity aligns with sex assigned at birth" (e.g., an individual assigned female at birth who identifies as a woman/girl; APA, 2015, p. 861).
Transgender person	"An umbrella term used to describe the full range of people whose gender identity and/or gender role do not conform to what is typically associated with their sex assigned at birth" (APA, 2015, p. 863).
Gender identity change efforts	"A range of techniques used by mental health professionals and non-professionals with the goal of changing gender identity, gender expression, or associated components of these to be in alignment with gender role behaviors that are stereotypically associated with sex assigned at birth" (Substance Abuse and Mental Health Services Administration, 2015, p. 64). The term is gradually replacing *conversion therapy* in the professional literature because efforts to change someone's gender identity or expression do not qualify as therapy.

Note. APA = American Psychological Association.

queer (LGBTQ) communities, and public opinion was already shifting in favor of antidiscrimination protections in housing and employment for lesbians and gay men. Lesbian and gay characters were starting to appear in movies and in the mainstream media. I remember thinking (naively) at the time that SOCE's days were numbered.

And numbered they are, although not in the way I had expected. SOCE and GICE are still alive and well; the Williams Institute (Mallory et al., 2018) estimates that nearly 700,000 people have undergone some form of SOCE, and nearly half of those people are minors. The report further indicates that 20,000 minors will be subjected to SOCE from a licensed mental health professional in the 30 states that do not currently prohibit the practice. When clergy and pastoral counselors engaging in SOCE are taken into account, the number rises to 57,000 youth. Furthermore, the rise of anti-SOCE and anti-GICE laws in many states and jurisdictions has generated a backlash that is playing itself out in the latest version of America's culture wars, emboldened by court decisions to permit business owners (and presumably health care workers) to refuse service to LGBT persons based on "religious freedom" (see Grey et al., Chapter 9, this volume).

In 1997, Jack Drescher and Ariel Shidlo published the first volume summarizing the research, effects, and ethical implications of SOCE. This important volume was a compendium of the history, research, and clinical and ethical implications. Since that time, the visibility of—and public and professional criticism against—SOCE has increased. Furthermore, gender nonconforming and transgender individuals—and the efforts to "convert" them to cisgender status—have become much more visible in the past 20 tears, as have the heretofore commonly employed but dangerous efforts to socially reprogram gender nonconforming children and adolescents. At the same time, the literature in this area has grown. Therefore, an updated resource summarizing the literature is appropriate at this time.

ORGANIZATION OF THE BOOK

This book is for mental health professionals; allied health care workers; educators and researchers; those involved in social, legal, and professional policymaking roles; and, of course, the public. It contains information that all parents should understand before subjecting their children to SOCE or GICE. Furthermore, this book is for individuals giving comment to broadcast, print, and social media. In the interest of accuracy and clarity, the book rests on valid scientific evidence to reach its conclusions. Clinical impressions and philosophical perspectives are also included, but they serve as secondary supports to the main focus, which is credible evidence. After all, for those who have been critics of SOCE and GICE, lack of empirical evidence due to numerous methodological problems with pro-SOCE/pro-GICE studies has been a central point in arguments debunking and demonstrating these methods' potential harms. The pro-SOCE literature relies heavily on testimonials, self-reports, and retrospective memories in the context of extreme social pressure. We have worked to ensure that the material in this book is based on credible evidence.

Some may disagree with this book's entire premise, believing that sexual orientation and expression are fluid for everyone over the course of the life-span. We disagree. It is true that some people may experience their sexuality as fluid, noting changes in sexual identity and sexual expression depending on a variety of factors. Bisexual individuals in particular are likely to experience the fluid nature of sexual orientation. For most people, however, sexual orientation does not change. Gender, as an identity variable, does not require any kind of treatment other than supportive.

This book does not address some of the more recent iterations of SOCE, also known as "conversion therapy lite." These methods are promoted by individuals who profess not to have a bias against same-sex attraction and behavior but simply want to market treatments intended to diminish patients' unwanted same-sex desire and enhance their heterosexual response and function. Unless a patient is already bisexual, these methods appear to suffer from the same lack of validation as traditional SOCE; they also risk harm to the patient and collateral damage to the individuals' heterosexual partners. It is little wonder, then, that anti-SOCE/anti-GICE laws have the purveyors of such methods anxious that their industry could be put out of business.

Some may ask the purpose of including SOCE and GICE in the same volume. The reasons are several. First, focusing on SOCE or GICE alone would ignore the underlying commonality in these two phenomena—that gender-related behavior consistent with the individual's birth sex is normative and anything else is unacceptable and should be changed. Second, high-lighting the dangers of GICE is critical at a time when thousands of youth are being forced into "treatments" that may lead to severe depression and suicide attempts (see Glassgold & Ryan, Chapter 4, this volume). Trans and gender nonconforming individuals—especially people of color—are being harassed, victimized, and murdered at significant rates (see Rivera & Pardo, Chapter 2, this volume). Finally, many in the LGB community have a history of transphobia for which to atone. The inclusion of GICE in this book is intended to indicate that all of us should be concerned about the discredited and potentially dangerous practices used in attempts to change sexual orientation and gender identity.

Part I. Change Efforts: The Evidence Base

In Part I, we address several fundamental questions: What variables are most significant in motivating individuals to seek SOCE? What does the record show about the efficacy and effects of SOCE and GICE? As sampling techniques have improved vastly in recent years, does the recent research on SOCE show anything new? What further research might be useful in this area?

Whether an adult chooses SOCE or whether parents force a young person into SOCE, one factor is frequently present in some form: adherence to a conservative antigay religious tradition, most typically evangelical Christianity or Orthodox Judaism. In choosing to pursue SOCE, adult participants often place a value on maintaining good standing in their families and religious communities that is equal to or greater than the value they place on their sexual orientation. For many, the sum total of their life experiences and their social worlds—and all of the attachments that implies—is jeopardized if they come out as gay and enter into same-sex friendships and romantic relationships. The unknown LGBT community for many is an unfamiliar place, difficult to navigate; thus, changing sexual orientation—or at least developing sexual heterocompetence—is a more palatable choice, especially if one believes that sufficient faith in God/Jesus will provide a "cure."

The situation for youth is somewhat different, as Judith M. Glassgold notes in her summary of SOCE research in Chapter 1 of this volume. Parents who oblige their children to undergo some form of SOCE place them at threefold risk for suicidal ideation and depression when compared to heterosexually identified youth. Youth are typically instructed in religion-based SOCE that if they work/pray/try hard enough, they will be relieved of their "burden." As with adults, preexisting shame about being gay exponentially increases when SOCE fails, because now there is added shame about not having worked hard enough. Glassgold notes that those youth who undergo SOCE from a religious person are at greater risk for negative outcomes than those who see a licensed mental health provider.

In summarizing the SOCE research, Glassgold indicates that American Psychological Association's (APA's) 2009 Task Force Report on the subject found no empirical basis for supporting SOCE as effective or safe. Almost all studies purporting to demonstrate support for SOCE are rife with methodological problems (e.g., studies based entirely on self-report and retrospective memory in an environment with extreme social desirability characteristics, lack of follow-up, no objective assessment of sexual orientation of subjects, sampling bias).

In Chapter 2, David P. Rivera and Seth T. Pardo explore the science and history of efforts to change gender identity, or GICE. Until very recently, the medical establishment misunderstood sexual orientation, transgender, and gender nonconforming persons and often assumed that treatment was in order. This perspective inaccurately conflated the concepts of sex, gender identity, and gender expression. The enshrinement of the gender binary was unquestioned, and gender nonconforming persons—especially youth—were pathologized and "treated" with interventions designed to force children into presenting and behaving in a manner consistent with their assigned birth sex, not their true identities. Rivera and Pardo document the various forms of stigma, family rejection, discrimination, harassment, and violence that trans persons encounter. However, since the World Health Organization's official position has changed to view gender fluidity and transition as normal variants of the human experience, the trend toward GICE has changed. Now, the literature is describing many more affirmative treatment approaches to support, not change, transgender individuals.

Part II. Minority Stress and Collateral Impact

The concept of minority stress, in which prejudicial attitudes and discriminatory behaviors lead to adverse health consequences, has broad applications for LGBTQ persons. It is implicated in behavioral health problems (substance use, smoking, obesity, high-risk sexual behaviors) and mental health issues (depression, anxiety, suicidality). The internalization of stigma has been shown to lead to all of the above (see Hendricks, Chapter 3), including participation in SOCE and GICE. In fact, it can be argued that there is a circular relationship between minority stress and the aforementioned issues: The greater the internal pressure derived from external stressors (social stigma, youth obliged to participate in SOCE/GICE), the more likely it is that an individual will be at risk for any of these issues.

For most who have undergone SOCE or GICE, there is probably no stronger motivating force than affiliation with an organized religion whose dogma forbids same-sex behavior or any noncisgender identity or presentation. People such as Mark, briefly described at the beginning of this introduction, often feel that they have no choice other than SOCE when they face the prospect of being dismissed from family and community and being hated by God, and when they are frightened at the idea of becoming part of the unfamiliar LGBT community. Furthermore, the clinical picture is sometimes unclear for practitioners: If sexual orientation and religious affiliation are both elements of what we consider to be "diversity," how is the relationship between them to be navigated when there is an internal conflict? Part II of this book addresses this complicated question.

In Michael L. Hendricks's chapter on minority stress and change efforts (Chapter 3), we see that the concept of minority stress is implicated in adverse health consequences for LGBT people, as are some of the dysfunctional coping strategies—such as internalized homophobia or substance use—employed to deal with the stress. Hendricks identifies the dangers associated with distal stressors (external events, such as harassment or violence) and proximal stressors (such as internalizing the abuse inflicted by others). He describes the strategy of concealment, which is both a coping mechanism and a stressor in and of itself. Hendricks further identifies a number of strategies to counteract the effects of minority stress and boost coping and resilience for LGBT individuals, including identity formation/revision along with the importance of developing a psychological sense of community.

We might adapt an old adage by saying that "minority stress begins at home," which is certainly true for youth who are forced into SOCE or GICE by their parents and other family members. In Chapter 4, Judith M. Glassgold and Caitlin Ryan address the central role played by families in SOCE/GICE (the authors use the acronym SOGIECE to reflect the inclusion of "expression" because many gender-atypical youth are detected by their behavioral presentation and expression). Youth from low socioeconomic status and/or conservative religious families are 3 times as likely to be forced into SOCE/ GICE, and this double whammy (receiving negative messages at home and undergoing external interventions) puts youth at greatest risk for suicidal ideation. When youth are led to believe that their secure place in the family and society—and in some cases, even in the afterlife—is contingent on their changing their sexual orientation or their gender identity and expression, they often feel that there is no way out other than to contemplate or even attempt suicide.

Glassgold and Ryan report that children obliged to undergo GICE are at significant risk for adverse mental health consequences, including suicide attempts. However, the question of how gender fluid and nonconforming children should be treated remains open for discussion. Most clinicians working in this area oppose GICE on both practical and ethical grounds. However, there is less agreement on how transgender and gender nonconforming (TGNC) youth should be treated. Some espouse a "wait and see" approach, in which the child's behavior is monitored, presumably during a period of exploring gender identity and presentation (de Vries & Cohen-Kettenis, 2012). In this model, youth are provided the freedom to explore gender and gender expression in safe environments, forestalling full social transition until the child is old enough to determine a stable gender identity. This model is supported in part by data showing that very few gender nonconforming children go on to claim a transgender identity in adolescence and adulthood.

A more recent model, known as the gender affirming model (Ehrensaft et al., 2017), is based on the notion that children at any age are capable of deciding on their gender. Children in this model of treatment are fully supported in social transition and gender expression and presentation, including the use of prepubertal hormone blockers, to ease full gender transition in later years. Although further research using this model is necessary, it has gained popularity among many clinicians and scholars working in the area. For example, research conducted at the University of Washington (Olson, 2016) indicates that gender nonconforming children who have been permitted to transition socially in prepubescent years report the same level of psychological adjustment as cisgender adolescents.

One of the greatest institutional sources of minority stress for LGBTQ individuals is organized religion. Long after the mental health establishment discontinued pathologization of same-sex behavior, scriptural texts—mostly rooted in conservative traditions—continue to be used as justification for discrimination against LGBTQ persons. So-called religious freedom exemptions from antigay discrimination protections are gaining support and traction. Psychologist and religious scholar Thomas G. Plante explains in Chapter 5 of this volume the bases on which major religious traditions have viewed nonheterosexual orientations and noncisgender identities.

Understanding the role of religion in addressing sexual orientation and gender identity for religious clients is essential for practitioners working with clients who are conflicted about their sexuality and/or gender. For some, more progressive religious traditions—or no religion at all—makes sense; however, for many, both sexual orientation/gender identity and inclusion in a conservative religious community are of equal importance. Plante describes the complexities of dealing with this profound relationship as he reviews strategies for helping conflicted sexual minority and gender diverse individuals, and for working with religious organizations and institutions.

Part III. Affirmative Approaches: Guidelines and Ethics

Parts I and II examine the evidence base and its implications for SOCE and GICE. Part III turns to formal recommendations for clinical practice, education and training, research, and further policy development.

In Chapter 6, Kristin A. Hancock and Douglas C. Haldeman review APA's practice guidelines for LGB individuals. APA adopted its first set of LGB guidelines in 2000, although with only passing reference to what was then known as conversion therapy. The APA's Council of Representatives adopted its first policy on conversion therapy in 1997. The policy consisted primarily of ethical considerations. It was updated in 2009 along with the publication of APA's (2009) landmark report *Appropriate Therapeutic Responses to Sexual Orientation*. This resolution was much more direct than the 1997 policy, in that the 2009 policy summarized the conclusion that there is no evidentiary support for conversion therapy and admonished mental health professionals not to make unsupportable claims about the efficacy of conversion treatments, minimize their potential dangers, or disseminate inaccurate information about sexual orientation. More recently, in 2021 APA adopted an updated resolution categorically opposing SOCE (APA, 2021c). At the same time, APA's first-ever resolution opposing GICE was adopted (APA, 2021b), as well as a revised version of the LGB Practice Guidelines (APA, 2021a; see Chapter 6, this volume, for further details).

In Chapter 7, Anneliese A. Singh, Raven K. Cokley, and Frank B. Gorritz explain the APA (2015) *Guidelines for Psychological Practice With Transgender and Gender Nonconforming Clients*. The authors highlight the unique minority stressors faced by TGNC individuals and make recommendations for fostering resilience and addressing trauma. These guidelines reference foundational knowledge regarding how to understand the unique stressors and stigma faced by most TGNC persons. They also reference developmental issues and make recommendations for trans-affirming practice.

In Chapter 8, psychological ethicist Linda F. Campbell delineates the ethical aspects of clinical, cultural, and subject matter competence necessary in the treatment of sexual minority and TGNC clients. Campbell considers the unique challenges faced by sexual minority and TGNC individuals. She also examines the role of their mental health professionals in meeting these challenges in the context of applicable ethical principles (e.g., informed consent, multiple relationships, confidentiality, recordkeeping). Traumatization from social stigma can lead individuals into ineffective care and maltreatment that promotes change efforts. Campbell explores the ethical aspects of psychotherapy services in light of requested or offered change efforts. She also discusses research on change effort outcomes, along with the methods that mental health professionals can use to inform clients of accurate information (and educate them about inaccurate information).

Part IV. Affirmative Approaches: Advocacy and International Issues

Recent research suggests a strong connection between public policy and mental health with respect to LGBT individuals. Those who live in more LGBT-friendly locales tend to do significantly better with mental health issues than their counterparts in more rural or politically conservative areas. Part IV ties together the previous three parts and demonstrates the ways in which research on SOCE/GICE can inform social policy, the public, and legislative and judicial processes.

In 2012, California senator Ted Lieu authored the first legislation prohibiting licensed mental health professionals from using SOCE with minors. Since then, 20 other states and the District of Columbia, as well as numerous local jurisdictions, have followed suit with their own statutes, otherwise known as Youth Mental Health Protection Acts. In addition to legislative prohibitions against SOCE and GICE, some states have considered regulatory bans because they are more readily adopted in states with conservative legislatures. Melissa J. Grey, Sam Brinton, and Douglas C. Haldeman summarize these and other issues in Chapter 9. A project by The Trevor Foundation to present Youth Mental Health Protection Acts in all 50 states is described.

Grey et al.'s chapter also features a brief chronology of landmark court rulings on LGBT issues, with a warning that despite the generally positive trajectory of judicial decisions on LGBT issues this is not a time for complacency. In the current political era, "religious freedom" laws seek to dismantle discrimination protections for LGBT persons in the name of personal religious beliefs. The only case thus far to be adjudicated in the courts concerned a homophobic baker refusing to make a cake for a same-sex couple; however, the implications for medical and emergency services are chilling for the LGBT community and beyond, especially given the recent conservative majority on the U.S. Supreme Court.

As mentioned earlier, in 2020 the United Nations Human Rights Council issued a report from its Independent Expert on Protection Against Violence Based on Sexual Orientation and Gender Identity (IESOGI) that states the following:

> All practices attempting conversion are inherently humiliating, demeaning and discriminatory. The combined effects of feeling powerless and extreme humiliation generate profound feelings of shame, guilt, self-disgust, and worthlessness, which can result in a damaged self-concept and enduring personality changes. The IESOGI is convinced that the decision to subject a child to conversion practices can never truly be in conformity with a child's best interests. Parents must make decisions for their children under the premise of informed consent, which entails knowing the practice's true nature, its inability to actually achieve "conversion," and the mounting evidence pointing towards its long-term physical and psychological harm. (p. 3)

American psychology has traditionally been focused primarily on research and practice within the United States, and LGBTQ psychology is no exception. In Chapter 10, on international issues, Sharon G. Horne and Mallaigh McGinley explore the development and influence of SOCE/GICE in transnational contexts. They describe the historical trajectory of SOCE/GICE and the impact of religious teachings and colonialism as they explore SOCE/GICE in several world regions. LGBT refugees throughout the world, especially in countries where same-sex behavior and/or cross-gender presentation are criminalized, constitute an international humanitarian refugee crisis. American LGBT psychology has a role to play in developing strategies to combat SOCE/GICE worldwide, as well as to provide support to the thousands of LGBT refugees and asylum seekers attempting to flee their homelands.

SOCE and GICE are the symptoms of a patriarchal constellation of medical, social, cultural, religious, and historical factors. That same-sex attraction and transgender identity call for interventions intended to change or control them is a vestige of heterocentric and cisgender privilege and power. Such thinking cannot outlast the clear trend toward equality that we have witnessed over the past few decades. Nevertheless, much work remains—work that will rely on a strong evidence base to continue. We hope that this book is helpful in that regard.

REFERENCES

American Psychological Association. (2009). *Report of the American Psychological Association Task Force on appropriate affirmative responses to sexual orientation.* https://www.apa.org/pi/lgbt/resources/therapeutic-response.pdf

American Psychological Association. (2015). Guidelines for psychological practice with transgender and gender nonconforming people. *American Psychologist, 70*(9), 832–864. https://doi.org/10.1037/a0039906

American Psychological Association. (2021a). *APA guidelines for psychological practice with sexual minority persons.* https://www.apa.org/about/policy/psychological-sexual-minority-persons.pdf?_ga=2.150671670.1093579335.1633297884-1820363891.1557865924

American Psychological Association. (2021b). *APA resolution on gender identity change efforts.* https://www.apa.org/about/policy/resolution-gender-identity-change-efforts.pdf

American Psychological Association. (2021c). *APA resolution on sexual orientation change efforts.* https://www.apa.org/about/policy/resolution-sexual-orientation-change-efforts.pdf

Davison, G. C. (1976). Homosexuality: The ethical challenge. *Journal of Consulting and Clinical Psychology, 44*(2), 157–162. https://doi.org/10.1037/0022-006X.44.2.157

de Vries, A. L., & Cohen-Kettenis, P. T. (2012). Clinical management of gender dysphoria in children and adolescents: The Dutch approach. *Journal of Homosexuality, 59*(3), 301–320. https://doi.org/10.1080/00918369.2012.653300

Ehrensaft, D., Giammattei, S. V., Storck, K., Tishelman, A. C., & Keo-Meier, C. (2017). Prepubertal social gender transitions: What we know what we can learn—a view from a gender affirmative lens. *International Journal of Transgenderism, 19*(2), 251–268. https://doi.org/10.1080/15532739.2017.1414649

Kraft-Ebbing, R. (1892). *Psychopathia sexualis.* F.A. Davis.

Mallory, C., Brown, C. N. T., & Conron, K. J. (2018, January). *Conversion therapy and LGBT youth.* The Williams Institute, UCLA School of Law. https://williamsinstitute.law.ucla.edu/demographics/conversion-therapy-and-lgbt-youth/

Olson, K. R. (2016). Prepubescent transgender children: What we do and do not know. *Journal of the American Academy of Child and Adolescent Psychiatry, 55*, 155–156.

Rosario, M., & Scrimshaw, E. W. (2014). Theories and etiologies of sexual orientation. In D. L. Tolman, L. M. Diamond, J. A. Bauermeister, W. H. George, J. G. Pfaus, & L. M. Ward (Eds.), *APA handbook of sexuality and psychology: Vol. 1. Person-based approaches* (pp. 555–596). APA Books. https://doi.org/10.1037/14193-018

Substance Abuse and Mental Health Services Administration. (2015). *Ending conversion therapy: Supporting and affirming LGBTQ youth* (HHS Publication No. 15-4928).

United Nations. (2020). *Report on conversion therapy by Independent Expert on Protection Against Violence and Discrimination Based on Sexual Orientation and Gender Identity.* https://undocs.org/A/HRC/44/53

PART I CHANGE EFFORTS: THE EVIDENCE BASE

1 RESEARCH ON SEXUAL ORIENTATION CHANGE EFFORTS

A Summary

JUDITH M. GLASSGOLD

Scientific research indicates that variation in same-sex sexual orientation is normal and part of the spectrum of human sexuality (American Psychological Association [APA], 2021; APA Task Force on Psychological Practice with Sexual Minority Persons, 2021). Despite this evidence, sexual orientation change efforts (SOCE) continue to be provided to adults, children, and adolescents (Green et al., 2020; Mallory et al., 2019). Given the continued practice of SOCE, it is important to review the evidence on its outcomes. In 2009, a comprehensive systematic review of the research on SOCE concluded that these efforts were unsuccessful at changing sexual orientation (APA Task Force on Appropriate Therapeutic Responses to Sexual Orientation [APA Task Force], 2009). Further, the review found harms specific to SOCE (APA Task Force, 2009). Since 2009, number of articles on SOCE have been published in professional journals, but there has not been a thorough review of this literature. This chapter reviews the scientific evidence to date on SOCE. Most of the research and practice is based on sources from the United States, and in certain instances international information is provided.

https://doi.org/10.1037/0000266-002

The Case Against Conversion "Therapy": Evidence, Ethics, and Alternatives,
D. C. Haldeman (Editor)

BACKGROUND ON SEXUAL ORIENTATION AND SOCE

Sexual orientation is a complex human characteristic involving attractions, behaviors, and emotions. *Sexual orientation* refers to an individual's patterns of sexual, romantic, and affectional arousal and desire for other persons associated with those persons' gender and sex characteristics. The research and clinical literature finds that same-sex sexual and romantic attractions, feelings, behaviors, and identities are normal and positive variations of human sexuality and are not indications of either mental or developmental disorders (APA, 2021; APA Task Force, 2009, p. 2). Sexual orientation is tied to physiological drives and biological systems that are beyond conscious choice and involves profound emotional feelings, such as "falling in love" (APA Task Force, 2009, p. 2).

The term *sexual orientation change efforts* in the United States describes methods based on psychotherapeutic techniques and theories (e.g., behavioral therapy, psychoanalysis, medical approaches) and religious and spiritual approaches (e.g., prayer, Bible study) that aim to change a person's same-sex sexual orientation to other-sex orientation (e.g., gay to straight), regardless of whether mental health professionals or lay individuals (including religious professionals, religious leaders, social groups, and other lay networks, such as self-help groups) are involved. In the United States, SOCE is usually provided in verbal form. In the past, SOCE included behavioral, verbal, and aversive methods. SOCE can be provided to all age groups and is delivered in individual, group, family, inpatient, outpatient, and residential settings. In international settings, SOCE can take on additional forms, including degrading forms of physical and verbal abuse; many of these practices are clandestine or are government sanctioned (Bishop, 2019; United Nations Independent Expert on Protection Against Violence and Discrimination Based on Sexual Orientation and Gender Identity [UNIESOGI], 2020).

Although SOCE takes diverse forms, it generally has the following elements: (a) foundational belief that same-sex attractions, behaviors, and orientations are unhealthy, development defects, mental illnesses, and undesirable compared with heterosexual attractions, behaviors, and orientations; (b) lack of accurate scientific information about same-sex attractions or lesbian, gay, bisexual, and transgender (LGBT) individuals, including outdated theories and inaccurate and negative stereotypes about causes of same-sex orientation; (c) purported negative health and social outcomes and fear-based messages about LGBT life outcomes; (d) encouragement of traditional sexual and gender roles and expressions in children, adolescents, and adults; and (e) prohibitions of certain sexual behaviors and gender nonconforming expression and identity (APA Task Force, 2009, p. 22; Fjelstrom, 2013; Flentje et al., 2013; UNIESOGI, 2020). SOCE directed at religious individuals usually includes information about same-sex orientation's incompatibility with faith doctrines and negative spiritual outcomes of LGBT identity and sexual orientation (APA Task Force, 2009, pp. 44–49; Beckstead & Morrow, 2004; UNIESOGI, 2020).

SOCE directed at children and youth usually includes additional elements: (a) family engagement in prohibiting and/or punishing same-sex and gender nonconforming behaviors and identity, (b) negative information about sexual orientation and gender identity diversity, and (c) encouragement of parental behaviors that are perceived as critical and rejecting by children and adolescents (Ryan et al., 2018).

PREVALENCE

The number of individuals in the United States currently treated with SOCE is difficult to measure and may vary by age, gender, generation, geographic location, and identity/faith. International estimates vary by age, region, and country (UNIESOGI, 2020). Although these estimates differ, scores of youth and adults appear to be exposed to SOCE in the United States. One sample of sexual minority U.S. adults (male/female/nonbinary) found that 7% reported undergoing SOCE (Blosnich et al., 2020); another U.S. survey of middle-aged and older cisgender men found that 17% reported undergoing SOCE (Meanley et al., 2020). In a study of 13- to 25-year-olds, Green et al. (2020) found that 4.2% of their sample (male/female/cisgender/transgender/ nonbinary) had been exposed to SOCE or gender identity change efforts (GICE) in their lifetime. Higbee et al. (2020) found that, in a sample of individuals from the southern United States, slightly more than 11% reported exposure to SOCE. This sample included cisgender (male, female) and nonbinary and transgender individuals. In a Canadian sample of sexual minority cisgender men, Salway et al. (2020) found a lifetime prevalence of 3.5% for individuals who received SOCE as of 2012.

A report from the Williams Institute (Mallory et al., 2019) estimated, based on information from a cross-sectional population sample, that 698,000 LGBT adults (ages 18–59) in the United States reported having received SOCE, and 350,000 LGBT adults received treatment as adolescents. The report predicted that 16,000 LGBT youth (ages 13–17) who are in the 32 states that currently (as of 2019) do not ban the practice will undergo conversion therapy from a licensed health care professional before they reach the age of 18. Another prediction is that 57,000 youth (ages 13–17) across all U.S. states will receive conversion therapy from religious or spiritual advisors before they reach age 18.

HISTORICAL ISSUES

Rise of Scientific Research and Depathologization of Homosexuality

SOCE was the predominant treatment provided to U.S. individuals with a same-sex orientation in the early to mid-20th century. Efforts to change sexual orientation through mental health treatment reflected the values of the times when same-sex sexual orientation was seen as immoral, criminal, and pathological; many individuals sought out SOCE to avoid discrimination and legal penalties (APA Task Force, 2009, pp. 21–25). The science of sexuality in the late 19th and early 20th centuries reflected these very same negative attitudes and stereotypes toward same-sex sexual orientation (APA Task Force, 2009, pp. 21–26).

As scientific measurement and analysis improved, scientific methods provided a pathway to rebut erroneous and stereotypic views (Gonsiorek, 1991). Further research using objective mental health measures and quality experimental designs found no basis for the assumption that homosexuality per se was a mental disorder (Gonsiorek, 1991; Haldeman, 1994). Based on the preponderance of scientific research, in 1973 homosexuality was removed from the diagnostic manuals used by mental health professionals (APA Task Force, 2009, pp. 21–26).

Once homosexuality was no longer a disorder, the diagnostic rationale for attempting to change sexual orientation was eliminated. Published critiques of SOCE emerged as the science of sexual orientation became more rigorous. These critiques found that there was no scientific basis for SOCE (Haldeman, 1994). The psychological constructs underlying SOCE were found to be unsustained by evidence and ultimately rejected for bias and illogic (APA Task Force, 2009, pp. 21–26; Drescher, 1998; Haldeman, 1994; Shidlo & Schroeder, 2002).

Resurgence of SOCE in the United States

However, in the late 20th century and early 21st century, conservative religious and social forces urged a renewal of SOCE as part of the rejection of the growing social acceptance of LGBT individuals (APA Task Force, 2009, p. 25; Grace, 2008). Scientific and ethical debates expanded (Drescher, 1998;

Haldeman, 2002), including a volume by Shidlo and Schroeder (2002) that provided theoretical, clinical, and ethical assessments and critiques of SOCE. Initial research was conducted with SOCE participants who appraised their experiences, and the research found little evidence of change and documented harms (Shidlo & Schroeder, 2002). Spitzer published a report that was advanced by proponents of SOCE as evidence of its effectiveness, creating a controversy in the professional community; serious objections were raised to this study's lack of sound research methodology (Zucker, 2003).[1] Critiques followed that analyzed the complex intersection of culture, science, and politics, including anti-LGBT stigma (Drescher & Zucker, 2006).

RESEARCH ISSUES

This chapter analyzes quality research published in peer-reviewed journals from 2009 to 2020. These dates were chosen to follow up on the systematic and comprehensive review of research on SOCE from 1960 to 2008 completed by the APA Task Force in August 2009.[2] The APA Task Force examined high-quality research published in peer-reviewed journals from 1960 to 2008. Results are presented in a similar format to that of the APA Task Force Report: efficacy, harms, and other outcomes in research on adults and then a separate section for research on children and adolescents.

Issues in Research Methodology

The APA Task Force (2009) found that serious methodology issues affected much of the research from the 1960s to 2008 that claimed that SOCE resulted in a change to sexual orientation (pp. 25–34). Some of these same methodological issues are relevant to the research from 2008 to 2020, so this section reviews key elements to quality research and methodological weaknesses common in SOCE research. The APA Task Force Report provides a thorough analysis of research issues (pp. 26–34).

Research investigates scientifically valid constructs in a field of study. To establish causal relations, a researcher exposes a population to a uniform intervention and then evaluates its effect. Well-constructed psychological

---

[1]Spitzer (2012) retracted his 2003 article claiming sexual orientation could be changed. He admitted that its methodological limitations meant that the results were not reliable and that the study could not determine whether sexual orientation could be changed.

[2]The author was the chair of the APA Task Force and a contributor and an editor of the report.

research demonstrates that the intervention is the only plausible explanation for an observed outcome, such as change in sexual orientation. Methodological limitations can undermine the certainty that observed changes in people's attitudes, beliefs, and behaviors are a function of the particular interventions to which they were exposed.

Although research design is specific to the research question, some general features of experimental research that can assess causal effects include (a) randomized assignment to the intervention/no intervention groups provides assurances that individual traits did not affect outcomes; (b) reliable and validated measures applied immediately prior to and immediately post treatment ensure that the impact of the intervention is measured; (c) expectations of the researcher and participant should not change the results, and patients and researchers are unaware who received an intervention; and (d) the intervention should be tested on a population that is significantly representative of the population impacted so that the results can be generalized to others.

Treatment research evaluates a uniform and defined intervention. Since the behavioral protocols of the 1960s, there is no defined SOCE treatment. There is also no cogent theory of SOCE, and practitioners use an amalgam of theories—many of which are now rejected—and religious prohibitions (APA Task Force, 2009, p. 11). SOCE theories overlap with stereotypes of human sexuality, do not have a research basis, and cannot be administered because of research ethics and human rights issues (e.g., theories that claim abuse can cause diverse sexual orientations; APA, 2021; APA Task Force, 2009, p. 46; Panozzo, 2013).

Other types of quantitative research can establish correlations or associations but cannot establish causality. These research types can use psychological tests and measures to assess traits or the prevalence of certain conditions in a population, or compare populations. As with experimental research, this research relies on valid measures and assessment tools, internal safeguards to prevent researcher or participant bias, and samples that are large enough to measure an effect and that are representative of the population. Qualitative research can explore in unstructured ways the perceptions and experiences of participants in order to develop hypotheses to be tested.

Measuring sexual orientation and sexual orientation identity is complicated but crucial to evaluating claims of SOCE effectiveness. Sexual behavior, sexual arousal/attraction, and sexual orientation identity are labeled and expressed in many ways by individuals, which makes reliance on self-appraisal unreliable (APA Task Force, 2009, pp. 30–31). Much of the literature since the 1980s that aims to evaluate whether SOCE changes sexual orientation relies on self-appraisal.

Studying Negative Effects and Harm

As psychological science has no standard method of studying the negative effects of psychotherapy or harms (Dimidjian & Hollon, 2010; Rozental et al., 2018), different methods are used. Some studies include the negative effects or harms as part of an evaluation of the effectiveness or benefits of an intervention. Other studies evaluate harm as part of larger studies of impact of events and treatments by comparing samples who experienced events or treatments with those who did not. Investigators can also record negative effects (e.g., negative emotional and physical side effects, perceptions of harm, high dropout rates). Mechanisms such as case studies, patient registries, and self-report portals and surveys are also valid means to report harms of a treatment (Chou et al., 2010).

Assessments of harm are especially lacking in treatments of children (Mercer, 2017). Given children's developmental vulnerability and lack of ability to consent to treatment, this deficiency is particularly concerning. In some instances, harmful therapies have resulted in serious adverse events that have led to legal action (Mercer, 2017). Current government standards for research on children are quite stringent and limit that could pose harm to children (Department of Health and Human Services, 2018). The lack of direct research necessitates a greater use of anecdotal or case study assessments as well as retrospective studies when researching harms in children and youth (Dimidjian & Hollon, 2010; Mercer, 2017).

In research from 2009 to 2020, participants are explicitly asked to evaluate their experiences, especially the benefits and harms of SOCE, as adults (Bradshaw et al., 2015; Dehlin, Galliher, Bradshaw, Hyde, & Crowell, 2015). Most studies examine associations between participation in SOCE as adults or as children and negative mental health effects directly using comparison between those who experienced SOCE and those who did not. This research compares psychological measures of mental health, vocational and educational achievement, and reports of suicidality and suicide attempts. The research explores efforts implemented by families on their children (Ryan et al., 2018) and those by practitioners and religious professionals (Blosnich et al., 2020; Green et al., 2020; Higbee et al., 2020; Salway et al., 2020) to change sexual orientation.

RESEARCH REVIEW 1960-2008

APA Task Force Report: Systematic Review of Research on Adults

Given the continuing controversy surrounding SOCE, the APA appointed a task force to undertake an evaluation of SOCE in adults, adolescents, and children. The APA Task Force published the APA Task Force Report, a rigorous systematic review of the research in peer-reviewed professional journals from the 1960s to 2008 that evaluated outcomes, such as effectiveness, harms, and benefits. The APA Task Force also reviewed high-quality qualitative research related to people's experiences of efforts aimed at altering their sexual orientation, including studies that aimed to understand participants' motivations and perspectives in undertaking SOCE.

Information About Adult Participants

The APA Task Force Report found studies that were limited to predominantly White men who experienced conflicts and distress related to same-sex attractions. These studies identified two distinct populations in the United States based on time periods. During the 1960s, 1970s, and 1980s, the vast majority of people who participated in studies were White men who wished to avoid the negative social, political, legal, and financial effects of anti-LGBT stigma and discrimination. Many of these individuals were court-mandated to receive treatment or fearful of losing their jobs and families because of discrimination (APA Task Force, 2009, pp. 44–53). Early research included verbal and behavioral techniques. The verbal techniques included cognitive approaches to reduce attractions. The behavioral techniques included behavioral conditioning techniques, masturbation reconditioning, and systematic desensitization, along with aversive stimuli such as electric shock, deprivation of food and liquids, smelling salts, and chemically induced nausea. These aversive treatments can no longer be provided because of ethical concerns (APA, 2017). Other techniques assessed in these studies were verbal psychotherapies, imaginary systematic desensitization, biofeedback, and hypnosis. Some studies combined both approaches (APA Task Force, 2009, pp. 65–80).

The second group of studies, from the 1990s through the 21st century, includes a U.S. adult population predominantly composed of White men who participate in traditional or conservative faiths (e.g., the Church of Jesus Christ of Latter-day Saints [LDS], Evangelical Christianity, Orthodox Judaism). These individuals had tried a variety of methods to change their sexual orientation in order to follow religious precepts, including psychotherapy, support groups, religious efforts, and self-study (APA Task Force, 2009, pp. 44–53).

The APA Task Force Report found that some of the research from the 1960s to the 1980s used experimental designs that allowed for causal conclusions on the impact of interventions. However, substantial deficiencies existed in the design and analysis of research from the 1980s to 2008 (APA Task Force, 2009, pp. 26–35). Because of these deficiencies, none of the research from the 1980s to 2008 can make credible causal claims. These deficiencies include (a) inconsistent or nonuniform treatment, or multiple treatments so that it is unclear what actually impacted the patient; (b) unreliable assessment and outcome measures, including subjective measures of sexual orientation; (c) inappropriate selection and performance of statistical tests; (d) retrospective recall, where participants recall treatment experiences from long ago, which increase subjective judgments in the reporting of results that vulnerable to reappraisal, omission, social desirability, and distortion; (e) high participant dropout rates; and (f) selective recruitment from SOCE providers or religious self-help groups that advocate for SOCE (APA Task Force, 2009, pp. 26–35; Panozzo, 2013).

Effectiveness

The APA Task Force Report concluded that the entire body of research from the 1960s to 2008 does not support any claims that SOCE can change sexual orientation. It made this finding based on the results of studies with accepted research designs from which one could draw conclusions (APA Task Force, 2009, pp. 35–43). Participants in the early research continued to experience same-sex attractions following SOCE and did not report significant change to other-sex attractions that could be empirically verified (APA Task Force, 2009, pp. 35–43).

Harms

The earliest research from the late 1960s through the early 1980s did document harms, such as adverse effects to individuals who received verbal and behavioral treatments.[3] The negative side effects included loss of sexual feeling, depression, suicidality, and anxiety. The high dropout rates seen in early treatment studies may also indicate harmful impacts (APA Task Force, 2009, pp. 41–43).

---

[3]These studies did not set out to assess harms but did report multiple negative effects from the treatments.

The APA Task Force review analyzed studies of religiously oriented SOCE (e.g., verbal forms, support groups, religious efforts). In these nonexperimental studies, participants perceive they have been harmed by SOCE. Some participants identified negative changes in relationships with family; increased negative self-esteem and self-worth; increased self-blame; and increased depression, anxiety, suicidality, and loss of faith (APA Task Force, 2009, pp. 50–52; Beckstead & Morrow, 2004). Individuals who failed to change their sexual orientation, while believing they should have changed as the result of such efforts, described their experiences as a significant cause of emotional and spiritual distress and negative self-image (APA Task Force, 2009, pp. 50–53).

Other Outcomes

The APA Task Force Report found that participants in qualitative research reported diverse evaluations of their experiences. Some participants felt that SOCE provided non-SOCE that they valued. For example, certain individuals reported that they had experienced less social isolation, found acknowledgment of their conflict and distress regarding faith and sexual orientation, and connected to similar individuals via groups efforts. Other individuals reported that SOCE helped them live in a manner consistent with their faith even if it did not change their sexual orientation (APA Task Force, 2009, pp. 44–53; Beckstead & Morrow, 2004).

However, these studies cannot be generalized to other populations and cannot predict individual responses to SOCE. Across studies it is unclear which specific individual characteristics and diagnostic criteria would, in advance of treatment, distinguish those individuals who will later perceive that they had been harmed by SOCE from those who do not report harms (APA Task Force, 2009, p. 43).

APA Task Force Report: Research on Children and Adolescents

The APA Task Force (2009) reviewed the literature on SOCE in children and adolescents and found no research demonstrating that SOCE has an impact on childhood or eventual adult sexual orientation (pp. 71–80). In published studies, one common treatment in children was reinforcing gender stereotypic behaviors and suppressing nonconforming gender expressions to prevent adult LGB attraction and identity. However, the studies provided no confirmation that teaching or reinforcing stereotyped gender-normative behavior in childhood or adolescence can alter future adult sexual orientation (APA Task Force, 2009, pp. 71–80).

Published accounts that describe inpatient facilities for adolescents designed to change their sexual orientation or the behavioral expression of their sexual orientation suggest that such approaches have the potential to increase isolation, self-hatred, internalized stigma, depression, anxiety, and suicidality by presenting fear-based inaccurate and stereotyped information (APA Task Force, 2009, pp. 71–80). These programs can violate ethical and practice guidelines by ignoring current scientific information on sexual orientation, by not providing treatment in the least-restrictive setting possible, and by not protecting client self-determination (APA, 2017; APA Task Force, 2009, pp. 71–80).

Conclusion

The APA Task Force concluded that SOCE had not been proven to be effective in changing sexual orientation in adults or youth. Some studies reported participant harms. Some participants report effects consistent with supportive/group therapy (e.g., reduction of isolation).

CURRENT SOCE RESEARCH 2009-2020

I completed a literature review that was similar in scope to that conducted by the APA Task Force, focusing on quality peer-reviewed literature in scientific journals published since 2008. The major works are listed in Table 1.1. The literature review did not find any experimental studies, such as a controlled trial of a specific intervention, which could assess a clear causal impact of SOCE on outcomes. Instead, most SOCE research from 2008 to 2020 falls into two broad categories that use retrospective reports: (a) studies of individuals who have undergone SOCE to explore their experiences (Bradshaw et al., 2015; Dehlin, Galliher, Bradshaw, Hyde, & Crowell, 2015; Fjelstrom, 2013; Flentje et al., 2014; Maccio, 2011; Weiss et al., 2010) and (b) studies that compare sexual minority individuals who have undergone SOCE with those who did not (Blosnich et al., 2020; Green et al., 2020; Higbee et al., 2020; Ryan et al., 2018; Salway et al., 2020).

Demographics

The first set of SOCE research explores the perceptions and experiences of specific populations, predominantly White men, most of whom are from conservative Christian faiths, including LGBT, ex-gay, ex-ex-gay, and those wishing to change their sexual orientation because of the perception that

TABLE 1.1. Research Relevant to SOCE 2009–2020

Year	Author(s)	N	Population	Research type	Research design	Key findings
2020	Blosnich et al.	1,518	Self-identified sexual minority individuals in nationally representative United States	Nonexperimental, SOCE one aspect of broader study	Questionnaire, quantitative	Association of SOCE to suicidal ideation controlling for demographics and adverse childhood events
2020	Green et al.	34,000	Self-identified sexual minority youth (ages 13–24) in the United States	Nonexperimental, SOCE one aspect of broader study	Questionnaire, quantitative	Association between SOCE and suicide risk
2020	Higbee et al.	475	Self-identified LGB adults from southern United States	Nonexperimental, SOCE one aspect of broader study	Questionnaire, quantitative	Association between SOCE and negative mental health
2020	Meanley et al.	1,237	Men enrolled in U.S. multicenter AIDS study (M age = 61.5)	Nonexperimental, SOCE one aspect of broader study	Quantitative	No association between HIV infection and SOCE
2020	Salway et al.	8,388	Adults in Canada (2011–2012)	Nonexperimental, SOCE one aspect of broader study	Questionnaire, quantitative	Prevalence of SOCE in Canada, association between SOCE and negative mental and physical health
2018	Ryan et al.	245	Young adults (ages 21–25) in U.S.	Nonexperimental	Questionnaire, quantitative	Parent-initiated SOCE associated with negative mental health risks
2015	Bradshaw et al.	1,612	Adults, current or former members of LDS Church	Nonexperimental	Questionnaire, quantitative and qualitative	Patient evaluation of SOCE–significant risk of harms, minimal if any change in sexual orientation

Year	Author	N	Sample	Design	Method	Focus
2015	Dehlin et al.	1,612	Adults, current or former members of LDS Church	Nonexperimental	Questionnaire, quantitative and qualitative	Patient report of prevalence, type, and effectiveness of SOCE
2013	Fjelstrom	15	Adults in Midwest United States	Nonexperimental	Qualitative, interviews	Patient perspective on sexual orientation and change efforts
2013	Flentje et al.	38	Self-identified ex-ex-gay adults	Nonexperimental	Questionnaire, qualitative and quantitative	Patient report of SOCE experience
2011	Maccio	37	LGB adults in the United States	Nonexperimental	Survey, quantitative	Patient report of results of SOCE pre/post: no change
2011	Jones and Yarhouse	100	Adults in the United States, members of Exodus	Nonexperimental, longitudinal	Survey, quantitative and qualitative	Patient reports of results of SOCE (behavior, attraction) and distress
2010	Karten and Wade	117	U.S. adult men recruited from SOCE providers	Nonexperimental	Quantitative	Motivation and perception of SOCE
2010	Maccio	263	LGB adults in the United States	Nonexperimental	Quantitative	Motivations and characteristics of SOCE participants compared with non-SOCE participants
2010	Ryan et al.	245	LGBT adults in the United States	Nonexperimental	Quantitative	Experiences of youth with family rejection (includes being sent to SOCE)
2010	Weiss et al.	267 ex-gay, 71 ex-ex-gay	Ex-gay and ex-ex-gay U.S. adults	Nonexperimental	Quantitative and qualitative analysis of messages	Motivation and experience with SOCE

Note. LDS = Church of Jesus Christ of Latter-day Saints; LGBT = lesbian, gay, bisexual, and transgender; SOCE = sexual orientation change efforts.

same-sex orientation is presented as inconsistent with faith, family, and community (Bradshaw et al., 2015; Dehlin, Galliher, Bradshaw, Hyde, & Crowell, 2015; Fjelstrom, 2013; Flentje et al., 2013; Karten & Wade, 2010; Maccio, 2010; Weiss et al., 2010). Given the lack of diversity of participants, the findings from one study cannot necessarily be generalized to other samples and cannot be seen as representative of all individuals who may have experienced SOCE.

The second set of studies uses cross-sectional samples that include broader samples of individuals, including youth (Green et al., 2020). This research provides information on the relationship of SOCE to later adverse health outcomes in samples of LGBT individuals. These studies use existing large samples or internet recruitment to include more demographically diverse participants (Blosnich et al., 2020; Green et al., 2020; Higbee et al., 2020; Salway et al., 2020). Some studies include women and people of color (Green et al., 2020; Higbee et al., 2020; Ryan et al., 2018). Results indicate that higher proportions of Hispanic/Latinx respondents, those from low-income families, and those from the South were found among those who underwent SOCE and GICE. Being raised in a family where religious critiques of same-sex sexual orientation and nonconforming gender is reported by those who report SOCE in youth (Green et al., 2020; Higbee et al., 2020). Salway and colleagues (2020) found that SOCE had been provided to adult Canadians across the country.

Reasons to Seek SOCE—Adults

Studies gathered information on the concerns of those adults who seek SOCE (Bradshaw et al., 2015; Dehlin, Galliher, Bradshaw, Hyde, & Crowell, 2015; Fjelstrom, 2013; Flentje et al., 2013; Maccio, 2010; Weiss et al., 2010). Additionally, the participants provided subjective assessments of their efforts so that these studies may assist psychotherapists serving this population (Bradshaw et al., 2015; Dehlin, Galliher, Bradshaw, & Crowell, 2015). Both male and female (religious and formerly religious) adult participants were reported to believe that their same-sex attractions and feelings were incompatible with their faith (Dehlin, Galliher, Bradshaw, & Crowell, 2015; Dehlin, Galliher, Bradshaw, Hyde, & Crowell, 2015; Fjelstrom, 2013; Maccio, 2010). These studies focus on understanding the self-perceptions of conflicts and cognitive dissonance of religious individuals who experience attraction and arousal to members of their own sex (Dehlin, Galliher, Bradshaw, Hyde, & Crowell, 2015; Fjelstrom, 2013; Flentje et al., 2013, 2014; Weiss et al., 2010). This dissonance appears to be related to distress among participants.

Maccio (2010) explored the role of faith, family, and community on why individuals choose to enter SOCE. Family pressure and the fear of family rejection are also motives for religiously conservative individuals to participate in SOCE (Maccio, 2010). Maccio (2010) found that the possibility that an individual would try SOCE increased with negative family reactions to a disclosure of same-sex orientation or expectations that family reactions would be negative. Certain individuals in one study experienced a desire for a heterosexual marriage—consistent with certain faith traditions—or to remain in a heterosexual marriage (Maccio, 2010; Weiss et al., 2010). The fear of rejection by a faith community or actual directions by a faith community to participate in SOCE play a role in participation in SOCE (Dehlin, Galliher, Bradshaw, Hyde, & Crowell, 2015; Maccio, 2010).

Internalized stigma was also a factor in pursuing SOCE. Bradshaw and colleagues explored underlying psychological motivations, and their research points to internalized stigma as a cause of distress in those who undertake SOCE. Participant attempts to change sexual orientation reflect a negative appraisal of same-sex attractions (Bradshaw et al., 2015). Minority stress—negative emotional repercussions from being a stigmatized population—appears to contribute to depression in LDS adult male populations (Crowell et al., 2015).

Effectiveness

As noted earlier, I was unable to identify any methodologically sound studies to evaluate whether SOCE changes sexual orientation. For example, none of the published studies were experiments in which specific treatments were adequately tested. The selection by practitioners or by existing organizations that support change efforts also raised issues of bias in sampling, as in these sample subjects were more likely to endorse sexual orientation change (e.g., Drescher & Zucker, 2006; Jones & Yarhouse, 2011; Karten & Wade, 2010). Claims that SOCE definitively changed sexual orientation in two studies were because of methodological and statistical flaws or unreliable because of methodological limitations (Linacre Quarterly, 2020; Panozzo, 2013; Spitzer, 2012).

Two studies that assess change efforts use methods that render their conclusions unreliable. A longitudinal study of members of a religiously based organization that aimed to examine change efforts had one third of participants drop out, imperfect statistical design, and subjective measures of change (Jones & Yarhouse, 2011). The participants in this study engaged in a variety of efforts over a number of years (e.g., support groups, psychotherapy from licensed practitioners, religious interventions, self-initiated efforts, and parent interventions). Although some participants felt that the treatment had benefited them, the impact (harm or benefit) of a specific type of effort is unknown. In another study, Maccio (2011) asked whether SOCE had impacted the sexual orientation of currently identified LGB participants. There was no change in subjective measures of sexual orientation (pre–post treatment) in retrospectively recalled experiences. Methodological concerns, including the retrospective nature of the assessment and the lack of specificity of treatment, mean that this study cannot provide definitive results.

In contrast to this research, Bradshaw et al. (2015) designed a study to remedy some of the flaws in prior research and to assess participant perceptions of SOCE to provide some in-depth information but without claiming causal results. In their 1,600-person sample of LDS members who had undergone SOCE, Bradshaw and collaborators found that same-sex attractions and arousal persisted despite the individuals' efforts to change (Bradshaw et al., 2015; Dehlin, Galliher, Bradshaw, & Crowell, 2015; Dehlin, Galliher, Bradshaw, Hyde, & Crowell, 2015). The vast majority of participants (95+%) reported little to no perceived change in sexual orientation change as a result of these efforts (Bradshaw et al., 2015; Dehlin, Galliher, Bradshaw, Hyde, & Crowell, 2015). Participants did note that they perceived some aspects of the efforts as helpful, such as social support; however, 42% reported that efforts were not at all helpful (Bradshaw et al., 2015). Other nonexperimental studies reported that SOCE participants did not report changes in sexual orientation (Fjelstrom, 2013; Flentje et al., 2013; Weiss et al., 2010).

Harms

A 2020 study from a nationally representative sample of LGB adults (Blosnich et al., 2020), which controlled for adverse childhood events often linked to mental health issues, found a significantly higher incidence of suicidal ideation and attempts in those who had experienced SOCE. Specifically,

> SOCE was associated with twice the odds of lifetime suicidal ideation, 75% increased odds of planning to attempt suicide, and 67% increased odds of suicide attempt resulting in moderate or severe injury (the last did not reach statistical significance at $p < .05$). (Blosnich et al., 2020, p. 1027)

The results of this study support concerns voiced by participants in all recent studies and suggest that SOCE has a significant association with suicide risk. Salway et al. (2020) reported that the study participants identified both negative mental and physical health effects. The negative mental health effects include suicide attempts and ideation, depression, isolation, and illicit drug use. Meanley and colleagues (2020) did not find differences in HIV-seroconversion status; this may be unsurprising because of the many factors related to transmission (e.g., community base rates, pharmacological advances).

Bradshaw et al.'s (2015) study found that 37% of participants reported efforts were moderately to severely harmful. Reported harms included decreased self-esteem, increased self-shame, increased depression and anxiety, the feeling that they had wasted time and money, increased distance from God and their faith institutions, worsening of family relationships, and increased suicidality. Religious participants reported these psychological harms as well as loss of faith, negative effects on family relations, and regret over the of waste of time and money (Bradshaw et al., 2015; Dehlin, Galliher, Bradshaw, Hyde, & Crowell, 2015). Religious efforts (e.g., prayer, religious study, religious retreats) were rated as more ineffective and damaging than SOCE provided by mental health professionals (Bradshaw et al., 2015). Individuals start SOCE with the expectation of change; those who expected a change in sexual orientation perceived greater harms by SOCE. These individuals reported a loss of self-esteem and loss of religious faith (Bradshaw et al., 2015). Other studies also report harms. Flentje and colleagues (2014) found similar self-reported harms, such as increased depression, anxiety, suicidality, shame, guilt, and self-hatred.

Other Outcomes

Some individuals did not experience change in sexual orientation but had diverse experiences and some of the following: reduced distress; acceptance by self and/or family; increased coping with conflict; and self-acceptance as lesbian, gay, bisexual, transgender, and questioning or queer (LGBTQ; Bradshaw et al., 2015; Dehlin, Galliher, Bradshaw, Hyde, & Crowell, 2015; Flentje et al., 2014). Efforts to isolate or compartmentalize sexual orientation from faith beliefs that condemn diverse sexual orientations were difficult and not maintained over time (Dehlin, Galliher, Bradshaw, & Crowell, 2015). Those who integrated their faith and sexual orientation or rejected their faith beliefs to accept their sexual orientation reported better psychological functioning (Dehlin, Galliher, Bradshaw, & Crowell, 2015). Some participants felt that certain types of SOCE—those conducted by professionals—did provide a forum for discussing psychological conflicts and were more beneficial than religious methods (Bradshaw et al., 2015).

POST-2009 STUDIES OF SOCE IN CHILDREN AND YOUTH

A review of published studies found no experiments evaluating SOCE or quasi-experiments that were conducted on children and youth. There is no research base for claims that SOCE can change sexual orientation in children and youth or that interventions in childhood affect an adult's sexual orientation.

The Family Acceptance Project has conducted a number of studies on families and the impact of their behavior on LGBTQ child and adolescent mental health (Ryan et al., 2009, 2010). A recent study by Ryan and collaborators (2018) evaluated the impact on adults' mental health and vocational achievement of family-implemented SOCE experienced in adolescence. Green and collaborators (2020) undertook a study of 13- to 25-year-olds in real time to assess suicidality. The team included two questions on SOCE and GICE. As part of a larger study, Higbee et al. (2020) evaluated young adults who had experienced SOCE as youths. Each of these studies provides information on mental health concerns and is examined next.

The Impact of Family-Implemented SOCE on Mental Health

Families often seek out SOCE when they are distressed about their child's sexual orientation and gender identity. Accepting behaviors from families appear to be helpful to the healthy development of children compared with behaviors that are critical and rejecting (Ryan et al., 2009, 2010). SOCE often encourages parents to engage in coercive, rejecting, and critical behaviors based on false claims that these behaviors can change or influence a child's gender identity or sexual orientation. The rejection of an adolescent's gender identity and expression is associated with poorer emotional, social, and vocational outcomes (Ryan et al., 2009). Research by Ryan, Russell, and collaborators indicates that children and adolescents perceive SOCE as family rejection (Ryan et al., 2010). Those youth who experienced such rejection faced increased negative mental health condition, including depression, suicidal thoughts, and suicide attempts (Ryan et al., 2010).

Ryan and collaborators examined the impact of family-implemented SOCE applied during adolescence on 245 young adults' mental health, social support, and economic status (Ryan et al., 2018). Family-implemented SOCE is where families attempt through parenting to change sexual orientation. Ryan and collaborators compared those who did not receive SOCE with those who received family-implemented SOCE and with those who received SOCE by a religious or mental health professional. Compared with LGBT-identified young adults who did not receive SOCE, those who did receive efforts delivered by mental health or religious professionals reported serious mental health harms, such as increased suicidal ideation and attempts and depressive symptoms; the rates of these serious mental health conditions were at least 3 times as high among those who received SOCE compared with those who did not. Those who reported family efforts to change their sexual orientation during childhood also noted harms, such as negative mental health symptoms; the rates were about twice as high as for those who did not receive SOCE.

Beyond the negative mental health effects, participants who received a form of SOCE in this study were found to have negative long-term effects such as lowered life satisfaction, less social support, lower socioeconomic status, and other serious difficulties in young adulthood that could affect them over the long term. Although this study used retrospective accounts and sampled only those who identified as LGBTQ, the harms experienced were significant and the differences between those who received and did not receive a form of SOCE were striking. Finally, the results indicated that some youth may be at higher risk of receiving SOCE. Youth whose gender expression was not consistent with social norms, whose parents were immigrants, or whose family had strong conservative religious beliefs were more likely to receive SOCE (Ryan et al., 2018). Half of the participants in this study identified as female.

Studies of SOCE in Minors and Young Adults

Green and collaborators (2020) assessed the impact of SOCE in a large study (34,000) of the experience of sexual minority youth and suicidal ideation and attempts. The researchers asked two questions relevant to SOCE: (a) "Has anyone tried to change your sexual orientation?" and if so, (b) "Have you ever undergone reparative therapy or conversion therapy?" (p. 1223). The researchers did control for a number of factors to isolate the impact of SOCE from other life events (e.g., discrimination, bullying), and compared those who had experienced SOCE with those who did not. Those who reported undergoing SOCE and/or GICE were more than twice as likely to report having attempted suicide and having multiple suicide attempts. Those who reported exposure to SOCE had almost 2 times greater odds of seriously considering suicide, more than 2 times greater odds of having attempted suicide, and 2½ times greater odds of multiple suicide attempts in the previous year. The study cannot determine causality, but the results do underscore a potential association, and the size of this study is certainly important. For example, the researchers reported that even after controlling for other events, SOCE was the strongest predictor of multiple suicide attempts.

The demographic characteristics of this survey expanded understanding of those groups affected. Cisgender male and female (two-thirds of sample) and transgender and gender nonconforming (one third of the sample) individuals were surveyed. LGBTQ individuals aged 13 to 17 were half the population. Young people with lower family incomes, who are from the South, and whose parents use negative religious themes reported higher frequencies of engaging in SOCE. Green and collaborators also found that more than three fourths of young people who underwent change efforts reported hearing their parents or caregivers use negative religious references about being LGBTQ, as compared with slightly less than half of those who did not undergo SOCE.

Studies of Adults Who Report SOCE as Minors

Higbee et al. (2020) examined a quantitative analysis of a convenience sample survey of adults who live in the southern United States. The study assessed various topics and included two questions on SOCE. The first question inquired if subjects had experienced SOCE as an adolescent. Women, Latinx, and non–gender conforming individuals reported a higher likelihood of SOCE, and most reported that SOCE was provided by a religious professional. Respondents who experienced conversion therapy as an adolescent have a significantly higher probability of experiencing a serious mental illness later in life. Additionally, those experiencing SOCE reported less religious observance later in life and lower educational attainment. This is consistent with Ryan et al.'s (2018) findings that SOCE is negatively associated with less education and lower overall socioeconomic status.

Higbee and collaborators found similar results to Green et al. (2020) in terms of demographics. Higbee et al. (2020) included respondents who were younger, transgender, nonbinary, lesbian, gay, another sexual orientation, Hispanic, less educated, and less religious at the time of taking the survey. This is an indication that SOCE is still being provided despite its rejection by professional associations and that the population that is exposed is quite diverse.

There are limitations to this and other work on adults who recall receiving change efforts as children or youth. The studies are based on recall of past efforts, and the limitations with retrospective recall have been described earlier in this chapter and in the 2009 APA Task Force Report (p. 29). These studies are with self-identified LGBTQ individuals who may perceive their experiences differently than those who do not so identify.

Summary of Research Related to Children

There are no reports of change to sexual orientation. There are reported harms from SOCE, such as an increase in suicidality and suicide attempts, as well as an increase in depression and anxiety, decreased religious beliefs, and lower educational and socioeconomic attainment. There are no reported benefits to the child or adolescent from SOCE (e.g., less isolation, social support).

SYNTHESIS OF RESEARCH FINDINGS

No methodologically adequate research provides evidence that SOCE can change SOCE in adults or children. There is evidence that SOCE is harmful and has negative mental health effects, such as depression, self-hatred, and suicidality in adults and youth (APA Task Force, 2009; Blosnich et al., 2020; Bradshaw et al., 2015; Dehlin, Galliher, Bradshaw, Hyde, & Crowell, 2015; Green et al., 2020; Higbee et al., 2020; Ryan et al., 2018; Salway et al., 2020).

The major studies are consistent. Green et al. (2020) found that youth aged 13 to 25 who reported being exposed to SOCE also reported that in the past 12 months they had seriously considered suicide; they were twice as likely to report having attempted suicide and having had multiple suicide attempts in the previous year. Ryan et al. (2018) found high rates of suicidality and suicide attempts in children who experienced family-implemented SOCE. Research on adults who participated in SOCE as youth shows evidence of long-term negative effects (Higbee et al., 2020; Ryan et al., 2018), such as negative mental health effects and vocational deficits when compared with young adults who did not experience SOCE. In a representative sample of LGBT adults who underwent SOCE, Blosnich and collaborators (2020) found significantly more suicidal ideation and attempts.

Adults who struggle with isolation and rejection from both the LGB and religious communities and participate in SOCE (e.g., psychotherapy, support groups, religious efforts) to reduce distress and conflicts. Although some see SOCE as consistent with religious prohibitions toward nonheterosexual sexual orientations, SOCE presents a high-risk effort for religious populations because of the potential loss of faith from such efforts. One of the greatest risks of harms is in the emotional repercussions of being told one should succeed in changing, when such a change cannot occur (Bradshaw et al., 2015; Dehlin, Galliher, Bradshaw, Hyde, & Crowell, 2015). The sense of failure is especially difficult for religious individuals who have such a great deal at stake (including their relationship with the divine and ties to family and community; see also APA Task Force, 2009; Beckstead & Morrow, 2004). For faith-based populations, interventions not associated with SOCE are generally safer and potentially more beneficial by clients (Bradshaw et al., 2015; Dehlin, Galliher, Bradshaw, Hyde, & Crowell, 2015).

Studies cannot predict how individuals will respond to SOCE—experience harms or relief from isolation. This uncertainty about how a client will respond to treatment makes avoiding harm more difficult and increases the ethical risks of providing SOCE (Drescher, 2015). The provision of an ineffective intervention with an association to harm is inconsistent with professional ethics and may pose extreme risks to children (American Psychiatric Association, 2013; APA, 2017; Mercer, 2017). There is no evidence that there are any positive aspects to SOCE that are unique to it. The positive elements reported by adult clients are similar to those offered religiously sensitive support groups and individual therapy and include social support and a forum for discussion of conflicts between spirituality and sexuality. Thus, SOCE could be replaced by such efforts without any negative effects to clients.

Although the earlier review by the APA Task Force found that most who had experienced SOCE were White men. The research conducted since 2008 finds that women, Latinx, and noncisgender individuals were sent to SOCE by family or experienced SOCE. SOCE is conducted by individuals by professionals and religious professionals, as well as by families.

FUTURE DIRECTIONS

Research

Given that variation in sexual orientation and gender identity are part of normal human development, it is clear that research focused on sexual orientation change is obsolete. This is particularly true for research on children, as federal guidelines for ethical research on children must minimize the potential for harm (Department of Health and Human Services, 2018). To increase the safety of children and adolescents, Mercer (2017) developed criteria for categorizing potentially harmful treatments for children; SOCE is such an effort and is unsupported by research or psychological constructs.

As noted in the APA Task Force Report, future directions in research can assist in developing psychotherapies that assist in integrating multiple diverse identities and reducing distress. Many therapies can assist those affected by prejudice and discrimination or denied appropriate treatment (Mercer, 2017;

Pachankis et al., 2015). Given that certain psychotherapy is effective in relieving mental health distress and not harmful, psychotherapists, families, and religious leaders should pursue these efforts and not SOCE (APA, 2021; APA Task Force on Psychological Practice with Sexual Minority Persons, 2021). A description of key efforts is provided in the next section.

Issues in Adult Psychotherapy

A growing body of clinical studies provides more information on individuals with strong faith beliefs who go through a process of identity development and integration (Bradshaw et al., 2015; Lefevor et al., 2020; Levy & Reeves, 2011; Pietkiewicz & Kołodziejczyk-Skrzypek, 2016; Rosenkrantz et al., 2016; Weiss et al., 2010; Yarhouse & Beckstead, 2011). These studies provide support that those who have conflicts between their religious identity and sexual orientation identity can develop satisfying, self-directed lives. Many reconcile faith and nonheterosexual identities; reduce mental health distress; and learn how to develop satisfying, self-directed lives with different sexual orientation identity outcomes. LGBTQ sexual orientation and faith can be positive forces in individuals' lives and enhance each identity (Bozard & Sanders, 2011; Rosenkrantz et al., 2016). Stigma plays a large role in identity integration for individuals (Sherry et al., 2010). For those from faith traditions that prohibit sexual orientation diversity, the most recent version of narrative sexual identity synthesis therapy (Yarhouse, 2019) focuses on reducing shame around same-sex attractions that can arise in those from traditional faiths reducing distress and enhancing emotional functioning.

As noted earlier, many studies are focused on the experience of White, cisgender Christian men. There is a small but growing literature on African American men (Lassiter, 2014; Pitt, 2010), Jewish clients (Slomowitz & Feit, 2015), and Muslim individuals (Jaspal & Cinnirella, 2010) with conflicts between faith, culture, and sexual orientation identities. One priority in future research to expand the diversity of the population studied.

For those negatively impacted by stigma, Pachankis and colleagues (2015) used a rigorous experimental design to evaluate an approach that reduces the negative mental health effects of minority stress on individuals addressing sexual orientation issues. Reducing minority stress and cognitive dissonance with respect to multiple identities can assist the client in resolving overt conflicts between faith and sexual orientation. The client's ultimate identity should be self-determined without a provider-imposed outcome (APA Task Force, 2009, p. 55; Bozard & Sanders, 2011; Haldeman, 2004; Lefevor et al., 2020; Pitt, 2010; Weiss et al., 2010).

Issues in Psychotherapy for Children and Youth

In response to growing concerns about potential harms caused by SOCE and GICE in children, the U.S. Substance Abuse and Mental Health Services Administration (SAMHSA) published a report based on these consensus findings. The report concluded that SOCE and GICE should not be offered to children and youth because of a lack of scientific evidence and risk of harms:

> Interventions aimed at a fixed outcome, such as gender conformity or other-sex sexual orientation, including those aimed at changing gender identity, gender expression, and sexual orientation are coercive, can be harmful, and should not be part of behavioral health treatments. Directing the child to be conforming to any gender expression or sexual orientation, or directing the parents to place pressure for specific gender expressions, gender identities, and sexual orientations [is] inappropriate and reinforce[s] harmful gender and sexual orientation stereotypes. (SAMHSA, 2015, p. 11)

SAMHSA (2015) developed recommendations for the treatment of children and youth that include the provision of

> accurate information on sexual orientation, gender identity, and expression; increase family and school support; and reduce rejection of sexual minority youth. Behavioral health practitioners identify sources of distress and work to reduce distress experienced by children and adolescents. Behavioral health professionals provide efforts to encourage identity exploration and integration, adaptive coping, and family acceptance to improve psychological well-being. (p. 12)

Specific treatment strategies relevant to specific concerns (sexual orientation, gender identity) and developmental age are presented in the report.

Human Rights Issues

The UNIESOGI undertook an examination of conversion therapy across all ages and among international populations. The UNIESOGI performed site visits to various countries and reviewed documents, reports, and research and took testimony from individuals (e.g., researchers and those who underwent SOCE), professional associations, and researchers. The report concluded that SOCE reflects stigmatizing cultural attitudes, political discrimination, and persecution (Bishop, 2019; UNIESOGI, 2020; Vezzosi et al., 2019). The UNIESOGI condemned SOCE as inappropriate for all ages and all nationalities, as harmful to mental and physical health, and as a violation of international law (UNIESOGI, 2020). With regard to children, the UNIESOGI report states, "The IESOGI is convinced that the decision to subject a child to conversion practices can never be in conformity with a child's best interests" (p. 3).

An additional concern expressed by the UNIESOGI is that sexual minorities are denied the opportunity to be a spiritual being when faith and diverse sexual orientations are framed as inconsistent (Madrigal-Borloz, 2020). Ongoing risks related to SOCE are stereotypes and government propaganda that demonize sexual minorities—deny individuals the rights of citizenship and place in society—and criminalize and pathologize diverse sexual orientations (UNIESOGI, 2020).

Preventing the Use of SOCE

Given SOCE's ineffectiveness and potential harms, reducing its occurrence is crucial. SOCE has been repudiated by all the major medical and mental health organizations (GLAD, n.d.) and banned for minors by many state and local governments in the United States (Movement Advancement Project, n.d.). Other countries have banned SOCE; for example, a ban on SOCE for all ages has been instituted through the Memorandum of Understanding on Conversion Therapy in the UK (version 2; 2019) to all professional health care organizations (Fitzsimons, 2020). As noted earlier, the UNIESOGI (2020) condemned the use of SOCE for any person.

Professional guidelines published by the APA for the treatment of LGB individuals and other international professional associations (i.e., Canada, United Kingdom, Western Europe, Australia, and New Zealand) urge the discontinuation of SOCE and recommend multicultural, affirmative approaches (e.g., APA Task Force on Psychological Practice with Sexual Minority Persons, 2021). Many international professional associations have adopted psychotherapy guidelines for LGBT and gender nonconforming individuals that reject SOCE (APA, n.d.).

Client participation in SOCE is a response to social stigma directed at LGBT individuals that results in social rejection and legal discrimination (Bishop, 2019; Haldeman, 2002; UNIESOGI, 2020). Thus, reducing discrimination and rejection associated with same-sexual orientation would reduce demand for SOCE (APA Task Force, 2009; UNIESOGI, 2020). Continued advocacy and the inclusion of LGBT rights as human rights are essential to provide protections to all individuals (e.g., Bishop, 2019; Clinton, 2011; Panozzo, 2013; UNIESOGI, 2020).

Bans on SOCE for children, youth, and adults as well as legal action against SOCE practitioners under consumer protection acts may provide some protection for clients and reduce stigma directed at LGBT individuals. However, most to the research cited in this chapter found that the majority of SOCE is often provided by religious providers or families who are often exempted from these laws. Given Bradshaw et al.'s (2015) finding that participants reported that religious therapy was more unhelpful, it is of great concern that U.S. law exempts religious efforts. Given this research, children and youth should be protected from these efforts, given their inability to provide informed consent. Adults in faith communities or whose family support SOCE may have difficulty in providing full informed consent. Further, many individuals from faith communities report a loss of faith from these efforts (Beckstead & Morrow, 2004). Given that there are multiple non-SOCE therapeutic approaches that address the concerns of faith communities, there is no rationale for SOCE to be provided for those from faith backgrounds.

Ryan et al. (2018) found that individualized behaviors or family-implemented interventions are some of the most practiced forms of SOCE in certain populations. This finding underscores that efforts to reduce SOCE must address these family practices, which are not addressed by legal bans on licensed practitioners. Such personal efforts may reflect particular faith beliefs, but they result in continued distress and suffering (Ryan et al., 2018).

As an alternative, broad family-based affirmative early education on sexual orientation and gender identity may reduce distress in families and children; such information could be tailored to specific communities (see Chapter 4, this volume). Therapeutic alternatives that combine spiritually sensitive practices and LGBT-affirmative alternatives can assist those in distress without the risk of harms (APA Task Force, 2009).

CONCLUSION

Consumers of psychotherapy of all ages deserve safe and effective treatment, and there is clear evidence that SOCE is not effective and persuasive evidence that SOCE is not safe (e.g., causes harm). All current research findings support the discontinuation of SOCE by clients, families, and practitioners because of risks of harm, including increased risk of depression, anxiety, suicidal ideation, and attempts. For children and adolescents, SOCE provided by professionals also has elevated risks of harm for this vulnerable population, such as increasing depression and suicidality. SOCE provided by parents can dramatically weaken the protective and nurturing functions of the family by enlisting the family in rejecting behaviors that can cause harm the child.

Instead of SOCE, treatment provided to adults, children, and adolescents who are distressed or whose parents are distressed can include well-established psychotherapy techniques designed to diminish self-stigma and integrate and reconcile religious and sexual orientation identities. Evidence-based approaches with available for clients in distress and providers in this area (e.g., Pachankis et al., 2015; Ryan et al., 2009). These approaches include the reduction of minority stress and cognitive dissonance to support the affirmation and integration of multiple identities (APA Task Force, 2009, p. 55; Bozard & Sanders, 2011; Haldeman, 2004; Lefevor et al., 2020; Pitt, 2010; Weiss et al., 2010). For children and adolescents, developmentally appropriate interventions that assist them in improving their mental health, reach key emotional and social milestones, and strengthen family support are recommended instead (SAMHSA, 2015).

There is no justification for providing SOCE to either adults or children in the United States or internationally (APA, 2021; UNIESOGI, 2020). Policymakers can increase efforts to encourage practitioners to adopt alternative approaches and discontinue SOCE. Further, ending the criminalization and pathologization of diverse sexual orientations is a priority worldwide to prevent the stigma and prejudice that is associated with client distress. Reducing the stigma surrounding diverse sexual orientations has reduced demand for SOCE to this point and can continue to do so (APA Task Force, 2009).

REFERENCES

American Psychiatric Association. (2013). *The principles of medical ethics with annotations especially applicable to psychiatry.* https://www.psychiatry.org/psychiatrists/practice/ethics

American Psychological Association. (n.d.). *IPsyNet guidelines and practice position statements.* https://www.apa.org/ipsynet/practice/guidelines

American Psychological Association. (2017). *Ethical principles of psychologists and code of conduct* (2002, Amended June 1, 2010, and January 1, 2017). https://www.apa.org/ethics/code/ethics-code-2017.pdf

American Psychological Association. (2021). *APA resolution on sexual orientation change efforts.* https://www.apa.org/about/policy/resolution-sexual-orientation-change-efforts.pdf

American Psychological Association Task Force on Appropriate Therapeutic Responses to Sexual Orientation. (2009). *Report of the American Psychological Association Task Force on Appropriate Therapeutic Responses to Sexual Orientation.* https://www.apa.org/pi/lgbt/resources/therapeutic-response.pdf

American Psychological Association Task Force on Psychological Practice With Sexual Minority Persons. (2021). *Guidelines for psychological practice with sexual minority persons.* https://www.apa.org/about/policy/psychological-sexual-minority-persons.pdf

Beckstead, A. L., & Morrow, S. L. (2004). Mormon clients' experiences of conversion therapy: The need for a new treatment approach. *The Counseling Psychologist, 32*(5), 651–690. https://doi.org/10.1177/0011000004267555

Bishop, A. (2019). *Harmful treatment: The global reach of so-called conversion therapy.* OutRight Action International. https://outrightinternational.org/sites/default/files/ ConversionFINAL_1.pdf

Blosnich, J. R., Henderson, E. R., Coulter, R. W. S., Goldbach, J. T., & Meyer, I. H. (2020). Sexual orientation change efforts, adverse childhood experiences, and suicide ideation and attempt among sexual minority adults, United States, 2016–2018. *American Journal of Public Health, 110*(7), 1024–1030. https://doi.org/10.2105/ AJPH.2020.305637

Bozard, R. L., Jr., & Sanders, C. J. (2011). Helping Christian lesbian, gay, and bisexual clients recover religion as a source of strength: Developing a model for assessment and integration of religious identity in counseling. *Journal of LGBT Issues in Counseling, 5*(1), 47–74. https://doi.org/10.1080/15538605.2011.554791

Bradshaw, K., Dehlin, J. P., Crowell, K. A., Galliher, R. V., & Bradshaw, W. S. (2015). Sexual orientation change efforts through psychotherapy for LGBQ individuals affiliated with the Church of Jesus Christ of Latter-day Saints. *Journal of Sex & Marital Therapy, 41*(4), 391–412. https://doi.org/10.1080/0092623X.2014.915907

Chou, R., Aronson, N., Atkins, D., Ismaila, A. S., Santaguida, P., Smith, D. H., Whitlock, E., Wilt, T. J., & Moher, D. (2010). AHRQ Series Paper 4: Assessing harms when comparing medical interventions: AHRQ and the effective health-care program. *Journal of Clinical Epidemiology, 63*(5), 502–512. https://doi.org/10.1016/j.jclinepi. 2008.06.007

Clinton, H. (2011, December 6). Hillary Clinton on gay rights abroad: Secretary of State delivers historic LGBT speech in Geneva. *The Huffington Post.* https://www. huffingtonpost.com/2011/12/06/hillary-clinton-gay-rights-speech-geneva_n_ 1132392.html

Crowell, K. A., Galliher, R. V., Dehlin, J., & Bradshaw, W. S. (2015). Specific aspects of minority stress associated with depression among LDS affiliated non-heterosexual adults. *Journal of Homosexuality, 62*(2), 242–267. https://doi.org/10.1080/ 00918369.2014.969611

Dehlin, J. P., Galliher, R. V., Bradshaw, W. S., & Crowell, K. A. (2015). Navigating sexual and religious identity conflict: A Mormon perspective. *Identity: An International Journal of Theory and Research, 15*(1), 1–22. https://doi.org/10.1080/ 15283488.2014.989440

Dehlin, J. P., Galliher, R. V., Bradshaw, W. S., Hyde, D. C., & Crowell, K. A. (2015). Sexual orientation change efforts among current or former LDS church members. *Journal of Counseling Psychology, 62*(2), 95–105. https://doi.org/10.1037/cou0000011

Department of Health and Human Services. (2018). 45 CFR 46. https://www.hhs. gov/ohrp/regulations-and-policy/regulations/45-cfr-46/index.html

Dimidjian, S., & Hollon, S. D. (2010). How would we know if psychotherapy were harmful? *American Psychologist, 65*(1), 21–33. https://doi.org/10.1037/ a0017299

Drescher, J. (1998). I'm your handyman: A history of reparative therapies. *Journal of Homosexuality, 36*(1), 19–42. https://doi.org/10.1300/J082v36n01_02

Drescher, J. (2015). Can sexual orientation be changed? *Journal of Gay & Lesbian Mental Health, 19*(1), 84–93. https://doi.org/10.1080/19359705.2014.944460

Drescher, J., & Zucker, K. J. (Eds.). (2006). *Ex-gay research: Analyzing the Spitzer study and its relation to science, religion, politics, and culture.* Harrington Park Press.

Fitzsimons, T. (2020, May 6). *Germany is fifth country to ban conversion therapy for minors.* NBC News. https://www.nbcnews.com/feature/nbc-out/germany-5th-country-ban-conversion-therapy-minors-n1203166

Fjelstrom, J. (2013). Sexual orientation change efforts and the search for authenticity. *Journal of Homosexuality, 60*(6), 801–827. https://doi.org/10.1080/00918369.2013.774830

Flentje, A., Heck, N. C., & Cochran, B. N. (2013). Sexual reorientation therapy interventions: Perspectives of ex-ex-gay individuals. *Journal of Gay & Lesbian Mental Health, 17*(3), 256–277. https://doi.org/10.1080/19359705.2013.773268

Flentje, A., Heck, N. C., & Cochran, B. N. (2014). Experiences of ex-ex-gay individuals in sexual reorientation therapy: Reasons for seeking treatment, perceived helpfulness and harmfulness of treatment, and post-treatment identification. *Journal of Homosexuality, 61*(9), 1242–1268. https://doi.org/10.1080/00918369.2014.926763

GLAD. (n.d.). Conversion therapy. https://www.glaad.org/conversiontherapy?response_type=embed

Gonsiorek, J. C. (1991). The empirical basis for the demise of the illness model of homosexuality. In J. C. Gonsiorek & J. D. Weinrich (Eds.), *Homosexuality: Research implications for public policy* (pp. 115–136). Sage. https://doi.org/10.4135/9781483325422.n8

Grace, A. P. (2008). The charisma and deception of reparative therapies: When medical science beds religion. *Journal of Homosexuality, 55*(4), 545–580. https://doi.org/10.1080/00918360802421676

Green, A. E., Price-Feeney, M., Dorison, S. H., & Pick, C. J. (2020). Self-reported conversion efforts and suicidality among US LGBTQ youths and young adults, 2018. *American Journal of Public Health, 110*(8), 1221–1227. https://doi.org/10.2105/AJPH.2020.305701

Haldeman, D. C. (1994). The practice and ethics of sexual orientation conversion therapy. *Journal of Consulting and Clinical Psychology, 62*(2), 221–227. https://doi.org/10.1037/0022-006X.62.2.221

Haldeman, D. C. (2002). Gay rights, patient rights: The implications of sexual orientation conversion therapy. *Professional Psychology, Research and Practice, 33*(3), 260–264. https://doi.org/10.1037/0735-7028.33.3.260

Haldeman, D. C. (2004). When sexual and religious orientation collide: Considerations for psychotherapy with conflicted gay men. *The Counseling Psychologist, 32*(5), 691–715. https://doi.org/10.1177/0011000004267560

Higbee, M., Wright, E. R., & Roemerman, R. M. (2020). Conversion therapy in the southern United States: Prevalence and experiences of the survivors. *Journal of Homosexuality.* Advance online publication. https://doi.org/10.1080/00918369.2020.1840213

Jaspal, R., & Cinnirella, M. (2010). Coping with potentially incompatible identities: Accounts of religious, ethnic, and sexual identities from British Pakistani men who identify as Muslim and gay. *British Journal of Social Psychology, 49*(4), 849–870. https://doi.org/10.1348/014466609X485025

Jones, S. L., & Yarhouse, M. A. (2011). A longitudinal study of attempted religiously mediated sexual orientation change. *Journal of Sex & Marital Therapy, 37*(5), 404–427. https://doi.org/10.1080/0092623X.2011.607052

Karten, E. Y., & Wade, J. C. (2010). Sexual orientation change efforts in men: A client perspective. *Journal of Men's Studies, 18*(1), 84–102. https://doi.org/10.3149/jms.1801.84

Lassiter, J. M. (2014). Extracting dirt from water: A strengths-based approach to religion for African American same-gender-loving men. *Journal of Religion and Health, 53*(1), 178–189. https://doi.org/10.1007/s10943-012-9668-8

Lefevor, G. T., Blaber, I. P., Huffman, C. E., Schow, R. L., Beckstead, A. L., Raynes, M., & Rosik, C. H. (2020). The role of religiousness and beliefs about sexuality in well-being among sexual minority Mormons. *Psychology of Religion and Spirituality, 12*(4), 460–470. https://doi.org/10.1037/rel0000261

Levy, D. L., & Reeves, P. (2011). Resolving identity conflict: Gay, lesbian, and queer individuals with a Christian upbringing. *Journal of Gay & Lesbian Social Services, 23*(1), 53–68. https://doi.org/10.1080/10538720.2010.530193

Linacre Quarterly. (2020). Retracted: Effects of therapy on religious men who have unwanted same-sex attraction. *Linacre Quarterly, 87*(1), 1–17. https://journals.sagepub.com/doi/10.1177/0024363918788559

Maccio, E. M. (2010). Influence of family, religion, and social conformity on client participation in sexual reorientation therapy. *Journal of Homosexuality, 57*(3), 441–458. https://doi.org/10.1080/00918360903543196

Maccio, E. M. (2011). Self-reported sexual orientation and identity before and after sexual reorientation therapy. *Journal of Gay & Lesbian Psychotherapy, 15*(3), 242–259.

Madrigal-Borloz, V. (2020, September 8). Presentation: *Lesbians & conversion therapy: Tracing its history, impact & ways to fight back!* ELC Eurocentralasian Lesbian Community. Facebook Live. https://www.facebook.com/ELC-Eurocentralasian-Lesbian-Community-1860721560840038

Mallory, C., Brown, C. N. T., & Conron, K. J. (2019, June). *Conversion therapy and LGBT youth: Update.* The Williams Institute, UCLA School of Law. https://williamsinstitute.law.ucla.edu/wp-content/uploads/Conversion-Therapy-Update-Jun-2019.pdf

Meanley, S. P., Stall, R. D., Dakwar, O., Egan, J. E., Friedman, M. R., Haberlen, S. A., Okafor, C., Teplin, L. A., & Plankey, M. W. (2020). Characterizing experiences of conversion therapy among middle-aged and older men who have sex with men from the Multicenter AIDS Cohort Study (MACS). *Sexuality Research & Social Policy, 17*(2), 334–342. https://doi.org/10.1007/s13178-019-00396-y

Memorandum of Understanding on Conversion Therapy in the UK, version 2. (2019). https://www.bacp.co.uk/events-and-resources/ethics-and-standards/mou/

Mercer, J. (2017). Evidence of potentially harmful psychological treatments for children and adolescents. *Child & Adolescent Social Work Journal, 34*(2), 107–125. https://doi.org/10.1007/s10560-016-0480-2

Movement Advancement Project. (n.d.). *Conversion "therapy" laws.* http://www.lgbtmap.org/equality-maps/conversion_therapy

Pachankis, J. E., Hatzenbuehler, M. L., Rendina, H. J., Safren, S. A., & Parsons, J. T. (2015). LGB-affirmative cognitive-behavioral therapy for young adult gay and bisexual men: A randomized controlled trial of a transdiagnostic minority stress approach. *Journal of Consulting and Clinical Psychology, 83*(5), 875–889. https://doi.org/10.1037/ccp0000037

Panozzo, D. (2013). Advocating for an end to reparative therapy: Methodological grounding and blueprint for change. *Journal of Gay & Lesbian Social Services, 25*(3), 362–377. https://doi.org/10.1080/10538720.2013.807214

Pietkiewicz, I. J., & Kołodziejczyk-Skrzypek, M. (2016). Living in sin? How gay Catholics manage their conflicting sexual and religious identities. *Archives of Sexual Behavior, 45*(6), 1573–1585. https://doi.org/10.1007/s10508-016-0752-0

Pitt, R. N. (2010). "Killing the messenger": Religious Black gay men's neutralization of anti-gay religious messages. *Journal for the Scientific Study of Religion, 49*(1), 56–72. https://doi.org/10.1111/j.1468-5906.2009.01492.x

Rosenkrantz, D. E., Rostosky, S. S., Riggle, E. D. B., & Cook, J. R. (2016). The positive aspects of intersecting religious/spiritual and LGBTQ identities. *Spirituality in Clinical Practice, 3*(2), 127–138. https://doi.org/10.1037/scp0000095

Rozental, A., Castonguay, L., Dimidjian, S., Lambert, M., Shafran, R., Andersson, G., & Carlbring, P. (2018). Negative effects in psychotherapy: Commentary and recommendations for future research and clinical practice. *BJPsych Open, 4*(4), 307–312. https://doi.org/10.1192/bjo.2018.42

Ryan, C., Huebner, D., Diaz, R. M., & Sanchez, J. (2009). Family rejection as a predictor of negative health outcomes in White and Latino lesbian, gay, and bisexual young adults. *Pediatrics, 123*(1), 346–352. https://doi.org/10.1542/peds.2007-3524

Ryan, C., Russell, S. T., Huebner, D., Diaz, R., & Sanchez, J. (2010). Family acceptance in adolescence and the health of LGBT young adults. *Journal of Child and Adolescent Psychiatric Nursing, 23*(4), 205–213. https://doi.org/10.1111/j.1744-6171.2010.00246.x

Ryan, C., Toomey, R., Diaz, R., & Russell, S. T. (2018). Parent-initiated sexual orientation change efforts with LGBT adolescents: Implications for young adult mental health and adjustment. *Journal of Homosexuality, 67*(2), 159–173. https://doi.org/10.1080/00918369.2018.1538407

Salway, T., Ferlatte, O., Gesink, D., & Lachowsky, N. J. (2020). Prevalence of exposure to sexual orientation change efforts and associated sociodemographic characteristics and psychosocial health outcomes among Canadian sexual minority men. *Canadian Journal of Psychiatry, 65*(7), 502–509. https://doi.org/10.1177/0706743720902629

Sherry, A., Adelman, A., Whidle, M. R., & Quick, D. (2010). Competing selves: Negotiating the intersection of spiritual and sexual Identities. *Professional Psychology, Research and Practice, 41*(2), 112–119. https://doi.org/10.1037/a0017471

Shidlo, A., & Schroeder, M. (2002). Changing sexual orientation: A consumers' report. *Professional Psychology: Research and Practice, 33*(3), 249–259. https://doi.org/10.1037/0735-7028.33.3.249

Slomowitz, A., & Feit, A. (2015). Does God make referrals? Orthodox Judaism and homosexuality. *Journal of Gay & Lesbian Mental Health, 19*(1), 100–111. https://doi.org/10.1080/19359705.2014.975583

Spitzer, R. L. (2012). Spitzer reassesses his 2003 study of reparative therapy of homosexuality. *Archives of Sexual Behavior, 41*(4), 757. https://doi.org/10.1007/s10508-012-9966-y

Substance Abuse and Mental Health Services Administration. (2015). *Ending conversion therapy: Supporting and affirming LGBTQ youth* (SMA15-4928). https://store.samhsa.gov/product/Ending-Conversion-Therapy-Supporting-and-Affirming-LGBTQ-Youth/SMA15-4928

United Nations Independent Expert on Protection Against Violence and Discrimination Based on Sexual Orientation and Gender Identity. (2020). *Report on conversion therapy*. https://www.ohchr.org/Documents/Issues/SexualOrientation/ConversionTherapyReport.pdf

Vezzosi, J. Í. P., Ramos, M. M., Almeida Segundo, D. S., & Costa, A. B. (2019). Crenças e atitudes corretivas de profissionais de psicologia sobre a homossexualidade [Beliefs and corrective attitudes of psychology professionals on homosexuality]. *Psicologia: Ciência e Profissão, 39*(3), 174–193. https://doi.org/10.1590/1982-3703003228539

Weiss, E. M., Morehouse, J., Yeager, T., & Berry, T. (2010). A qualitative study of ex-gay and ex-ex-gay experiences. *Journal of Gay & Lesbian Mental Health, 14*(4), 291–319. https://doi.org/10.1080/19359705.2010.506412

Yarhouse, M. A. (2019). *Sexual identity and faith*. The Templeton Foundation.

Yarhouse, M. A., & Beckstead, L. (2011). Using group therapy to navigate and resolve sexual orientation and religious conflicts. *Counseling and Values, 56*(1–2), 96–120. https://doi.org/10.1002/j.2161-007X.2011.tb01034.x

Zucker, K. J. (2003). The politics and science of "reparative therapy." *Archives of Sexual Behavior, 32*(5), 399–402. https://doi.org/10.1023/A:1025691310172

2

GENDER IDENTITY CHANGE EFFORTS

A Summary

DAVID P. RIVERA AND SETH T. PARDO

A recent Williams Institute report estimates that 16,000 young people will receive some type of "conversion therapy" from a licensed health care professional before reaching 18 years of age (Williams Institute, 2019). This statistic takes into consideration the growing number of states and municipalities (20 states to date) that have prohibited these practices with young people and makes clear the significant magnitude and reach of these so-called therapies with respect to the lives of queer and transgender people. The American Psychological Association's (APA's, 2021) Resolution on Gender Identity Change Efforts (GICE; APA, 2021) summarizes the evidence regarding the significant harm associated with GICE and takes a stance opposing GICE because of these associated harms. In this chapter, we illuminate the background and proliferation of GICE, which is a more accurate name for these practices, as well as issues salient to gender identity development for transgender and gender nonbinary people. Our analysis suggests that these harmful practices are reflections of distorted historical and contemporary notions of optimal gender identity development embedded in society.

https://doi.org/10.1037/0000266-003
The Case Against Conversion "Therapy": Evidence, Ethics, and Alternatives,
D. C. Haldeman (Editor)

51

Commonly labeled *conversion therapy*, GICE refers to a variety of practices enacted by health care practitioners and others (often religious counselors) with the ultimate goal of altering gender identity or gender expression to conform with social norms for gender identification and expression (SAMHSA, 2015). Definitions of GICE included in local or state policy in the United States, documentation by social justice organizations, and in the scientific literature are largely consistent in language and scope and have much in common. For example, the language from a Kent, Ohio, local resolution states that GICE may include any professional effort in a therapeutic context that aims to keep a person identified with the gender originally assigned at birth regardless of their assertion of having a gender identity that is different than the gender assigned at birth (City of Kent, Ohio, 2019). Similarly, in the Commonwealth of Massachusetts (2019), the General Laws Section 275 about GICE defines GICE as

> any practice by a health care provider that attempts or purports to impose change of an individual's sexual orientation or gender identity including, but not limited to, efforts to change behaviors or gender expressions or to eliminate or reduce sexual or romantic attractions or feelings towards individuals of the same sex.

Moreover, the Human Rights Campaign (n.d.) reported that "conversion" therapies or "reparative" therapies are targeted toward lesbian, gay, bisexual, transgender, and queer youth and are practices that seek to change their sexual or gender identities to fit within a heteronormative and gender normative status quo. In addition, in a recent systematic review, Kinitz et al. (2021) defined sexual orientation and gender identity and expression change efforts (SOGIECE) as a "set of scientifically discredited practices that aim to deny and suppress the sexual orientations, gender identities, and/or gender expressions of sexual and gender minorities" (p. 1). As summarized in this 2021 publication,

> "Conversion therapy," sometimes referred to as "reparative therapy," "reintegrative therapy," or "reorientation therapy," refers to a set of pseudo-scientific, discredited practices that aim to deny and suppress the sexual orientations, gender identities, and/or gender expressions of sexual and gender minorities. (p. 2)

These so-called therapeutic efforts are often based on the misuse of psychological theory and practices. Examples of GICE include the use of aversive operant conditioning techniques (e.g., pairing a homoerotic image with an electric shock), cognitive restructuring, and psychoanalytic processing of formative experiences. GICE may also include more subtle talk "therapies" that encourage, for example, trans women or more femininely identified persons who were assigned male at birth to override any feelings of having a more female or effeminate gender identity or expression to take on identities that are more aligned with their gender assigned at birth—that is, to take on identities as more masculine men. However, these interventions lack sufficient empirical evidence to label them as safe, acceptable, ethical, and therapeutic (SAMHSA, 2015).

Although many cultures throughout history have validating and strength-based narratives for transgender and gender nonbinary people, the medical and helping fields have a counterhistory that includes pathologizing transgender individuals and those who disclose concerns related to gender identity (Barkai, 2017; Stryker, 2017). A wide-reaching example of the medical pathologization of transgender and gender nonbinary people is the inclusion of gender identity disorders in previous editions of the American Psychiatric Association's *Diagnostic and Statistical Manual of Mental Disorders (DSM)*. This systemic and institutionalized form of transphobia and cisgenderism is informed by the larger Western and U.S.-based medical-model narratives that (a) favor binary definitions of gender, (b) conflate gender with physical sex markers, (c) favor masculinity and characteristics historically attributed to men over femininity and characteristics historically attributed to women, (d) create systems that privilege cisgender people, and (e) actively discriminate against transgender people. This history helped to create the context for the development and proliferation of GICE, which rests on the notion that any gender identity that is discordant with sex assigned at birth is disordered and that a cisgender identity is healthier, preferable, and superior to a transgender identity.

Recognizing that intentional and unintentional inaccuracies in terminology and definitions of gender-related phenomena contribute to the misunderstanding and pathologization of transgender and gender nonbinary people, it is necessary to articulate the meaning of gender terms used in this chapter. *Gender identity* refers to a person's experience of gender, including one's view of oneself as a woman, man, genderqueer, gender nonbinary, or any other gender. Although *gender* refers to the trait characteristics and behaviors culturally associated with biological sex (Fausto-Sterling, 2000), in some cases gender may be distinct from the physical markers of biological sex (e.g., genitals, chromosomes), which are generally used to assign sex at birth. Gender identity is also distinct from *gender role or expression*, which refers to the socialization and behaviors ascribed to one gender or another via cultural and social influences. *Cisgender* refers to individuals who identify with the sex they were assigned at birth (e.g., an individual assigned female at birth who identifies as a woman). *Transgender* refers to individuals who identify differently from the sex they were assigned at birth, or people for whom the sex assigned at birth is an incorrect or incomplete description of themselves. This chapter uses a broad definition of transgender to include transgender women, transgender men, genderqueer, nonbinary individuals (i.e., people who identify as other than a woman or a man), and any people who articulate a gender identity different from societal expectations based on their sex assigned at birth. Some transgender individuals seek gender-affirming medical care (e.g., hormone therapy, surgery), whereas others do not. Similarly, some transgender people seek to change their gender and/or their name on legal documents, whereas others do not. This chapter applies to all transgender people, regardless of their desire to seek social, medical, or legal transition.

SEX-GENDER INCONGRUENCE IS A NORMAL HUMAN VARIATION

Following several recent reports from large professional organizations (APA, 2015; Knudson et al., 2010; SAMHSA, 2015), it is increasingly understood that gender identities and expressions that are incongruent with the sex assigned at birth and stereotyped cultural norms are normal human variations. The trajectory to this modern understanding that transgender and gender nonbinary identities and expressions are normative human variations was not direct, and it represents a paradigm shift for many.

Historically and theoretically (Bem, 1981, 1983), newborns assigned male at birth learned that they were expected to identify as boys and to ultimately take on societal gendered roles traditionally assumed by men. Similarly, newborns assigned female at birth were expected to identify as girls and to take on societal gender roles traditionally assumed by women. It followed that in circumstances when a gender identity developed discordantly from sex assigned at birth, the medical, psychological, and theoretical literatures discussed transgender (and transsexual) presentations as pathological (Bahlburg, 2009; Meyer-Bahlburg, 2009; Zucker, 2010).

In 1980, the *DSM-III* (American Psychiatric Association, 1980) introduced the diagnostic categories of "transsexualism" within a diagnostic group called "gender identity disorders," and large professional organizations recognized that sex–gender discordance was a risk factor for poor mental health outcomes. Today, nearly 4 decades later, the *DSM-5* includes "gender dysphoria" instead of gender identity disorder as the main entry for sex–gender discordance (American Psychiatric Association, 2013). On one hand, this shift in diagnostic labeling better limits the interpretation that gender expansiveness or divergence from sex–gender congruent identity and behavioral norms is disordered or pathological in itself. On the other hand, the continued inclusion of gender dysphoria in the *DSM* may continue to misrepresent the source of the discontent (or at least part of the discontent) as a mental health disorder and not as a medical condition (World Health Organization, 2018a). In fact, for the 2018 revisions of the *International Statistical Classification of Diseases and Related Health Problems* (*ICD*) by the World Health Organization, gender incongruence was reclassified from a mental health condition to a sexual health condition (World Health Organization, 2018b). The rationale was that,

> while evidence is now clear that [gender incongruence] is not a mental disorder, and indeed classifying it in this can cause enormous stigma for people who are transgender, there remain significant health care needs that can best be met if the condition is coded under the ICD. (World Health Organization, 2018c)

Moreover, there are a handful of criteria for gender dysphoria of which two must be observed for at least 6 months to warrant a diagnosis. These criteria include "a marked incongruence between one's experienced/expressed gender and primary and/or secondary sex characteristics" and "a strong conviction that one has the typical feelings and reactions of the *other* gender" (American Psychiatric Association, 2016, para. 5). As discussed elsewhere (Diamond et al., 2011), it is important to highlight here that since the first diagnostic entries emerged, and still today, inherent in the *DSM*'s entries for transsexualism, gender identity disorder, and gender dysphoria is an underlying framework that there are only two sexes (male and female) and that medically acceptable treatments for gender dysphoria should aim to bring one's assigned sex at birth in better alignment with the "other" gender. In many ways, these diagnoses perpetuate misunderstanding and mistreatment of transgender and gender nonbinary people, which can lead to the intentional and unintentional practices associated with GICE.

STIGMA IN HEALTH CARE SETTINGS

Concerns about the mental health of transgender persons are not entirely misplaced; however, it is important to review these concerns in the appropriate social context. First, interviews dating back at least 20 years with gender nonbinary youth revealed themes of feeling threatened in the world and fear of losing caregivers as a result of their cross-gender identifications (Coates et al., 1991; Zucker & Bradley, 1995). Second, accounts of physical and emotional violence, health care discrimination, and elevated rates of substance use to cope with the stigma and discrimination were on the rise, and higher on average than in cisgender comparison groups (White Hughto et al., 2015, 2017). Third, ample research demonstrates how stigma, discrimination, and rejection are associated with suicide and depression (Bockting et al., 2013). Moreover, as suggested by minority stress theory, stigma, discrimination, and rejection are in and of themselves forms of external social harm that may become internalized and result in psycho-emotional harm (Bockting et al., 2013; Egan & Perry, 2001; Hendricks & Testa, 2012; Meyer, 2003; Nadal et al., 2012; Sandfort et al., 2007; Toomey et al., 2010).

Despite the evidence suggesting that the mental health concerns among trans and gender nonbinary identified persons may have originated from coping with stigma and discrimination from the outside world, early work that examined associated psychopathologies among children and youth with cross-gender identity and behavior reported that, on average, boys who had been diagnosed with Gender Identity Disorder were "significantly more disturbed" (p. 874) than the cisgender siblings who were assessed as control participants (Bradley & Zucker, 1997). Moreover, behavioral assessments completed with validated measures, such as the Child Behavioral Checklist, were summarized as revealing "significant behavioral difficulties" (Bradley & Zucker, 1997, p. 874). In addition, one publication (Bailey, 2003) described a typology for trans women that was based on research by Blanchard (2005). The author argued that some trans women sought medical gender-affirmation surgeries because of a type of paraphilia and not because of gender dysphoria (details of the controversy can be found elsewhere; see Dreger, 2008a, 2008b). Although this more recent work was criticized for overgeneralizing specific cases and was accused of violating professional ethics (McCain, 2003), the pattern of pathologization within the medical and psychological professional communities between the 1950s and the early 2000s was clear.

On the basis of reports such as those just discussed, clinicians sought methods to provide greater congruence between the child's gender-related behavior and social norms. These GICE techniques are thought by some to be a desirable treatment protocol. Although these techniques are commonly called *conversion therapies*, the term is inaccurate and misleading, as these techniques lack sufficient empirical evidence to render them as accepted forms of therapy (Hill et al., 2010; SAMHSA, 2015). Moreover, GICE has its roots in a history that is founded on the notion that any gender identity that is not concordant with sex assigned at birth is disordered and that a cisgender identity is healthier, preferable, and superior to a transgender identity. Moreover, although GICE aims to change the identified patient (i.e., the person who displays a disordered gender identity, or the atypical gendered behavior that is of concern to the patient or to others), the data suggest that the root causes of patients' distress are in fact the social stigma, stress, violence, and discrimination with which they must cope, and not trans identity or gender nonbinary behavior (Bockting et al., 2013; Russell et al., 2012; Stotzer, 2012).

A growing body of research that is focused on more affirming psychological practices is helping treatment providers better understand that the invalidation and rejection by others (e.g., families, therapists) of transgender identity and diverse gender expressions are forms of discrimination, stigma, and victimization that result in psychological distress (APA, 2015; Hidalgo et al., 2015; Landolt et al., 2004; Menvielle & Tuerk, 2002; Price et al., 2019; Singh et al., 2011, 2014; White Hughto & Reisner, 2016). For example, the U.S. Transgender Survey, one of the largest surveys to examine the experiences of transgender people in the United States (more than 27,000 respondents), reported that trans people experience pervasive mistreatment and violence (James et al., 2015).

The report's executive summary presents notable statistics. At home, "one in ten (10%) of those who were out to their immediate family members reported that a family member was violent towards them because they were transgender, and 8% were kicked out of the house because they were transgender" (James et al., 2015, p. 2). At school, "the majority of respondents who were out or perceived as transgender while in [grade] school (K–12) experienced some form of mistreatment, including being verbally harassed (54%), physically attacked (24%), and sexually assaulted (13%) because they were transgender . . . [and] 17% experienced such severe mistreatment that they left a school as a result" (p. 2). At work, nearly one-third of the respondents who had a job reported "being fired, denied a promotion, or experiencing some other form of mistreatment in the workplace due to their gender identity or expression, such as being verbally harassed or physically or sexually assaulted at work" (p. 2).

Approximately one third of the study sample reported verbal harassment or health care treatment refusals. In contrast, a recent U.S. survey of adults in the general U.S. population conducted between January and February 2019 (Pew Research Center, 2019) revealed that approximately 13% of all African American respondents reported that they regularly faced discrimination. Thus, the disparities highlighted here suggest that stigma and discrimination are a serious concern. Although it is difficult to identify the impact of the pathologization of transgender identity and nonconforming behavior following their classification as a mental disorder in 1980, the predictive associations between stigma, discrimination, and violence toward transgender individuals and psychological harm are clear.

TREATMENTS FOR GENDER IDENTITY

Initial interventions for gender atypical presentation and behavior in children and adolescents have their roots in psychoanalytic hypotheses, largely focusing on correcting a particular family constellation (e.g., absent or detached father, overintimate relationship with mother). This view was particularly advanced by Robert Stoller (1985), who viewed cross-gender presentation and behavior in boys as the result of an overclose relationship with their mother. Stoller's program served as the basis for Richard Green's works *Sexual Identity Conflicts in Children and Adults* (1974) and *The "Sissy Boy Syndrome" and the Development of Homosexuality* (1987). Green's methods involved augmenting contact with fathers, including typical "masculine" activities, and requesting that mothers should step back. Green's attempt at social engineering with his young patients included encouraging both parents to praise boys for engaging in traditional male behaviors (e.g., playing sports, roughhousing, presenting as "masculine") and shaming them mercilessly for effeminate or cross-gender behaviors. These methods were intended to extinguish atypical gender behaviors as well as prevent eventual homosexual orientation. In fact, these methods often did more harm than good, resulting in a feeling of betrayal (by parents) and depression over the fact that the goals of the "treatment" were impossible.

Green's methods were adopted by Dr. Kenneth Zucker at the Center for Addiction and Mental Health in Toronto (Zucker & Bradley, 1995; Zucker et al., 2012) but modified so that the focus was primarily on preventing a child from developing an eventual transgender identity. Zucker called his approach the "living in your own skin" model, in which behavior and presentation were modified to conform to gender role expectations associated with one's natal sex. His methods included behavioral modification of cross-gender play interests, encouraging greater engagement on the part of the same-sex parent (and less of the opposite-sex parent), as well as psychodynamic therapy. Therapeutic programs based on this model have subsequently been banned in the province of Ontario.

Zucker went on to consult with a Dutch group that developed a different approach to gender variant children, often known as the "watchful waiting" approach (Steensma & Cohen-Kettenis, 2011). In this approach, children are encouraged to explore cross-gender interests and behaviors in private, but the approach stops short of encouraging full social transition in public. Theirs was also the first program to make prepubertal hormone blockers available to more easily facilitate gender transition at a later time. The rationale for waiting to encourage full, public social transition was based on research showing that the vast majority of gender atypical children do not eventually claim a transgender identity but rather identify as gay or lesbian (Steensma & Cohen-Kettenis, 2011). The Dutch program allowed children the freedom to explore a cross-gender identity in private without the added risk of social rejection. It is possible, however, that there may be a cost associated with waiting for some gender variant children. Further research on this issue is needed.

A study at the University of Washington concluded that prepubertal gender variant children who were permitted full social transition were equal to their peers in social, emotional, and cognitive development (Olson et al., 2016). These data support the most recent approach for addressing gender issues in children, the "gender affirming model" of Diane Ehrensaft (2016; Ehrensaft et al., 2018). In this model, it is the child—not parents or therapists—who has authority over the child's gender identity and expression. Every effort is made to support the child in establishing their own gender identity, whether or not the child eventually decides to embark on a social or medical transition. Although further research on this model will be useful, it is important to note that recent data show that people who were coerced into some form of GICE are at significantly elevated risk for depression and suicide attempts (see Chapter 4, this volume). A longitudinal study that examines the effects of pubertal hormone blockers on youth is underway at four major sites of pediatric gender care (Hidalgo et al., 2013). Sites in this study adhere to the major tenets of the gender-affirmative model, which affirm that gender variations in and of themselves are not pathological. Rather, it is an inhospitable social climate that causes distress for gender variant children.

STIGMA, DISCRIMINATION, VIOLENCE, AND PSYCHOLOGICAL HARM

The literature increasingly reveals both the prevalence and consequences of stigma and discrimination against transgender and gender nonbinary people. This research has identified meaningful connections between stigma and its resultant harm. When the connections between stigma and harmful consequences are not apparent, stand-alone statistics of consequences such as compromised mental health, substance abuse, and employment disparity rates can add to the overpathologization of transgender and nonbinary people. For example, if we compare rates of psychological distress between the transgender respondents in the U.S. Transgender Survey and the general U.S. population, we see that rates of serious psychological distress reported by trans respondents (39%) were 8 times higher than rates recorded in the general U.S. population (5%). Also, suicide attempt rates were 10 times higher in the trans respondents than in the general U.S. population (4.6%; James et al., 2015). Some have argued that these correlates are not empirically rigorous enough to conclude that transgender people are not inherently mentally ill, thus suggesting that GICE is warranted to ensure the well-being of trans people. However, it is clear that these statistics, in isolation and out of context, can lead to the false assumption of compromised well-being for trans and nonbinary people. Furthermore, relying on comparison and simple statistical models to understand disparities experienced by transgender and nonbinary people can lead to the propagation of inappropriate and harmful interventions, such as GICE.

However, theoretically motivated research with trans samples that test the minority stress model (Hendricks & Testa, 2012; Meyer, 2003) hypothesizes that "the stress associated with stigma, prejudice, and discrimination will increase rates of psychological distress" (Bockting et al., 2013, p. 943). Bockting and colleagues (2013) also noted that the sources of social stigma and discrimination commonly faced by transgender and gender nonconforming individuals can be found in social structures and norms outside of the person (e.g., actual experiences of discrimination). In addition, stigma and discrimination may become internalized after chronic exposure (e.g., anticipated stigma). Either way, the effects of minority stress are hazardous for one's mental health, and making this connection explicit can help decrease stigma and pathology (Testa et al., 2017). For example, Bockting and colleagues found that when compared with a cisgender sample, transgender respondents had "disproportionately high rates of depression, anxiety, somatization, and overall psychological distress" (p. 948) and that these patterns were not a result of an inherent gender dysphoria or gender disorder. Rather, and as hypothesized by the minority stress model (Hendricks & Testa, 2012; Meyer, 2003), the reported distress was a direct result of both actual and anticipated stigma. Other studies found similar correlations between gender-related abuse and symptoms of depression (Nemoto et al., 2011). Using the minority stress model (Hendricks & Testa, 2012; Meyer, 2003) to understand the nature of mental health disparities for transgender and gender nonbinary people is critical to the development of therapeutic interventions that incorporate the influence of social determinants on mental health and other contextual issues.

Studying the impact of environmental stressors on health is necessary across all contexts, including health care settings. Not only does the stress from these contexts have the potential to influence the quality of health, but it also serves as a significant barrier to transgender and gender nonbinary people accessing competent care. Results from the National Transgender Discrimination Survey illustrate the harmful impact of health care–based stigma (Reisner et al., 2015); gender minority–related stressors, particularly actual and anticipated stigma in health care settings, were associated with substance use to cope with mistreatment in health care settings. Moreover, substance use as a coping strategy was associated with delaying both needed health care and preventative care. This study also found that when trans masculine persons were refused care in the past, they subsequently delayed seeking medical care even when it was necessary for an illness or injury. This finding further supports the need to study the contextual antecedents of health outcomes in developing a complete understanding of the causes of health disparities for transgender and nonbinary people.

It is most important to point out that (a) the invalidation or rejection by others (e.g., families, therapists) of transgender identity and/or diverse gender expressions are forms of discrimination, stigma, and victimization; and (b) stigma, discrimination, and rejection are, in and of themselves, forms of external social harm that may become internalized and result in psychoemotional harm. GICE causes harm by reinforcing antitransgender stigma and discrimination and by creating social pressure on an individual to conform to an identity and/or presentation that may not be consistent with that person's sense of self.

WHERE DO WE GO FROM HERE? DEVELOPING THE CASE FOR GENDER-AFFIRMING PRACTICES

Although the story of GICE is incomplete, the known evidence drafts a narrative suggesting overwhelmingly that these practices cause much more harm than good. As health care professions consider how to best move forward regarding GICE in working with transgender and gender nonbinary people, it is necessary to examine the various premises used both in favor of and in opposition to GICE. The debates and rhetoric regarding GICE are often based on several premises: (a) religious, moral, and societal norms for gender identification and expression; (b) empirical bases for GICE-induced harm; (c) empirical bases for therapeutic intervention; and (d) limits to scope of practice for clinicians and consumer fraud. However, a robust, direct exploration of these premises is largely missing from the empirical research.

The religious, moral, and societal norms for gender identification and expression create the basis for the pathologization of people with transgender and gender nonbinary identities and expressions (see Chapter 5). Just as religious doctrine is often used to deem same-sex attractions as sinful and immoral, it is also used to stigmatize people who defy social norms for gender identity and expression. For example, the binaries that constrict gender can, in part, be traced to biblically based doctrines that create a strict delineation between men and women and their roles and places in society. From our perspective, when pro- or anti-GICE rhetoric focuses on religious and moral issues and norms, it can create a debate vacuum in which the religious or moral argument supersedes and ignores scientific inquiry and evidence. We cannot ignore religious and moral perspectives, but we must expand the conversation to include scientific inquiry and professional consensus in our efforts to destigmatize noncisgender identities and expressions.

The reasons for the dearth of empirical research regarding GICE and GICE-related phenomena likely hinge on ethical considerations (see Chapter 8). Given the "do no harm" mandate honored by the helping professions, competent researchers presumably avoid direct tests of GICE and related outcomes because of the assumed harmful nature of these practices. This in turn creates a catch-22 situation. A "damned if you do, damned if you don't" scenario emerges that restricts researchers' ability to ethically test the impact of GICE on real people. It is highly unlikely that institutional review boards would approve a GICE study that potentially exposes people to more risks than benefits, and competent researchers are likely to harshly criticize the nature of the research design, leaving the field in the "damned if you don't" position: Without the empirical base supporting GICE harm, it is more difficult to disprove the efficacy and benefits of GICE.

In the absence of a substantial empirical base regarding GICE and GICE-related phenomena, opponents of GICE rely on other methods for providing evidence for the harmful nature of these practices. A convincing method follows the logic presented earlier in this chapter. First, there is movement to conceptualize the distress and dysphoria symptoms experienced by transgender and gender nonbinary people as emerging from extrinsic factors, such as societal and interpersonal stigma and discrimination, as opposed to intrinsic factors. This shift is essential in that it shifts the focus to the social climate in which gender norms support gender binaries and cisgender identities and expressions. Conceptualizing symptomatology emerging from social pressure and discord, as opposed to inherent, intrinsic factors, also helps to tamp down the religious and moral premises that focus on the individual rather than on how the individual is reacting to society. In this way, GICE opponents reject these practices because the focus is on the individual as disordered rather than society as disordered. In essence, the problem is more about the stigma, discrimination, and rejection that noncisgender people experience in society and the resultant psycho-emotional harm that includes distress and dysphoria symptoms.

The shift in focus to external factors that can induce symptomatology allows for an inclusion of societal stigma and discrimination in the GICE narrative. As mentioned earlier, there is a close, if not perfect, parallel between the gender-related bias, discrimination, and forced gender conformity experienced by transgender people and the GICE practices that favor gender-role conformity and rejection of a transgender identity and expression (Gagné & Tewksbury, 1998). Without the ability to directly test the impact of GICE on individuals in real time, this parallel helps in developing evidence for the harmful impact of GICE.

Along with the recommendation to shift pathology away from the individual, opponents of GICE may focus on (a) developing a gender-expansive paradigm for understanding gender identity and expression, (b) nurturing the strengths of transgender and gender nonbinary people, and (c) creating empirically validated gender-affirming and culturally relevant practices. These efforts have led to the establishment of the APA's (2015) *Guidelines for Psychological Practice With Transgender and Gender Nonconforming People* (see Chapter 7, this volume), as well as methods for promoting resilience among gender expansive people (e.g., Breslow et al., 2015; Singh et al., 2014). The ethical dilemmas inherent in experimentally investigating the effects of GICE, considered alongside the recent shift in focus to a resilience promotion model over outdated pathologization models, already have begun to suggest that resilience promotion models improve mental health outcomes and increase individual well-being (Austin & Craig, 2015; de Vries et al., 2014; Haas et al., 2010; Sevelius, 2013; White Hughto & Reisner, 2016). As we work toward a gender paradigm that depathologizes the lived experiences of transgender and gender nonbinary people, we will likely find that remedying institutionalized oppressions, such as removing gender dysphoria from the *DSM*, is a necessary component of this paradigm shift.

RESOURCES

1. *Affirmative Care for Transgender and Gender Nonconforming People: Best Practices for Front-Line Healthcare Staff.* https://www.lgbthealtheducation. org/wp-content/uploads/2016/12/Affirmative-Care-for-Transgender-and-Gender-Non-conforming-People-Best-Practices-for-Front-line-Health-Care-Staff.pdf

2. *Conversion Therapy and LGBT Youth Update* (Williams Institute). https://williamsinstitute.law.ucla.edu/wp-content/uploads/Conversion-Therapy-LGBT-Youth-Update-June-2019.pdf

3. *Guidelines for Psychological Practice With Transgender and Gender Nonconforming People* (American Psychological Association). https://www.apa.org/practice/guidelines/transgender.pdf

REFERENCES

American Psychiatric Association. (1980). *Diagnostic and statistical manual of mental disorders* (3rd ed.).

American Psychiatric Association. (2013). *Diagnostic and statistical manual of mental disorders* (5th ed.). https://doi.org/10.1176/appi.books.9780890425596

American Psychiatric Association. (2016, February). *What is gender dysphoria?* https://www.psychiatry.org/patients-families/gender-dysphoria/what-is-gender-dysphoria

American Psychological Association. (2015). Guidelines for psychological practice with transgender and gender nonconforming people. *American Psychologist, 70*(9), 832–864. https://doi.org/10.1037/a0039906

American Psychological Association. (2021). *APA resolution on gender identity change efforts*. https://www.apa.org/about/policy/resolution-gender-identity-change-efforts.pdf

Austin, A., & Craig, S. L. (2015). Transgender affirmative cognitive behavioral therapy: Clinical considerations and applications. *Professional Psychology, Research and Practice, 46*(1), 21–29. https://doi.org/10.1037/a0038642

Bahlburg, H. F. L. (2009). From mental disorder to iatrogenic hypogonadism: Dilemmas in conceptualizing gender identity variants as psychiatric conditions. *Archives of Sexual Behavior, 39,* 461–476. https://doi.org/10.1007/s10508-009-9532-4

Bailey, J. M. (2003). *The man who would be queen.* Joseph Henry Press.

Barkai, A. R. (2017). Troubling gender or engendering trouble? The problem with gender dysphoria in psychoanalysis. *Psychoanalytic Review, 104*(1), 1–32. https://doi.org/10.1521/prev.2017.104.1.1

Bem, S. L. (1981). Gender schema theory: A cognitive account of sex typing. *Psychological Review, 88*(4), 354–364. https://doi.org/10.1037/0033-295X.88.4.354

Bem, S. L. (1983). Gender schema theory and its implications for child development: Raising gender-aschematic children in a gender-schematic society. *Signs: Journal of Women in Culture and Society, 8*(4), 598–616. https://doi.org/10.1086/493998

Blanchard, R. (2005). Early history of the concept of autogynephilia. *Archives of Sexual Behavior, 34*(4), 439–446. https://doi.org/10.1007/s10508-005-4343-8

Bockting, W. O., Miner, M. H., Swinburne Romine, R. E., Hamilton, A., & Coleman, E. (2013). Stigma, mental health, and resilience in an online sample of the US transgender population. *American Journal of Public Health, 103*(5), 943–951. https://doi.org/10.2105/AJPH.2013.301241

Bradley, S. J., & Zucker, K. J. (1997). Gender identity disorder: A review of the past 10 years. *Journal of the American Academy of Child & Adolescent Psychiatry, 36*(7), 872–880. https://doi.org/10.1097/00004583-199707000-00008

Breslow, A. S., Brewster, M. E., Velez, B. L., Wong, S., Geiger, E., & Soderstrom, B. (2015). Resilience and collective action: Exploring buffers against minority stress for transgender individuals. *Psychology of Sexual Orientation and Gender Diversity*, *2*(3), 253–265. https://doi.org/10.1037/sgd0000117

City of Kent, Ohio. (2019). Ordinance No. 2019-70: Adopting chapter 723 "sexual identity or gender identity change efforts." https://www.kentohio.org/DocumentCenter/View/7163/2019-077-Adopting-723-Gender-Identity-Change-Efforts

Coates, S., Friedman, R., & Wolfe, S. (1991). The etiology of boyhood gender identity disorder: A model for integrating temperament, development, and psychodynamics. *Psychoanalytic Dialogues*, *1*(4), 481–523. https://doi.org/10.1080/10481889109538916

Commonwealth of Massachusetts. (2019). General Laws Section 275. https://malegislature.gov/Laws/GeneralLaws/PartI/TitleXVI/Chapter112/Section275

de Vries, A. L., McGuire, J. K., Steensma, T. D., Wagenaar, E. C., Doreleijers, T. A., & Cohen-Kettenis, P. T. (2014). Young adult psychological outcome after puberty suppression and gender reassignment. *Pediatrics*, *134*(4), 696–704. https://doi.org/10.1542/peds.2013-2958

Diamond, L. M., Pardo, S. T., & Butterworth, M. R. (2011). Transgender experience and identity. In S. Schwartz, K. Luyckx, & V. Vignoles (Eds.), *Handbook of identity theory and research* (pp. 629–647). Springer. https://doi.org/10.1007/978-1-4419-7988-9_26

Dreger, A. D. (2008a). The controversy surrounding *"The man who would be queen"*: A case history of the politics of science, identity, and sex in the internet age. *Archives of Sexual Behavior*, *37*(3), 366–421. https://doi.org/10.1007/s10508-007-9301-1

Dreger, A. D. (2008b). Response to the commentaries on Dreger (2008) [Commentary]. *Archives of Sexual Behavior*, *37*, 503–510. https://doi.org/10.1007/s10508-008-9348-7

Egan, S. K., & Perry, D. G. (2001). Gender identity: A multidimensional analysis with implications for psychosocial adjustment. *Developmental Psychology*, *37*(4), 451–463. https://doi.org/10.1037/0012-1649.37.4.451

Ehrensaft, D. (2016). *The gender creative child: Pathways for nurturing and supporting children who live outside gender boxes*. The Experiment.

Ehrensaft, D., Giammattei, S. V., Storck, K., Tishelman, A. C., & Keo-Meier, C. (2018). Prepubertal social gender transitions: What we know, what we can learn—A view from a gender affirmative lens. *International Journal of Transgenderism*, *19*(2), 251–268. https://doi.org/10.1080/15532739.2017.1414649

Fausto-Sterling, A. (2000). *Sexing the body: Gender politics and the construction of sexuality*. Basic Books.

Gagné, P., & Tewksbury, R. (1998). Conformity pressures and gender resistance among transgendered individuals. *Social Problems*, *45*(1), 81–101. https://doi.org/10.1525/sp.1998.45.1.03x0158b

Green, R. (1974). *Sexual identity conflict in children and adults*. Basic Books.

Green, R. (1987). *The "sissy boy syndrome" and the development of homosexuality*. Yale University Press. https://doi.org/10.2307/j.ctt1ww3v4c

Haas, A. P., Eliason, M., Mays, V. M., Mathy, R. M., Cochran, S. D., D'Augelli, A. R., Silverman, M. M., Fisher, P. W., Hughes, T., Rosario, M., Russell, S. T., Malley, E., Reed, J., Litts, D. A., Haller, E., Sell, R. L., Remafedi, G., Bradford, J., Beautrais, A. L., . . . Clayton, P. J. (2010). Suicide and suicide risk in lesbian, gay, bisexual, and transgender populations: Review and recommendations. *Journal of Homosexuality, 58*(1), 10–51. https://doi.org/10.1080/00918369.2011.534038

Hendricks, M. L., & Testa, R. J. (2012). A conceptual framework for clinical work with transgender and gender nonconforming clients: An adaptation of the minority stress model. *Professional Psychology, Research and Practice, 43*(5), 460–467. https://doi.org/10.1037/a0029597

Hidalgo, M. A., Ehrensaft, D., Tishelman, A. C., Clark, L. F., Garofalo, R., Rosenthal, S. M., & Olson, J. (2013). The gender affirmative model: What we know and what we aim to learn. *Human Development, 56*(5), 285–290. https://doi.org/10.1159/000355235

Hidalgo, M. A., Kuhns, L. M., Kwon, S., Mustanski, B., & Garofalo, R. (2015). The impact of childhood gender expression on childhood sexual abuse and psychopathology among young men who have sex with men. *Child Abuse & Neglect: The International Journal, 46*, 103–112. https://doi.org/10.1016/j.chiabu.2015.05.005

Hill, D. B., Menvielle, E., Sica, K. M., & Johnson, A. (2010). An affirmative intervention for families with gender variant children: Parental ratings of child mental health and gender. *Journal of Sex & Marital Therapy, 36*(1), 6–23. https://doi.org/10.1080/00926230903375560

Human Rights Campaign. (n.d.). *The lies and dangers of reparative therapy.* https://www.hrc.org/resources/the-lies-and-dangers-of-reparative-therapy

James, S. E., Herman, J., Keisling, M., Mottet, L., & Anafi, M. (2015). *2015 U.S. Transgender Survey (USTS).* Inter-university Consortium for Political and Social Research.

Kinitz, D. J., Salway, T., Dromer, E., Giustini, D., Ashley, F., Goodyear, T., Ferlatte, O., Kia, H., & Abramovich, A. (2021). The scope and nature of sexual orientation and gender identity and expression change efforts: A systematic review protocol. *Systematic Reviews, 10*(1), Article 14. https://doi.org/10.1186/s13643-020-01563-8

Knudson, G., De Cuypere, G., & Bockting, W. (2010). Recommendations for revision of the *DSM* diagnoses of gender identity disorders: Consensus statement of The World Professional Association for Transgender Health. *International Journal of Transgenderism, 12*(2), 115–118. https://doi.org/10.1080/15532739.2010.509215

Landolt, M. A., Bartholomew, K., Saffrey, C., Oram, D., & Perlman, D. (2004). Gender nonconformity, childhood rejection, and adult attachment: A study of gay men. *Archives of Sexual Behavior, 33*(2), 117–128. https://doi.org/10.1023/B:ASEB.0000014326.64934.50

McCain, R. S. (2003, November 25). University investigates ethics of sex researcher. *The Washington Times.* https://www.washingtontimes.com/news/2003/nov/24/20031124-103155-8053r/

Menvielle, E. J., & Tuerk, C. (2002). A support group for parents of gender-nonconforming boys. *Journal of the American Academy of Child & Adolescent Psychiatry, 41*(8), 1010–1013. https://doi.org/10.1097/00004583-200208000-00021

Meyer, I. H. (2003). Prejudice, social stress, and mental health in lesbian, gay, and bisexual populations: Conceptual issues and research evidence. *Psychological Bulletin, 129*(5), 674–697. https://doi.org/10.1037/0033-2909.129.5.674

Meyer-Bahlburg, H. F. (2009). Variants of gender differentiation in somatic disorders of sex development: Recommendations for Version 7 of the World Professional Association for Transgender Health's Standards of Care. *International Journal of Transgenderism, 11*(4), 226–237. https://doi.org/10.1080/15532730903439476

Nadal, K. L., Skolnik, A., & Wong, Y. (2012). Interpersonal and systemic microaggressions toward transgender people: Implications for counseling. *Journal of LGBT Issues in Counseling, 6*(1), 55–82. https://doi.org/10.1080/15538605.2012.648583

Nemoto, T., Bödeker, B., & Iwamoto, M. (2011). Social support, exposure to violence and transphobia, and correlates of depression among male-to-female transgender women with a history of sex work. *American Journal of Public Health, 101*(10), 1980–1988. https://doi.org/10.2105/AJPH.2010.197285

Olson, K. R., Durwood, L., DeMeules, M., & McLaughlin, K. A. (2016). Mental health of transgender children who are supported in their identities. *Pediatrics, 137*(3), e20153223. https://doi.org/10.1542/peds.2015-3223

Pew Research Center. (2019). *Race in America 2019.*

Price, M., Olezeski, C., McMahon, T., & Hill, N. (2019). A developmental perspective on victimization faced by gender-nonconforming youth. In H. Fitzgerald (Ed.), *Handbook of children and prejudice: Integrating research, practice, and policy* (pp. 447–461). Springer. https://doi.org/10.1007/978-3-030-12228-7_25

Reisner, S. L., Pardo, S. T., Gamarel, K. E., White Hughto, J. M., Pardee, D. J., & Keo-Meier, C. L. (2015). Substance use to cope with stigma in healthcare among U.S. female-to-male trans masculine adults. *LGBT Health, 2*(4), 324–332. https://doi.org/10.1089/lgbt.2015.0001

Russell, S. T., Sinclair, K. O., Poteat, V. P., & Koenig, B. W. (2012). Adolescent health and harassment based on discriminatory bias. *American Journal of Public Health, 102*(3), 493–495. https://doi.org/10.2105/AJPH.2011.300430

Sandfort, T. G., Melendez, R. M., & Diaz, R. M. (2007). Gender nonconformity, homophobia, and mental distress in latino gay and bisexual men. *Journal of Sex Research, 44*(2), 181–189. https://doi.org/10.1080/00224490701263819

Sevelius, J. M. (2013). Gender affirmation: A framework for conceptualizing risk behavior among transgender women of color. *Sex Roles, 68*(11–12), 675–689. https://doi.org/10.1007/s11199-012-0216-5

Singh, A. A., Hays, D. G., & Watson, L. S. (2011). Strength in the face of adversity: Resilience strategies of transgender individuals. *Journal of Counseling and Development, 89*(1), 20–27. https://doi.org/10.1002/j.1556-6678.2011.tb00057.x

Singh, A. A., Meng, S. E., & Hansen, A. W. (2014). "I am my own gender": Resilience strategies of trans youth. *Journal of Counseling and Development, 92*(2), 208–218. https://doi.org/10.1002/j.1556-6676.2014.00150.x

Steensma, T. D., & Cohen-Kettenis, P. T. (2011). Gender transitioning before puberty? *Archives of Sexual Behavior, 40*(4), 649–650. https://doi.org/10.1007/s10508-011-9752-2

Stoller, R. (1985). *Presentations of gender.* Yale University Press.

Stotzer, R. L. (2012). *Comparison of hate crime rates across protected and unprotected groups—An update.* Williams Institute on Sexual Orientation Law and Public Policy.

Stryker, S. (2017). *Transgender history: The roots of today's revolution.* Seal Press.

Substance Abuse and Mental Health Services Administration. (2015). *Ending conversion therapy: Supporting and affirming LGBTQ youth.*

Testa, R. J., Michaels, M. S., Bliss, W., Rogers, M. L., Balsam, K. F., & Joiner, T. (2017). Suicidal ideation in transgender people: Gender minority stress and interpersonal theory factors. *Journal of Abnormal Psychology, 126*(1), 125–136. https://doi.org/10.1037/abn0000234

Toomey, R. B., Ryan, C., Diaz, R. M., Card, N. A., & Russell, S. T. (2010). Gender-nonconforming lesbian, gay, bisexual, and transgender youth: School victimization and young adult psychosocial adjustment. *Developmental Psychology, 46*(6), 1580–1589. https://doi.org/10.1037/a0020705

White Hughto, J. M., & Reisner, S. L. (2016). A systematic review of the effects of hormone therapy on psychological functioning and quality of life in transgender individuals. *Transgender Health, 1*(1), 21–31. https://doi.org/10.1089/trgh.2015.0008

White Hughto, J. M., Reisner, S. L., & Pachankis, J. E. (2015). Transgender stigma and health: A critical review of stigma determinants, mechanisms, and interventions. *Social Science & Medicine, 147*, 222–231. https://doi.org/10.1016/j.socscimed.2015.11.010

White Hughto, J. M., Rose, A. J., Pachankis, J. E., & Reisner, S. L. (2017). Barriers to gender transition-related healthcare: Identifying underserved transgender adults in Massachusetts. *Transgender Health, 2*(1), 107–118. https://doi.org/10.1089/trgh.2017.0014

Williams Institute. (2019). *Conversion therapy and LGBT youth update.*

World Health Organization. (2018a). *International classification of diseases.* https://www.who.int/health-topics/international-classification-of-diseases

World Health Organization. (2018b). *International statistical classification of diseases and related health problems* (11th ed.). https://icd.who.int/

World Health Organization. (2018c, June 18). *WHO: Revision of ICD-11 (gender incongruence/transgender)—Questions and answers (Q&A)* [Video]. YouTube. https://www.youtube.com/watch?v=kyCgz0z05Ik&feature=youtu.be

Zucker, K. J. (2010). The *DSM* diagnostic criteria for gender identity disorder in children. *Archives of Sexual Behavior, 39*(2), 477–498. https://doi.org/10.1007/s10508-009-9540-4

Zucker, K. J., & Bradley, S. J. (1995). *Gender identity disorder and psychosexual problems in children and adolescents.* Guilford Press.

Zucker, K. J., Wood, H., Singh, D., & Bradley, S. J. M. D. (2012). A developmental, biopsychosocial model for the treatment of children with gender identity disorder. *Journal of Homosexuality, 59*(3), 369–397. https://doi.org/10.1080/00918369.2012.653309

PART II MINORITY STRESS AND COLLATERAL IMPACT

3 MINORITY STRESS AND CHANGE EFFORTS

MICHAEL L. HENDRICKS

Minority stress is a theoretical model that was first proposed by Meyer (1995, 2003) to suggest that prejudice and stigma lead to adverse health consequences experienced by sexual minorities (i.e., lesbian, gay, and bisexual [LGB] persons). Meyer's model purported that sexual minorities experience more stress than their heterosexual counterparts because of prejudice and stigma related to their minority status. Embedded into social structures, this stress is pervasive and repeatedly disaffirms the sexual minority aspects of the individual's identity. It is this disaffirmation process that ultimately leads to health disparities.

In 2012, Hendricks and Testa proposed an adaptation of Meyer's model, applying minority stress theory to transgender and gender nonconforming individuals. Hendricks and Testa found a high degree of similarity between the health disparities among sexual minority people and gender minority people, though most studies at that time (reviewed in Hendricks & Testa, 2012) found higher rates of anxiety, depression, and suicide, among other adverse health consequences, for gender minority populations. Hendricks and Testa also noted differences between the two groups in how they manage

https://doi.org/10.1037/0000266-004
The Case Against Conversion "Therapy": Evidence, Ethics, and Alternatives,
D. C. Haldeman (Editor)

presentation of their minority status. For example, although individuals in both groups may choose not to divulge their minority status to various people or in various settings, gender minority people have the additional complication of having to decide whether to disclose not only their status as a gender minority person but also their gender history—including sex assigned at birth vis-à-vis current gender identity and presentation.

To account for these differences, Hendricks and Testa (2012) made modifications to Meyer's model. In one key modification, the authors incorporated elements of Joiner's (2010) interpersonal theory of suicide. This was deemed necessary to explain the extraordinarily high rates of suicide attempts found in numerous studies of gender minority people (which were among the highest attempts rates found in any population). Because minority stress is a social or interpersonal experience, it was necessary to find an explanation for elevated attempt rates that addressed suicide from that perspective. Joiner's theory provided exactly that.

Both models delineate processes by which minority stress erodes an individual's ability to effectively cope with the range of stressors normally encountered in life. Both models also suggest ways in which connection to a community of like others somehow provides benefits from which individuals may derive or devise coping strategies that serve to counter the adverse effects of stress, including minority stress. In this way, the minority stress models have two sides: One side of the model focuses on the adverse consequences of minority stress; the other side focuses on coping strategies that mitigate those adverse consequences and may even lead to resilience.

Although neither model directly addresses the question of sexual orientation change efforts (SOCE) or gender identity change efforts (GICE), both models indicate the ways in which social stressors ultimately lead to adverse mental health consequences (including anxiety, depression, and suicidal risk). In particular, an essential characteristic of minority stress is that it exacts its harm to the individual because it disaffirms a key aspect of the individual's core identity. The fact that this aspect of identity is socially marginalized in society both augments the negative impact it has on the individual and serves to perpetuate and sustain the onslaught of minority stress. SOCE and GICE, because they aim to change the individual's sexual orientation or gender identity—essential aspects of identity—are inherently disaffirming of the individual's identity and, thereby, the individual.

The minority stress models, on the other hand, suggest socially based channels through which lesbian, gay, bisexual, transgender, and questioning or queer (LGBTQ) people may manage to mitigate minority stress, increase social support, and develop coping and resilience that lead to improved health consequences. Ultimately, both models propose that sexual and gender minority people are able to achieve resilience through a process of acceptance and normalization of their minority status. SOCE and GICE are rooted in a pathologization of sexual and gender identity that is anything other than cisgender and heterosexual and seeks to deprive those who undergo SOCE or GICE of affirmation of the self and support of a community that potentially enhances their resilience and sense of well-being. The procedures involved in SOCE and GICE are antithetical to the very processes and resources that, in the minority stress models, lead to better health outcomes.

The purpose of this chapter is to introduce the reader to the minority stress models for sexual minorities and gender minorities, to demonstrate how and why these models argue strongly for creating and sustaining affirmative approaches and environments for sexual and gender minority individuals in order to reduce the health disparities these communities experience, and to explain how these models stand in opposition to SOCE and GICE. Both of these models and their various components have been successfully tested numerous times in the research literature. Their strength stands in stark contrast to the lack of empirical and ethical support for SOCE and GICE covered in other chapters of this book. Additionally, and particularly in light of the intense disaffirming effects of SOCE and GICE, this chapter suggests an expansion of the specific processes by which the minority stress models may facilitate the development of coping strategies in the face of minority stress that can ultimately lead to resilience.

Throughout this chapter's description of the minority stress models and of their subsequent expansion, themes of belongingness, affirmation, and resilience are highlighted. It is precisely the contrast between these aspects of the minority stress models and the profound lack of these elements in SOCE and GICE that are most salient.

FUNDAMENTALS OF MINORITY STRESS THEORY

A minority stress model was first proposed in 1995 by Ilan H. Meyer, who asserted that sexual minority (i.e., gay, lesbian, and bisexual) people encounter and are subjected to greater levels of stress because of social structures, such as prejudice, that result in subtle and overt discrimination and that this additional stress leads to adverse health consequences. Meyer refined the model in 2003. Meyer's model was perhaps a bit prescient, given that solid empirical evidence that LGB people did indeed experience adverse health consequences first appeared in 1999 but was not established until well into the 2000s (for a review, see Cochran et al., 2016).

In his model for LGB people, Meyer offered three foundational character-istics of minority stress: It is unique to stigmatized persons and adds to the general stressors experienced by everyone, and so it requires more adaptation that is not required by those who are not stigmatized. Minority stress is also chronic (meaning that it is pervasive and persistent) and arises from social and cultural structures that are stable aspects of a society. Prejudice, for example, is endemic in our culture. Although everyone encounters it, its adverse impact is experienced most directly by those who are the object of that prejudice. Finally, minority stress is socially based and stems from social processes, institutions, and structures beyond the individual rather than the person's biological, genetic, or other nonsocial characteristics. What consti-tutes stressors in the model is addressed next.

The model describes two net effects of minority stress and explains how each may arise. It is important to understand that one does not exist without the other; both are important and interrelated aspects of the model. The first comprises pathways to increased pathology, including substance use, mood and anxiety disorders, and suicidal behaviors. A recent indication of the level of psychopathology among LGBTQ youth, for example, was provided by The Trevor Project (Green et al., 2019) in its report of a 2018 survey of more than 34,000 respondents ages 13 to 24. This study found that 71% of respondents reported having had a period of at least 2 weeks during the past year when they felt sad or hopeless, and 39% reported having seriously contemplated suicide in the past year. More than half of the transgender and gender non-binary respondents indicated suicide contemplation in the same time frame. More recently, The Trevor Project's 2020 report of more than 40,000 LGBTQ youth found that 40% had seriously contemplated suicide in the previous year (59% among gender minority youth), 40% engaged in self-harm, and 10% reported having undergone "conversion therapy" (with 78% of those having been subjected to this "therapy" before age 18). Of particular note, youth who reported they had been in "conversion therapy" were more than twice as likely to attempt suicide than youth who had not been in "conversion therapy."

The other net effect of minority stress is resilience that arises from the development of coping strategies. Although social support and coping are basic elements of all stress models, the foundation for this side of Meyer's, as well as Hendricks and Testa's, minority stress model is rooted in Allport's (1954) assertion that members of minority groups respond to prejudice with what amounts to coping and resilience. In this way, the stress that results from minority status is directly associated not just with stress (negative effects) but also with positive coping that ameliorates the impact of stress and helps minority members cope with the adverse effects of minority stress (Meyer, 2015). Coping results from resources found within the minority group, such as group solidarity and cohesiveness, that ultimately serve as protective factors.

The minority stress models, then, account for both the negative consequences of processes that stem from prejudice and discrimination and the potential for the development of coping strategies that can lead to resilience and, ultimately, a reduction in adverse health outcomes. To better understand how all of this works and the impact that minority stress may have on individuals, it is necessary to examine the processes that make up the stress aspect of the models and the interaction between the individual and that person's community that potentially affords the benefits of coping.

STRESS PROCESSES

The minority stress model has four basic processes of stress, which are organized from the most distal from the individual to the most proximal to the individual. *Distal* stressors are those that are readily observable to anyone present; *proximal* processes occur internally, and the individual may not even be conscious of them. Although the distal–proximal distinction helps to organize stress processes based on the origin of the stress, an important aspect of the models is that repeated exposure to even the most distal processes ultimately has an effect on the individual by contributing to more proximal processes.

The most distal process in the model consists of environmental or external events that are observable to any person present who is aware of what is occurring. These events include discrimination, harassment, assaults, and bullying—essentially, the manifestations of prejudice. That is, they are directed at the individual because of the perception that the individual is a member of a sexual or gender minority group, and the actions taken are manifestations of prejudice or other negative thoughts or beliefs about the minority group or its members on the part of the person or persons engaging in the activity. Research has demonstrated a direct relationship between these external, environmental events and adverse health consequences. For example, Testa et al. (2012) found that trans individuals who were subjected to violence related to their gender identity or expression were more than 3 times as likely to subsequently attempt suicide. Similarly, Goldblum et al. (2012) found that trans individuals who had been subjected to bullying or violence in school were more than four times as likely to later attempt suicide.

Moving from distal to proximal, the next stress process consists of the minority individual's anticipation and expectation of external events that develops as a result of the regularity of the external events. In this way, the minority person becomes more alert and attuned to such events, anticipates various situations in which they might occur, and even expects them to occur at some point. As a result of this awareness and expectation, the minority individual develops a vigilance for such events. This vigilance causes the minority individual to approach the world differently, having internalized the expectation that these events will occur. In this process, social attitudes and prejudice become salient when the individual cognitively appraises them and attributes to them a level of psychological importance. In this sense, the negative attitudes of others "matter." Because they matter, they can be hurtful and harmful. A recent example of this process is the fear and anxiety that many LGBTQ individuals (and especially adolescents and young adults) experienced in the first 2 years of the Trump administration, as previous executive orders that had offered even nominal protection from discrimination were rescinded. Because these individuals had experienced discrimination and harassment, their anticipation that losing these protective measures would result in increased discrimination increased anxiety and depression.

The next most proximal stress process is the internalization of negative societal attitudes and prejudices, frequently described as internalized homo- and trans-negativity—or, previously, as internalized homophobia and transphobia. In this process, minority individuals accept the negative attitudes toward them based on their minority status, essentially "buying into" those attitudes, and thereby hold many of the same negative views of their minority status that are expressed in negative societal attitudes. At this point, external events may serve to reinforce this internalized negativity, but it exists with or without such events. Examples of internalized negativity are replete in "coming out" stories, especially among individuals who come out sometime after young adulthood. Their accounts frequently include descriptions of their own shame about their sexual orientation or gender identity.

The most proximal process is concealment of the individual's marginalized identity. This process is unique to marginalized people whose stigmatized identity can be hidden, and it applies directly to sexual and gender minority people. This process is generally not applicable to most racial and ethnic minority persons. Although concealment may be adaptive in some respects (e.g., it may allow the individual to avoid harm in a specific situation), the psychological damage is not insignificant. Concealment leads to the psychological damage of maintaining a secret about oneself, which is frequently documented in the literature under the umbrella term of living "in the closet." It also essentially robs the individual of the benefits of the coping and resilience side of the model, which requires connection to one's community. If individuals maintain concealment of their marginalized identity, they are unlikely to seek out this community, and the community will unlikely be able to locate them in order to reach out with resources.

Two aspects of concealment are important. First, both sexual and gender minority people may attempt to conceal or reveal their minority status with different groups or situations. For example, older LGBTQ people, faced with the prospect of requiring relocation to an assisted living environment, may choose not to disclose their minority status in this new environment. Second, gender minority individuals who have completed a gender transition may choose not to disclose their gender history, instead living "stealth" in their affirmed gender. In this way, they may choose not to affiliate with other members of the transgender community. Some such individuals are perceived by those around them not only in their affirmed gender but also as being cisgender. This may allow them to avoid experiences of prejudice and discrimination associated with the most distal stress process in the minority stress model, but it also makes connection with other trans individuals more challenging and may even foster internalized negative views related to their gender history or gender identity.

COPING AND RESILIENCE

The minority stress model also describes the ways by which sexual and gender minority people may acquire coping skills for effectively dealing with the stress processes just noted, thereby mitigating the adverse health consequences of minority stress. As previously mentioned, Allport (1954) proposed that minority group members (who are subjected to prejudice and discrimination) ultimately develop coping strategies by associating their minority status with positive coping, which leads to the mitigation of the negative effects of stress and resilience. This process begins with finding and identifying with other individuals who have the same minority status—in essence, *finding one's community*. Essential to the facilitation of the development and identification of "community" is the validation and affirmation the community provides to its members—especially with regard to the aspect(s) of identity around which the community is formed. The minority group then coalesces around the minority identity, creating a sense of group solidarity and cohesion that ultimately serve as protective factors in weathering the onslaughts of minority stress. From this group or community, individuals are able to learn from others and acquire coping strategies that help to address minority stress in healthier ways.

An example of the process of finding, identifying with, and benefiting from one's community can be observed among the drag queen community. Aspects of this were portrayed in the movie *Paris Is Burning* (Livingston, 1990) and are shown more widely in the television show *RuPaul's Drag Race* (Bailey et al., 2009–2021). Within the drag community, collectives of individuals, often referred to as "houses," formalize their connections with one another. Typically, each house will have a "mother," who is usually one of the older, more experienced drag queens and provides structure, lines of authority and mentoring, and physical and social support to her "children" in a "motherly" fashion. In turn, the other members of the house support the mother, in a sort of matriarchal structure.

The structure of these houses and their denizens provide the member drag queens with affirmation of their sexuality as well as their art, support in and for their exploration of their identity (often in a blended, intersectional manner), and explicit and implicit instruction on how to exhibit strength (sometimes referred to as "fierceness") and self-assurance. Initially, the house provides a safe space for personal expression and exploration; ultimately, it prepares individuals for not only public performance but coping with an often hostile world outside the drag scene. In this way, the house affirms the minority identity of its members, and this affirmation offers protection against potential assaults on that identity.

The group cohesion that forms in minority communities facilitates the development of a within-group identity in which the individual members derive their sense of who they are based in part on their minority status. Individuals can then engage in a reappraisal of the self to "like others" in which the minority status is not viewed as a detractor. The result is often a validation of the self as a member of the minority group and a positive view of the self.

The minority stress model pairs the processes of forming a minority identity with finding community. The model proposes that exposure to and engagement with others of one's own minority status lead to the formation and development of a minority identity, which ultimately may lead to increased self-esteem and psychological health as individuals are able to recast their sense of self-worth. Development of a strong minority identity is described in several prominent models and includes a crucial step of engagement with social and informational resources related to one's minority group. The immersion stage, in which access to social resources in one's minority group is crucial, is an important step in developing a sense of self-esteem. Similarly, models of LGB identity development highlight the importance of a period of engagement with resources related to LGB people and issues; this period of engagement is important for psychological health. So, in both racial minority and sexual minority populations, access to people from and information about one's minority group are related to resilience.

In addition to being a means for developing one's minority identity, exposure to and involvement in a minority community with which one identifies may act as a resilience factor by building a sense of belonging. (This is an essential aspect of the "house" model for drag queens, as just described.) Various movements in psychology have described sense of belongingness as a fundamental human psychological need, whereas thwarted belongingness and alienation are consistently linked to distress and have been implicated in suicide attempts and completions (Joiner, 2010).

In an adaptation of the model for transgender and gender nonconforming persons, Hendricks and Testa (2012) further asserted that connection to the minority community creates a sense of belonging, which satisfies a basic psychological need. Indeed, thwarted belongingness has been strongly implicated in negative mental health outcomes and increased suicide (Joiner, 2010; Van Orden et al., 2010). Given the demonstrated importance of belongingness in Joiner's interpersonal theory of suicide and the ostracism experienced by many trans people, this addition to minority stress theory was appropriate. Support for the importance of belongingness can be found in the research literature (e.g., Klein & Golub, 2016; Testa et al., 2014).

But by what psychological process (or processes) does belonging to a community of like others lead to increased health outcomes?

PSYCHOLOGICAL SENSE OF COMMUNITY

Sense of community in a mostly physical sense has long been proposed and examined in its role in a variety of human activities, including at least some with psychological implications. In this regard, "community" has typically carried a geospatial component, with membership in a community being defined, at least in part, by physical proximity (e.g., Hill, 1996). At the same time, a sense of belonging to some group has been experienced by most people, perhaps most notably with regard to family. Although community may indeed carry an aspect related to physical location, aspects of belonging and acceptance also seem to be part of the experience of belonging to a community.

Omoto and Snyder (2002) proposed that all of the important dimensions of a sense of community are essentially psychological in nature, and so they proposed the concept of a psychological sense of community (PSOC) and delineated psychological processes that ultimately lead to beneficial psychological effects. They further explained this construct in a chapter published in 2010 that explored why volunteers who provided assistance during the AIDS crisis withstood the stigma that came from being associated with anything related to HIV/AIDS during this crisis and how they ultimately benefited from their volunteer efforts. They found a sense of belongingness experienced by volunteers that transcended geospatial location and indeed seemed to have little to do with physical proximity to other members of the volunteer group. They defined PSOC as "fundamentally a feeling of belonging, connection, confidence, and esteem that is attached to a psychologically identifiable community or grouping" (Omoto & Snyder, 2002, p. 858). PSOC sounds remarkably like the communities of sexual and gender minorities that form and provide coping strategies, self-esteem, and self-worth.

Omoto and Snyder (2002, pp. 857–858) described a number of psychological benefits that accrue from membership/belongingness in a community, including the following:

- *Increased confidence that social support is available.* A greater sense of a community composed of people who care about the individuals in the group results in greater levels of optimism in facing personal problems, physical health problems, stigmatization, and social isolation.

- *Increased self-esteem.* Self-esteem is bolstered by a collective self-esteem and valued social identity (i.e., being a member of a group that wants its members). By valuing its members, the group confers social consensus and validation, along with positive regard and belongingness that leads to a collective self-esteem. This collective self-esteem reaffirms the worth of the individual, both as an individual and as a community member.

- *Modeling of upward social comparison.* Although members come to appreciate and benefit from the accomplishments of other members, they also may feel motivated to increase their contribution to the group and to succeed in ways that are important to the group.

- *Acquisition of problem-solving skills derived from community modeling and support for solving problems through collective action.* Communities possess more and different resources (than any one individual), and these resources become accessible with membership. Such resources include more specialized collective material and psychological resources.

- *Improved psychological functioning as members feel understood because of increased empathy and shared suffering.* Accepted and embraced within the community, members' identity is affirmed and supported, which allows them to "do more" and try harder, confident that their attempts will be appreciated and supported.

- *Psychological empowerment stemming from increased resources, confidence, and esteem provided by a sense of community.* As members of the community feel safer in their attempts to do more with supportive feedback from the group, they develop increased self-assurance and esteem that is rooted in the sense of belongingness.

Whereas Omoto and Snyder (2002) envisioned these processes to be particularly germane to communities of volunteers, their focus was on groups or communities of individuals lending their efforts to address the AIDS crisis—during a time when any affiliation with HIV/AIDS carried its own stigma. PSOC may help to explain how LGBTQ people derive very real and positive benefits from establishing and maintaining membership in communities of LGBTQ members.

Essentially, being a member of a community in which there is a common identity or cause conveys a sense of belonging coupled with affirmation of the individual. From that belongingness and affirmation stems a range of benefits that extend well beyond the tangibles that are frequently associated with a community in close physical proximity. In this way, PSOC helps to explain the social and interpersonal processes that ultimately lead to coping and resilience.

Having a connection to community does not erase the stress processes described in the minority stress model. Nor does it mean that the environmental and external events simply stop. However, by acquiring coping strategies from the community, by experiencing greater self-esteem and self-confidence in addressing those events with minimized negative impact, and by greatly reducing the extent of the more proximal processes of internalized negativity and concealment, the individual can achieve a much healthier state of mind, can address the external events (or not) as dictated by the circumstances, and can withstand the assaults of the distal stress processes with much less psychological impact.

In addition, it is worth noting that most LGBTQ people were not born into or did not grow up in a household composed primarily of LGBTQ parents and siblings. (And, in most cases, even if there does turn out to be a sibling who is also LGBTQ, that fact is typically not learned until at least middle adolescence.) Thus, there is typically no family member with whom the LGBTQ person inherently resonates and who can serve as guide and mentor from the perspective of having lived the life of a hidden minority. For this reason, establishing a connection with one's community is vitally important. In this community the LGBTQ individual stands to benefit from at least some of the informal and formal lessons that cannot be derived from growing up in a cisgender and heterosexual family. The concept of PSOC is especially helpful here: Whereas families of origin typically benefit from physical proximity—a benefit that conveys a connection that survives children growing up and moving away from the family home—LGBTQ communities may never have that benefit or may have only a limited amount of it. For example, some people may need to travel quite a distance to reach a support group. Others may live in areas where the only community to which they have access is an online community. PSOC asserts that these communities hold the potential of offering all of the same essential benefits of membership that a neighborhood-based community might afford, meaning that physical or geospatial proximity is not necessary to forming and becoming part of a community. Indeed, this has been made more apparent with the recent dramatic increased use of the internet to achieve virtual interpersonal interactions.

CONCEALMENT REVISITED

As noted earlier, concealment is the most proximal stress process in the minority stress model, applying to sexual and gender minority people in ways that typically do not apply to racial and ethnic minority people. When individuals remain in the closet, they cannot avail themselves of their community—they cannot reach their community, and their community cannot see them for who they are and are thus unable to offer the benefits of membership in that community. With the additional understanding of the essential elements of a community offered by PSOC, the profundity of this separation from one's own community becomes starker still.

Perhaps the most important aspect of membership in any community is belongingness. When individuals are in the closet and therefore not actual members of the community in which they might otherwise hold membership, the chasm between the individual and that person's potential community that could offer a sense of belongingness hinders identity formation (formation of the sexual and/or gender identity) and thwarts any transference of community benefits to the individual. Without the consensual validation and valuation of the individual by others, the individual is left to manage alone the "slings and arrows" of the stress processes, with no help from those who can offer it.

It needs to be noted that what it means to disclose or to be in the closet, and the community resources that are available, vary with culture. In many places, coming out is not safe, and the individual may need to carefully determine when disclosing a sexual or gender minority status is acceptable, safe, and perhaps helpful and when coming out would not be safe at all and may even be dangerous and disempowering.

As noted earlier, some individuals may wish to or need to return to the closet. Although the return to the closet may occur at any time, it typically does so as individuals enter their elder years or become disabled and face the need for care and care providers who are perceived to be intolerant or nonaffirming of the individual's stigmatized identity. In such cases, they may lose connection to their community, which can lead to a recurrence of the adverse health consequences associated with the stress processes of minority stress theory. The same results may also occur with individuals who begin a process of trying to change or inhibit their sexual or gender identity.

THE ROLE OF INTERSECTIONALITY

Although the primary focus of this chapter is on sexual and gender minority identities, it is vitally important to keep in mind that every individual has multiple social identities that encompass every social aspect of being human, including sex, race and ethnicity, level of education, immigration status, financial status, religion, relationship status, and ability/disability status. In 1989, Crenshaw introduced the concept of intersectionality to assist in understanding the relationships among the various identities that individuals possess, many of which had been overlooked by feminist theory and critical race theory.

It is important to first understand that within each identity domain there are privileged identities and marginalized or stigmatized identities. In fact, it is the multiplicity of identities that provide the structural and political foundation that creates privilege. Because the intersections between and among systems of oppression do not merely add to minority stress and marginalization but instead reinforce each other, the magnitude of stigma associated with multiple minority identities is the result of a synergistic effect. Because of this, marginalized identities must be addressed in combination to truly understand their impact. In effect, individuals who bear multiple marginalized identities suffer greater minority stress than the proverbial sum of their components might suggest.

Minority communities are also not free of prejudice and stigma toward other minority categories, exemplified by the racism and sexism that exist within LGBT communities. Having minority status in one domain does not immunize people against prejudice against minority members in another domain. Because of this, individuals who identify as a racial minority and a sexual minority may feel uncomfortable and experience minority stress within each of these identity communities—each group stigmatizing the other identity. Indeed, even within sexual minority and gender minority communities, there are those who discount (and therefore do not affirm) those with identities that do not fit neatly within an arbitrary binary system. Because of this, bisexual and gender nonbinary people may experience minority stress even within the community they seek for affirmation and support.

As is true of social science research generally, the extent to which studies that test the minority stress models and their components are sufficiently inclusive of other marginalized identities within their participant pools varies widely. Whereas some studies ensured a capacity for comparisons across certain demographic groups (in some cases by oversampling for minority participants), other studies, although moderately representative of the general population, do not include sufficient numbers of marginalized groups to allow for such comparisons. Many of those in the latter group are studies conducted via online recruitment and participation (e.g., The Trevor Project studies). Studies in the former group typically employed deliberate oversampling strategies to ensure an ability to make comparisons (e.g., Goldblum et al., 2012; Testa et al., 2012).

The question of intersectionality has been explored in studies with sufficient representation of participants across various demographic groups, and the findings have confirmed the synergistic hypothesis just noted. For example, in Goldblum et al. (2012), marginalized race/ethnicity was significantly associated with higher rates of suicide attempts, with participants who identified as multiracial reporting the highest rates of attempt (57.1%). This result does not mean that those gender minority individuals with more privileged racial identities reported suicide attempts at a level more on par with the general population. Indeed 23.0% of White participants reported a suicide attempt. Similar disparities in suicide attempt rates were found in this study between those assigned female at birth and those assigned male at birth (32.1% vs. 26.5%), and those reporting low and middle socioeconomic status and those reporting higher socioeconomic status (30.5% vs. 9.1%).

Several scientific journals (including a number of American Psychological Association journals and the journals of American Psychological Association Divisions) have fairly recently begun to insist on reporting results across a number of intersectional identities. Just as important, however, will be the ability to analyze data in terms of multiplicities of marginalized identities in order to fully understand the full (and real) impact of marginalization on health disparities. The hope is that this will correct the current paucity of such analyses and enrich the understanding of the real effect of intersectionalities, not just on health disparities but also on how and whence individuals with multiple marginalized identities access models for and develop coping strategies that may ultimately lead to resilience.

IMPLICATIONS FOR SOCE AND GICE

In essence, minority stress theory describes stress processes that result from possession of a stigmatized minority status and lead to negative health and social outcomes, on one hand, and a pathway to improved health and social outcomes through connection to a community of like-minded individuals, on the other. When individuals are able to establish a connection with their community, the psychological and other health benefits can be profound. The benefits that accrue are attributable to the level and processes of support described by both minority stress theory and by PSOC. The most important element of the coping and resilience benefits of the minority stress models is connection to a community of like individuals. It is through this connection, first suggested by Allport (1954) and later refined and articulated by Omoto and Snyder (2002, 2010), that sexual and gender minorities are able to withstand the onslaught of the distal and proximal processes of minority stress.

SOCE and GICE essentially separate individuals from the community from which they could derive these benefits and instead assert the notion that their identity is a form of pathology. Indeed, attempts to change someone's sexual orientation or gender identity are necessarily *dis*affirming of the individual's marginalized identity. It might then be expected that those who enter SOCE and GICE protocols would experience the negative effects of minority stress and none or few of the benefits of coping that results from the community connection on the other side of the model. This problem is not inconsequential. In a recent report, the Williams Institute estimated that nearly 700,000 LGBT adults had undergone some form of SOCE or GICE, and about half of them had experienced these approaches as adolescents (Mallory et al., 2019). But what is the actual harm of SOCE and GICE?

The 2019 and 2020 studies conducted by The Trevor Project provide a direct answer to this question. In the 2019 report (data collected in 2018), two-thirds of the respondents (ages 13–24) reported that someone had at one point tried to convince them to change their sexual orientation or gender identity. The youth who entered SOCE or GICE were more than twice as likely to have attempted suicide in the past year, compared with those who did not enter SOCE or GICE (Green et al., 2019). In the 2020 report (data collected mostly in 2020), 58% of respondents reported that someone had tried to convince them to change their sexual orientation or gender identity; among them, 19% attempted suicide, whereas 8% of those who had not experienced this attempted suicide. Additionally, the 2020 report indicated that 10% of respondents reported having received a more formal version of SOCE or GICE; of the 10%, 28% of those also reported a suicide attempt, and 12% of those who had not undergone SOCE or GICE reported a suicide attempt (The Trevor Project, 2020). Because most of those who are likely to enter SOCE or GICE are adolescents or young adults (those who are still under the authority and direction of their parents or guardians), this study seems to provide a direct answer to the question of what harm might come from not only depriving a youth of access to the LGBTQ community (an *un*affirming approach) but also *dis*affirming that youth's sexual and/or gender identity.

Change efforts are inherently disaffirming and devaluing and, in most cases, do not lead ultimately to actual change in sexual orientation or gender identity but rather to behaviors that are tantamount to retreating into the closet or returning to the stress-causing process of concealing a stigmatized identity. Therefore, change efforts would be expected to lead to negative social and health consequences and increases in health disparities, similar to (or possibly worse than) those experienced by individuals who have not found their community. The reader is also referred to Chapters 1 and 2 in this volume, which address in great detail the research on the effects of SOCE and GICE.

Unlike change efforts, minority stress theory makes it clear that the pathway to improved health and social outcomes and a decrease in health dispari-ties (as compared with the general population) is finding one's community, engaging with that community, establishing a sense of belonging, completing the process of identity formation around the stigmatized identity, and reaping the benefits that the community of LGBTQ people offers. In contrast to SOCE and GICE, both the model developed by Meyer and the model developed by Hendricks and Testa are very well supported in the literature. The key to healthier outcomes is an approach that affirms the individual's marginalized identity; that supports, validates, and values individuals for who they are; and that embraces the whole person. This approach provides LGBTQ indi-viduals with coping skills, improves their self-esteem, and possibly gives them individual incentive to do better. None of these outcomes are possible with SOCE and GICE.

REFERENCES

Allport, G. W. (1954). *The nature of prejudice*. Addison-Wesley.

Bailey, F., Barbato, R., & RuPaul. (Executive Producers). (2009–2021). *RuPaul's drag race* [TV series]. World of Wonder Productions.

Cochran, S. D., Björkenstam, C., & Mays, V. M. (2016). Sexual orientation and all-cause mortality among US adults aged 18 to 59 years, 2001–2011. *American Journal of Public Health, 106*(5), 918–920. https://doi.org/10.2105/AJPH.2016.303052

Crenshaw, K. (1989). Demarginalizing the intersection of race and sex: A Black feminist critique of antidiscrimination doctrine, feminist theory and antiracist politics. *University of Chicago Legal Forum, 1989*(1), Article 8.

Goldblum, P., Testa, R. J., Pflum, S., Hendricks, M. L., Bradford, J., & Bongar, B. (2012). The relationship between gender-based victimization and suicide attempts in transgender people. *Professional Psychology, Research and Practice, 43*(5), 468–475. https://doi.org/10.1037/a0029605

Green, A. E., Price-Feeney, M., & Dorison, S. H. (2019). *National estimate of LGBTQ youth seriously considering suicide*. The Trevor Project.

Hendricks, M. L., & Testa, R. J. (2012). A conceptual framework for clinical work with transgender and gender nonconforming clients: An adaptation of the minority stress model. *Professional Psychology, Research and Practice, 43*(5), 460–467. https://doi.org/10.1037/a0029597

Hill, J. L. (1996). Psychological sense of community: Suggestions for future research. *Journal of the American Medical Association, 24*(4), 431–438. https://doi.org/10.1002/(SICI)1520-6629(199610)24:4<431::AID-JCOP10>3.0.CO;2-T

Joiner, T. (2010). *Myths about suicide*. Harvard University.

Klein, A., & Golub, S. A. (2016). Family rejection as a predictor of suicide attempts and substance misuse among transgender and gender nonconforming adults. *LGBT Health, 3*(3), 193–199. https://doi.org/10.1089/lgbt.2015.0111

Livingston, J. (Director). (1990). *Paris is burning* [Film]. Off-White Productions.

Mallory, M., Brown, T. N. T., & Conron, K. J. (2019, June). *Update: Conversion therapy and LGBT youth*. The Williams Institute. https://williamsinstitute.law.ucla.edu/demographics/conversion-therapy-and-lgbt-youth/

Meyer, I. H. (1995). Minority stress and mental health in gay men. *Journal of Health and Social Behavior, 36*(1), 38–56. https://doi.org/10.2307/2137286

Meyer, I. H. (2003). Prejudice, social stress, and mental health in lesbian, gay, and bisexual populations: Conceptual issues and research evidence. *Psychological Bulletin, 129*(5), 674–697. https://doi.org/10.1037/0033-2909.129.5.674

Meyer, I. H. (2015). Resilience in the study of minority stress and health of sexual and gender minorities. *Psychology of Sexual Orientation and Gender Diversity, 2*(3), 209–213. https://doi.org/10.1037/sgd0000132

Omoto, A. M., & Snyder, M. (2002). Considerations of community: The context and process of volunteerism. *American Behavioral Scientist, 45*(5), 846–867. https://doi.org/10.1177/0002764202045005007

Omoto, A. M., & Snyder, M. (2010). Influences of psychological sense of community on voluntary helping and prosocial action. In S. Sturmer & M. Snyder (Eds.),

The psychology of prosocial behavior: Group processes, intergroup relations, and helping (pp. 223–243). Wiley-Blackwell. https://doi.org/10.1002/9781444307948.ch12

Testa, R. J., Jimenez, C. L., & Rankin, S. (2014). Risk and resilience during transgender identity development: The effects of awareness and engagement with other transgender people on affect. *Journal of Gay & Lesbian Mental Health, 18*(1), 31–46. https://doi.org/10.1080/19359705.2013.805177

Testa, R. J., Sciacca, L. M., Wang, F., Hendricks, M. L., Goldblum, P., Bradford, J., & Bongar, B. (2012). Effects of violence on transgender people. *Professional Psychology, Research and Practice, 43*(5), 452–459. https://doi.org/10.1037/a0029604

The Trevor Project. (2020). *2020 National Survey on LGBTQ Youth Mental Health.* http://www.thetrevorproject.org/survey-2020

Van Orden, K. A., Witte, T. K., Cukrowicz, K. C., Braithwaite, S. R., Selby, E. A., & Joiner, T. E., Jr. (2010). The interpersonal theory of suicide. *Psychological Review, 117*(2), 575–600. https://doi.org/10.1037/a0018697

THE ROLE OF FAMILIES IN EFFORTS TO CHANGE, SUPPORT, AND AFFIRM SEXUAL ORIENTATION, GENDER IDENTITY, AND EXPRESSION IN CHILDREN AND YOUTH

4

JUDITH M. GLASSGOLD AND CAITLIN RYAN

Although families play a central role and have an enduring influence on their children's health, emotional development, and well-being, most of what is known about sexual orientation change efforts (SOCE) has been learned through research with adults. Moreover, less information has been available on gender identity change efforts (GICE) with children and adolescents. This chapter provides a summary of research and clinical observations related to sexual orientation and gender identity and expression change efforts (SOGIECE) and affirmative approaches to support a child's sexual orientation, gender identity, and expression (SOGIE) in ethnically, racially, and culturally diverse families, with an emphasis on socially and religiously conservative families. The chapter concludes with recommendations for integrating family-oriented services, education, and guidance that support lesbian, gay, bisexual, transgender, and questioning or queer (LGBTQ) and gender diverse children and adolescents into all settings where children, youth, and families are served.

https://doi.org/10.1037/0000266-005
The Case Against Conversion "Therapy": Evidence, Ethics, and Alternatives,
D. C. Haldeman (Editor)

EFFECTS AND PREVALENCE OF SOGIECE AMONG YOUTH

SOGIECE,[1] also known as *conversion therapy*, present significant health risks to children and youth (American Psychological Association [APA], 2009; Substance Abuse and Mental Health Services Administration [SAMHSA], 2015). Research indicates that SOGIECE do not change sexual orientation but have the potential to seriously harm mental and physical health, which includes increasing the risk of depression, suicidal ideation, and suicide attempts (APA, 2009; Blosnich et al., 2020; SAMHSA, 2015). For transgender adults, GICE are associated with adverse mental health outcomes and a 2-times-greater likelihood of attempted suicide, compared with peers who have not experienced GICE (Turban et al., 2020). Because of potential harms, the major U.S. mental and physical health associations reject these efforts (for a list, see Chapter 9, this volume, and Movement Advancement Project, 2021; APA, 2009; SAMHSA, 2015).

A recent report from the Williams Institute at the University of California, Los Angeles indicates that a substantial number of children and youth are estimated to be exposed to these efforts, representing a significant public health risk (Mallory et al., 2018). This report was based on data from the Generations Project, a cross-sectional sample of the U.S. population, and found the following:

- Of the 698,000 LGBT adults (ages 18–59) in the United States who are estimated to have experienced conversion interventions, 350,000 LGBT adults received the interventions during adolescence.

- There were 16,000 LGBT youth (ages 13–17) who had received conversion interventions from a licensed health care professional in the 33 states that currently do not ban the practice (as of 2018).[2]

- There were 57,000 youth (ages 13–17) across all states who had received conversion interventions at some point in their lives from religious or spiritual advisors (Mallory et al., 2018).

Children and youth from conservatively religious families are especially vulnerable to exposure to conversion interventions (APA, 2009; Mallory et al., 2018; Ryan et al., 2010; Ryan, Toomey, et al., 2018). The Williams Institute

---

[1]Efforts to change gender expression are explicitly included in some forms of conversion therapy in children to target gender presentation as a way to change sexual orientation and gender identity.

[2]Although more states have approved bans on sexual orientation and gender identity change efforts (SOGICE), these projections are based on 2018 numbers.

estimates that 3 times as many children and youth receive religion-oriented SOGIECE than receive efforts from licensed professional mental health counselors (Mallory et al., 2018). These intervention efforts are applied by religious leaders, in support groups and youth programs; they are also carried out in families and by parents, caregivers, and guardians (APA, 2009). Past reports by LGBTQ advocacy groups conclude that religious organizations that believe homosexuality is a mental illness or an adverse developmental outcome may target families and their children for SOGIECE (Cianciotto & Cahill, 2006; Kennedy & Cianciotto, 2006).

In addition to mental and physical health risks, SOGIECE negatively impact children, youth, and families in other ways. SOGIECE may also harm parents' relationships with their children by increasing rejection, alienation, and other harmful behaviors. Parents and guardians may be misled into wasting time, financial resources, and energy (APA, 2009; SAMHSA, 2015). Parents and children may be given inaccurate information about sexual orientation and gender identity and are prevented from receiving affirming interventions that assist parents in supporting their children (APA, 2009; Ryan et al., 2010). Such affirmative interventions aim to prevent family rejection; to help families provide supportive environments; and to integrate the child's sexual orientation and gender identity into the family's cultural, religious, and social worlds (Ryan, 2019a, in press; Ryan et al., 2010; SAMHSA, 2014).

FAMILIES AND CONVERSION EFFORTS

Role of Families in Child Development

Given young children's emotional, physical, social, and economic dependence, families normatively provide key protective and nurturing functions. Through parental emotional responses such as empathy and affection, children ideally develop similar attributes, as well as emotional intelligence, self-esteem, the ability to form intimate and other social relationships, trust, behavioral self-mastery, coping skills, cognitive and executive functions, and educational and vocational skills and goals.

Impact of Family Responses

Family and caregiver responses to a child's, adolescent's, and young adult's SOGIE have a strong relationship to a child's health risks and well-being. Research conducted by the Family Acceptance Project (FAP; Ryan et al.,

2009, 2010; Ryan, Toomey, et al., 2018; SAMHSA, 2014) identified more than 100 specific behaviors that parents and caregivers use to express acceptance and rejection of their child's LGBTQ identity. Rejecting behaviors focus on trying to change, prevent, minimize, or deny a child's sexual orientation, gender identity, or expression. These behaviors include making children pray or attend religious services to change or suppress their identity, not allowing children to learn about or talk about their LGBTQ identity, not letting them have an LGBTQ friend, excluding children from family events and activities because of their SOGIE, and taking children to a therapist or religious leader for conversion interventions (Ryan, 2019d; Ryan et al., 2009). Ryan et al. (2010) identified a range of specific accepting behaviors that help families protect against health risks for their children (including suicidality) and promote their well-being. These behaviors include supporting their child's sexual orientation and gender expression, advocating for their children when others mistreat them because of their SOGIE, requiring family members to treat their LGBTQ child with respect, and finding an adult role model to give their child a positive sense of their future (Ryan, 2009, 2019b, 2019c).

Family Role in SOGIECE

FAP's research also found that parents and caregivers play a larger role in conversion efforts than has been previously understood (Ryan, Toomey, et al., 2018). These behaviors include parents both directly engaging in change efforts within their home and serving as gatekeepers to take their children to mental health practitioners and religious leaders with the goal of changing their children's SOGIE through conversion interventions.

In a study on sexual orientation change experiences (Ryan, Toomey, et al., 2018), the FAP found that more than half of LGBTQ young adults (53%) reported SOCE during adolescence both by their parents and by therapists and religious leaders. Both home-based parent and external sexual orientation conversion interventions by therapists and religious leaders contribute to multiple health and adjustment problems in young adulthood. These adolescents' symptoms include higher levels of depression and suicidal behavior, as well as lower levels of self-esteem, lower social support and life satisfaction, and lower levels of education and income in young adulthood, compared with those for LGBTQ young people who did not experience conversion efforts. Findings show the following:

- Rates of attempted suicide by LGBTQ young people whose parents and caregivers tried to change their sexual orientation were more than double

(48%) the rate for LGBTQ young adults who reported no conversion attempts (22%).

- Suicide attempts were nearly triple for LGBTQ young people who reported both home-based efforts to change their sexual orientation by parents and caregivers and intervention efforts by therapists and religious leaders (63%).

- Levels of depression in LGBTQ young adults were more than double (33%) for LGBTQ young people whose parents tried to change their sexual orientation compared with levels for those who reported no conversion experiences (16%); the levels were more than triple (52%) for LGBTQ young people who reported both home-based efforts to change their sexual orientation by parents and external SOCE by therapists and religious leaders.

- Sexual orientation change experiences during adolescence by both parents/ caregivers and therapists and religious leaders were associated with lower young adult socioeconomic status—specifically, less educational attainment and lower weekly income.

- LGBTQ adolescents from highly religious families and those from families with lower socioeconomic status were most likely to experience both home-based and external conversion efforts, whereas those who were gender nonconforming and who were from immigrant families were more likely to experience external conversion efforts initiated by parents and caregivers.

These findings underscore the explicit role of parents and caregivers in engaging in SOGIECE, through *family-rejecting behaviors* that overlap with external SOGIECE by therapists and religious leaders where parents also function as gatekeepers (Ryan, Toomey, et al., 2018).[3] More important, these findings expand the frame to focus on the broader role of family-rejecting behaviors that contribute to health risks, impaired adjustment, family conflict, and greater likelihood of removal or expulsion from the home (Ryan et al., 2009). Because LGBTQ youth cannot escape family-rejecting behaviors (e.g., Ryan, 2009; Ryan & Rees, 2012), approaches to prevent and ameliorate SOGICE must address the home, social, cultural, and religious influences on families and caregivers that precipitate SOGICE.

---

[3]Blosnich et al. (2020) also found a strong association between suicidal ideation and attempts and conversion therapy in their representative sample of adults.

CRITICAL ISSUES FOR FAMILIES OF TRADITIONAL FAITHS AND CULTURES

Psychology and traditional faiths can have contrasting views about same-sex orientation and gender diversity. Psychological research has found that sexual orientation and gender diversity are normal aspects of human diversity (APA, 2009). Although many traditional faiths adhere to beliefs that focus on the sanctity of heterosexual unions and traditional gender roles, it is important to note that there is a spectrum of religious beliefs about these issues (APA, 2009, pp. 17–20; see also Chapter 5, this volume).

Mental health approaches that address traditional faith concerns and child psychology still have key gaps, especially regarding issues related to the development of sexuality and gender (APA, 2009, pp. 17–20; Yarhouse & Tan, 2005). This absence of outreach and dialogue has left many of these family issues to faith leaders and traditional interpretations of religious beliefs that reject diversity in sexual orientation and gender identity. However, recent research and practice have developed evidence-informed, faith-based family guidance materials to help families learn to support their child's sexual orientation and gender diversity in the context of a variety of religious and cultural values (see Kleiman & Ryan, 2009, 2013; Ryan & Rees, 2012). These approaches for families and appropriate therapeutic responses are positive evidence-informed alternatives to conversion efforts and are explored in the following sections.

Issues for Parents and Families

Some families internalize the values and attitudes of their religion that characterize homosexuality and gender diversity negatively and as something to avoid and reject (Maslowe & Yarhouse, 2015; Yarhouse & Tan, 2005). Families then may perceive their child's potential or expressed sexual orientation and gender diversity as irreconcilable with their faith. For these families, the presence of children who are not heterosexual or cisgender can precipitate a crisis of epic proportions that may disrupt not only their belief system but also their ties to their community, heritage, ancestors, and the afterlife. Families then may experience shifts or losses in their core identity, role, purpose, and sense of order (Maslowe & Yarhouse, 2015; Ryan et al., 2009).

Families may fear for their children's future and moral well-being in the present as members of their family and community as well as in the afterlife (APA, 2009; Ryan et al., 2009, 2010; Ryan & Rees, 2012). As a result, parents and extended family members may attempt to change their child's SOGIE to enforce heterosexual and cisgender identities to make them acceptable to their vision of the divine order and the precepts of their faith and cultural community. Parents often do not realize that their attempts to change their child's SOGIE to save them from expulsion from the family and religious community and from being separated from their family for eternity have a terrible psychological cost for the child and the family (Ryan, 2015; Ryan et al., 2009, 2010). Family-based and external SOGIECE has the potential to disrupt the nurturing and protective functions of families within child development (Ryan, in press; SAMHSA, 2014).

Families may also experience their own fears of rejection and exclusion because of feelings of shame about their child as well as fear of judgment by religious leaders, other adherents, and the divine (Cates, 2007; Ryan et al., 2009). For many who come from faiths where there is a long historical overlap between faith, community, and family (e.g., the Church of Jesus Christ of Latter-day Saints, certain traditional Hasidic or Orthodox Jewish communities, Amish and traditional communities), a child's nonconformity with these aspects of faith will result in the family's rejection by their community, faith, eternity—the entire world as they know it. The sense of loss due to isolation from extended family and community can be tremendous (Kleiman & Ryan, 2013; Ryan et al., 2009, 2010).

These spiritual struggles may have mental health consequences for the parents as well as their children (Maslowe & Yarhouse, 2015; e.g., FAP, n.d.). The struggle to reconcile same-sex orientation and gender diversity with traditional faiths has been described as causing extreme emotional distress and conflict within a couple and with their children (Maslowe & Yarhouse, 2015). These spiritual struggles were sometimes associated with anxiety, panic disorders, depression, and suicidality, regardless of the level of religiosity or the perception of religion as a source of comfort and coping (APA, 2009, pp. 44–52).

Issues for Children and Youth

Children and youth who recognize the incompatibility of their feelings and identity with faith, family, and community may experience a variety of feelings, such as anger, confusion, religious disillusionment (anger toward God), fear, shame, and distress because of the conflict (Cates, 2007; Hatzenbuehler et al., 2012; Page et al., 2013; Yarhouse & Tan, 2005). Conflicts between SOGIE and faith, primarily the challenge of integrating diverse sexual orientations and gender identities into a religiously sanctioned life (i.e., one that provides an option for positive self-esteem and religion-sanctioned sexuality and family life), may be a significant challenge for children especially as they enter adolescence and young adulthood and recognize the disconnect between their feelings and sanctioned roles (APA, 2009, pp. 71–80; Cates, 2007; Hatzenbuehler et al., 2012; Page et al., 2013; Yarhouse & Tan, 2005). Such conflicts can have negative mental health effects (Hatzenbuehler et al., 2012; Page et al., 2013). For example, studies indicate that identity conflict in youth that results from dissonance between religious beliefs and LGBTQ identity was associated with higher risk of suicide (Gibbs & Goldbach, 2015; Hatzenbuehler et al., 2012; Page et al., 2013). Children and youth may become more isolated if they lack information and support from their family and community on alternatives other than to change or try to repress their SOGIE.

Therapeutic Approaches for Families

The disruption of cultural and religious faith by a child's SOGIE can threaten a family's coping skills and their ability to love and nurture a child (Ryan et al., 2009). A family's struggle with accepting or supporting a child's SOGIE can disrupt many of the important emotional and caregiving bonds and erode connectedness, which can lead to serious harm for their LGBTQ or gender diverse child. For example, parental rejection, criticism, fear, and even rage can overwhelm nurturing and affirming behaviors and responses to children (Ryan et al., 2010). Restoring a family's coping skills in the midst of this complex personal and religious crisis, particularly the family's ability to love and support their child, is a primary goal of affirmative family support interventions such as the FAP (Ryan et al., 2010, in press).

The FAP was launched in 2002 to fill a major gap in research, practice, and policy with LGBTQ children and youth—the need to understand how families respond to their LGBTQ children and to develop an evidence-based family support model to decrease rejection and increase support to prevent health risks and promote well-being grounded in family, cultural, and religious values. FAP used a participatory framework to conduct a range of studies that included families, LGBTQ youth, providers, educators, and religious leaders.

The FAP has generated multiple resources, including peer-reviewed publications, multilingual family education and guidance materials, and assessment tools and measures to help diverse families learn to support their LGBTQ children—even when they believe that being LGBTQ or gender diverse is wrong—through educating and assisting families to focus on their love for their child and understanding the negative health impact of rejecting behaviors and the positive impact of supportive, accepting, and affirming behaviors (see the FAP website at https://familyproject.sfsu.edu). FAP's family support work has been provided in several languages and with children and families from a wide range of ethnic, racial, and religious backgrounds. FAP's family support model includes not only community engagement strategies but also psychoeducation, counseling, skill building, peer support, and training to increase the ability of diverse parents, caregivers, foster parents, and guardians to communicate with, advocate for, and learn to support and provide affirmative parenting for LGBTQ and gender diverse children and adolescents (Ryan, in press).

FAP's family support model was designed to be integrated across systems of care in behavioral health, in family services, in out-of-home care, in primary care, and by school-based and pastoral care providers and religious leaders. FAP's team has been developing a series of family guidance resources to be used by families that are "Best Practice" resources for suicide prevention included in the Best Practice Registry for Suicide Prevention (Kleiman & Ryan, 2013; Ryan, 2009; Ryan & Rees, 2012) and strategies and resources to engage and help diverse families to move from rejection and struggle to support of their LGBTQ children (Kleiman & Ryan, 2009, 2013; Ryan, 2009, 2019b, 2019c, 2019d; Ryan & Rees, 2012; SAMHSA, 2014).

Recently, FAP integrated key components of FAP's family support model into trauma-focused cognitive behavior therapy to help modify this therapy for use with LGBTQ children and youth (Cohen et al., 2019). This modification resulted in significant improvement in posttraumatic stress symptoms for LGBTQ youth (Cohen, 2019; Cohen & Ryan, 2021). Family-rejecting behaviors are traumatic and in the context of other adverse experiences can contribute to complex trauma (Cohen & Ryan, 2021). As a result of the COVID-19 pandemic, loss of external support, and confinement with parents, families, and caregivers who reject their child's LGBTQ identity and gender diversity, risk is increased for LGBTQ children and adolescents (Cohen & Ryan, 2021; Salerno et al., 2020).

FAP calls for agencies, providers, religious leaders, and faith-based groups to educate parents, families, and caregivers on how their behaviors affect their LGBTQ children's risk and well-being. FAP's family support principles and core guidance strategies have been disseminated by the U.S. SAMHSA (2014) as a practice guide. A key component of FAP's approach is aligning FAP's research findings and behavioral framework with the family's cultural and religious values. This alignment includes incorporating underlying religious and spiritual values such as compassion, mercy, love, and respect into FAP's psychoeducation and family guidance approach that encourages support and acceptance of LGBTQ children and youth (Fortuna et al., 2020; Ryan, 2020, in press; Ryan et al., 2010).

Working with diverse families in a range of settings, Ryan and colleagues have found that diverse parents, caregivers, and families can learn to support their LGBTQ children when guidance and support are provided in ways that resonate for them (Ryan, 2014, 2020; Ryan, Sampson, et al., 2018; SAMHSA, 2014). Families that completed the integrated FAP program increased positive attitudes and support for their LGBTQ children, and their children remained in the home at 6- and 12-month follow-ups (Ryan, Sampson, et al., 2018). FAP has been useful for families that have LGBTQ children and youth after a child protective services investigation found their children to be at risk for removal for abuse and neglect.

FUTURE DIRECTIONS: FROM PREVENTING HARM TO PROMOTING WELL-BEING

Lack of Services for Families

Although family intervention models have been developed by the FAP (Ryan, 2014, 2019b, 2019c, 2019d) and the gender affirmative model (Keo-Meier & Ehrensaft, 2018) to increase family support for children and youth with diverse SOGIE and to prevent conversion efforts, a lack of family-oriented services in mainstream settings is a major barrier to reducing risk and promoting the well-being of these children and youth. Historically, families of LGBTQ youth were seen as rejecting and incapable of learning to support their LGBTQ children. As a result, services emerged over several decades to serve LGBTQ children and youth either individually—such as adults—or through peer support, but not in the context of their families (Ryan, 2014). Similarly, therapeutic and community services that engage diverse parents and caregivers and help them learn to support their LGBTQ children are also lacking.

Lack of Anticipatory Guidance

One harmful outcome of the historical pathologizing of same-sex sexual orientation and gender diversity is that information and services that support parents and children are omitted from the standard, normative health, mental health, and educational services that children and their families receive (Ryan, 2014). In contrast, most parents have access to resources about other aspects of child development, such as physical milestones, language development, cognitive development, and emotional development.

The absence of these resources, combined with the lack of therapy services, means that parents lack nonstigmatizing, culturally grounded information on

SOGIE—a lost opportunity to help parents and caregivers understand that SOGIE is part of normative development and to support positive development of sexual orientation and gender identity in their children (Ryan, 2014). Parents have few resources for anticipatory guidance on any aspect of SOGIE and thus have limitations for learning to support and care for their children in culturally affirming ways. Much of the education in these areas comes from social media and cultural institutions that may provide inaccurate, distorted, and incomplete information.

Transition From Stigma Remediation to Normalization

Scientific research has established that LGBTQ children and youth are negatively affected by the social stigma directed at LGBTQ individuals. For example, many LGBTQ youth are at higher risk for mental health challenges such as suicide, anxiety, and depression (di Giacomo et al., 2018; Hatzenbuehler & Pachankis, 2016; Russell & Fish, 2016; Toomey et al., 2018). LGBTQ children and youth may also have negative educational and vocational outcomes that are positively impacted by increasing supports and changing climate to be inclusive and affirming (Russell & Fish, 2016; SAMHSA, 2015). These risks seem to decline when LGBTQ youth live in states and communities with more LGBTQ-affirming policy protections (Raifman et al., 2017).

In response to this extensive literature on the public health harms of anti-LGBTQ stigma on mental and physical health and well-being of youth and adults (Hatzenbuehler & Pachankis, 2016; Russell & Fish, 2016) most schools and public health efforts have focused on protecting LGBTQ youth from harm, such as those from bullying, exclusion, and invisibility in schools (APA, n.d.; Ryan, 2014). In this framework, LGBTQ children and youth are not seen as the problem. Rather, the problem is society that stigmatizes them, makes them invisible, constricts access to normative supports, and ignores their sexual orientation and gender identity development.

A more comprehensive plan—and one that aims to prevent stigma and promote well-being—is to integrate normalizing approaches to support a child's SOGIE into mainstream public health and wellness programs that are offered to all children and families from birth through adulthood. Doing so essentially means integrating these issues into mainstream well-baby, well-child and adolescent, and well-young-adult curricula offered to parents and others by health care professionals. Likewise, support for positive development of sexual orientation and gender diversity must be integrated into every educational, health, and social policy venue. Such integration would generate a revolution in pediatric care, child development, social services, and educational policy (Ryan, 2014). This inclusion reinforces the inherent normalcy of the full range of diverse sexual orientations, gender identities, and expressions. This public health policy frame assists families in supporting their LGBTQ children through information that resonates with their values and beliefs. Inclusion in normative health information shifts the discourse on SOGIE from morality to health and well-being, and it provides guidance and support in the context of underlying health values (Ryan, 2014, 2019a, in press).

Given the health costs of family rejection, which includes conversion efforts, widespread public access to accurate, culturally appropriate family support information and guidance is a public health imperative. For many families, public settings are the primary venues in which they access information about health, children's rights, child development, and childcare. These public settings include schools, public health and mental health services, and government and community agencies—literally all places where children, youth, and families are served. Schools, for example, provide access for parents to information on children's health and development needs. Yet schools are a largely untapped source for guidance, information, support, and referrals for diverse families with LGBTQ and gender diverse children and youth (Ryan & Chen-Hayes, 2013).

The need for normalizing SOGIE diverse children has increased as LGBTQ and gender diverse children self-identify and are identified at increasingly younger ages. FAP routinely provides family support services for gay, transgender and gender diverse children younger than age 10. Because LGBTQ lives have not been seen as a normal developmental outcome, parents have not known how to react or have reacted negatively. By normalizing SOGIE development in children and focusing on the negative physical and mental health consequences of rejection, and the wellness-promoting impact of family acceptance, parents can learn and then focus on assisting their child with appropriate and affirmative developmental milestones (Ryan et al., 2010). This normalizing approach includes a public education campaign to educate parents, caregivers, providers, and religious leaders about the impact of family-rejecting and family-accepting behaviors and screening for these same behaviors as a routine part of assessment and care, as is increasingly done for Adverse Childhood Experiences. However, screening for Adverse Childhood Experiences does not include SOGIE and, in particular, does not include the specific family-rejecting and family-accepting behaviors that FAP has identified and measured in their research and that have been found to be predictive of risk and well-being for LGBTQ young people.

Agencies, institutions, and congregations can begin to address this gap by integrating FAP's evidence-based, multilingual approach into their work. One option is to use FAP's *Healthy Futures* posters (see Figure 4.1; Ryan,

FIGURE 4.1. Healthy Futures Acceptance Poster for Use in Conservative Settings

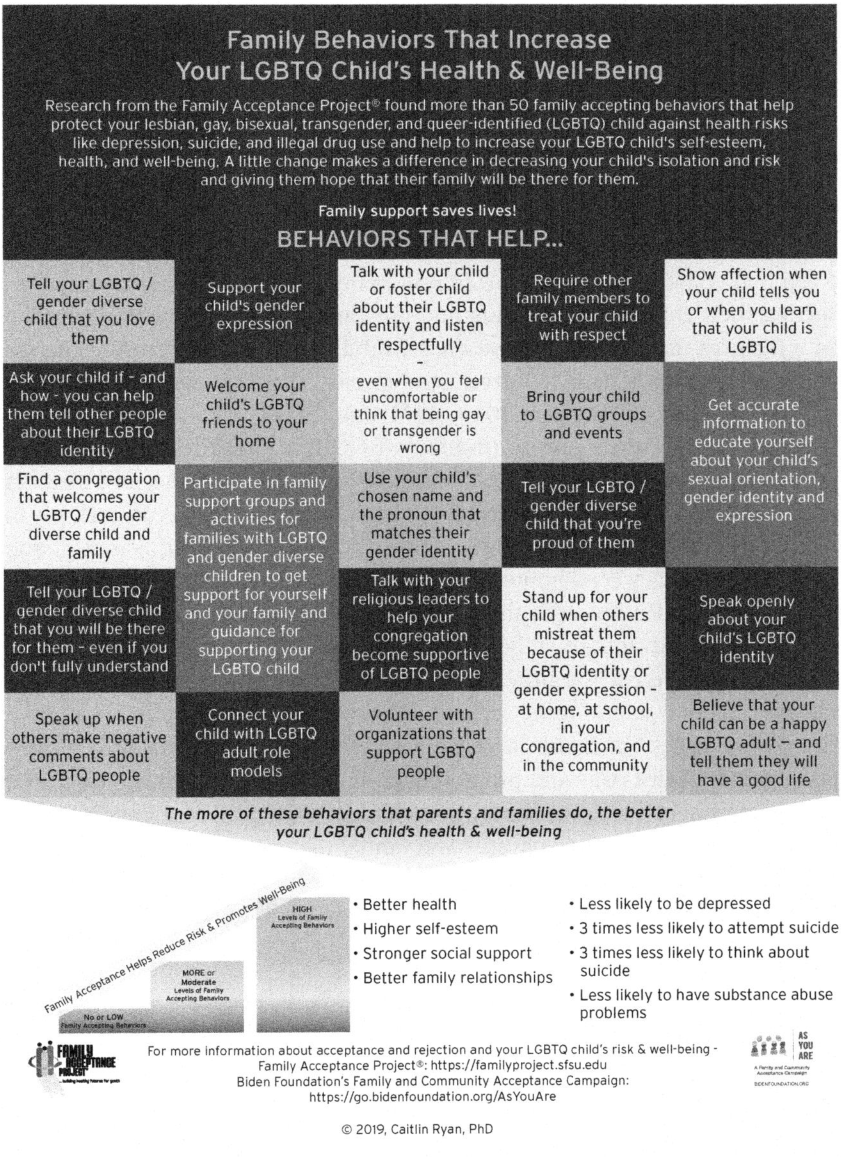

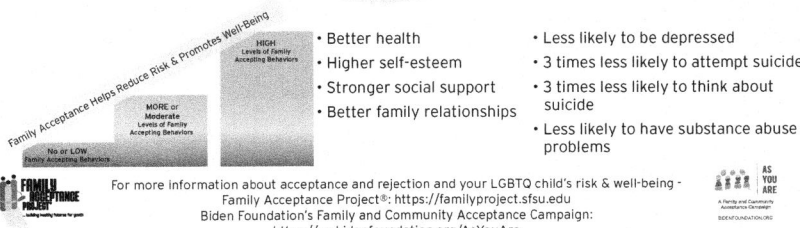

Note. Copyright by the Family Acceptance Project. Reprinted with permission. Camera-ready artwork available to download in four sizes with poster guidance and three versions of each poster in 10 languages from https://familyproject.sfsu.edu/poster.

2019b, 2019c, 2019d, 2019e), which tell the visual "story" of family rejection and acceptance on one page in all settings where children, youth, and families are served; at home; and in public spaces such as libraries, community centers, transportation settings, and public housing. These posters are available with a poster guidance in English and Spanish, and they are forthcoming in Chinese, Hindi, Korean, Japanese, Punjabi, Tagalog, and Vietnamese. As FAP's work has demonstrated, many parents, caregivers, and families are shocked to learn that behaviors they engage in to protect their children, to help them "fit in" and be respected by others, are instead experienced by their children as instilling shame and as trying to change, prevent, and deny their identities, which causes significant harm (Ryan, 2020; Ryan et al., 2009, 2010). Ryan and colleagues have reported that many families believe they are protecting their children by isolating and preventing them from being exposed to influences that parents believe are harmful, which instead prevents access to the very support that children need to ease their isolation and distress (Cohen & Ryan, 2021; Ryan, 2014; SAMHSA, 2014).

Providing accurate and normalizing SOGIE information also supports a normative parental function: advocating for a child's well-being. Parents and caregivers traditionally advocate for their children's needs and are in a key position to nurture, care for, and protect their children. Parental and caregiver advocacy is an important family-accepting behavior identified and measured in FAP's research that helps caregivers to decrease their LGBTQ child's risk and promote well-being (Ryan, 2009). Advocacy—standing up for one's children when others mistreat them because of their SOGIE in families, schools, community settings, and congregations—helps strengthen the parent–child bond and increases connectedness while helping to protect against health risks and promote well-being. These bonds are fractured when a parent or caregiver sends their child for SOGIECE from professionals or religious groups. When parents and family members lack access to or are denied accurate information about how to care for their child, they cannot be their child's advocate or understand how their behaviors affect their child's risk and well-being.

CONCLUSION

The primary policy response to protect children and adolescents from SOGIECE has been to regulate licensed practitioners through legislation or regulations (APA, 2009; SAMHSA, 2015; see also Chapter 9, this volume). However, this policy response does not address the efforts by parents and by nonlicensed practitioners, including religious leaders (Blosnich et al., 2020;

Mallory et al., 2018). Parents often attempt to change their child's SOGIE through behavioral interventions that include identified harmful, rejecting behaviors (Ryan et al., 2009, 2010; Ryan, Russell, et al., 2010). To protect children and youth, public policy interventions must address the role of the family in SOGIECE.

Potential interventions to reduce family SOGIECE, including therapeutic and educational resources on SOGIE for children and parents, are essential from childhood to young adulthood. Mainstreaming SOGIE-positive information into public education and health practices, through well-child education and school curriculum, is essential to promote the health and well-being of children and youth. Mental health practitioners can provide guidance for families on ways to support their LGBTQ children and thus prevent conversion efforts—in and out of the home. SOGIE-affirmative, culturally consistent, and religiously consistent education and intervention services for children's health and mental health are possible and enable families to support their LGBTQ children (Ryan, 2014). Such an approach is represented by the FAP and other therapeutic and educational efforts linked to overarching cultural and faith values such as compassion, love, hope, and welcome (APA, 2009; Ryan, 2015, in press; Ryan et al., 2010; SAMHSA, 2014; Yarhouse & Tan, 2005). FAP's family support model, in particular, provides access to culturally relevant peer support and includes family/parent support partners, a trained workforce of parents and caregivers with lived experience whose children have been served in behavioral health, out-of-home and related service systems, many of whom share cultural and faith-based experiences and language needs (SAMHSA, 2017). Peer support is essential to decrease the isolation that diverse parents with LGBTQ children experience and to provide the culturally grounded parenting guidance and support that caregivers routinely receive intergenerationally, so as to parent non-LGBTQ children and youth (Ryan, 2019a, in press).

The goal for providers is to model acceptance, reconciliation, and dialogue by incorporating family-based education and clinical services into clinical practices. Many professionals have found such parental faith-based rejection of diverse children challenging. Professionals cannot give up on families or see parental confusion, conflict, and rejection as so heinous as to be unforgivable and warranting condemnation and rejection. Those professional responses would be acts of despair and hopelessness—antithetical to appropriate clinical practice and the essential hopefulness of psychotherapy—and would mirror the mindset of those who reject LGBTQ children and youth. Instead, mental health providers can adopt an affirmative approach that includes teaching parents and caregivers empathy and compassion for their

LGBTQ and gender diverse children. This requires practitioners to have compassion for parents, caregivers, and families as well.

REFERENCES

American Psychological Association. (2009). *The report of the American Psychological Association Task Force on Appropriate Therapeutic Responses to Sexual Orientation.* https://www.apa.org/pi/lgbt/resources/therapeutic-response.pdf

American Psychological Association. (n.d.). *The Respect Online course.* https://www.apa.org/pi/lgbt/programs/safe-supportive/training/respect-online-course.aspx

Blosnich, J. R., Henderson, E. R., Coulter, R. W. S., Goldbach, J. T., & Meyer, I. H. (2020). Sexual orientation change efforts, adverse childhood experiences, and suicide ideation and attempt among sexual minority adults, United States, 2016–2018. *American Journal of Public Health, 110*(7), 1024–1030. https://doi.org/10.2105/AJPH.2020.305637

Cates, J. A. (2007). Identity in crisis: Spirituality and homosexuality in adolescence. *Child & Adolescent Social Work Journal, 24*(4), 369–383. https://doi.org/10.1007/s10560-007-0089-6

Cianciotto, J., & Cahill, S. (2006). *Youth in the crosshairs: The third wave of ex-gay activism.* National Gay and Lesbian Task Force.

Cohen, J. A. (2019). Trauma-focused cognitive behavioral therapy (TF-CBT) for LGBTQ youth. *Journal of the American Academy of Child & Adolescent Psychiatry, 58*(10), S29. https://doi.org/10.1016/j.jaac.2019.07.124

Cohen, J. A., Mannarino, A. P., Wilson, K., & Zinny, A. (2019). *Trauma-focused cognitive behavioral therapy LGBTQ implementation manual.* Allegheny Health Network.

Cohen, J. A., & Ryan, C. (2021). The Trauma-Focused CBT and Family Acceptance Project: An integrated framework for children and youth. *Psychiatric Times, 38*(6), 15–17. https://www.psychiatrictimes.com/view/the-trauma-focused-cbt-and-family-acceptance-project

di Giacomo, E., Krausz, M., Colmegna, F., Aspesi, F., & Clerici, M. (2018). Estimating the risk of attempted suicide among sexual minority youths: A systematic review and meta-analysis. *JAMA Pediatrics, 172*(12), 1145–1152. https://doi.org/10.1001/jamapediatrics.2018.2731

Family Acceptance Project. (n.d.). *Family videos.* San Francisco State University. https://familyproject.sfsu.edu/family-videos

Fortuna, L., Ryan, C., & Telingator, C. (2020). Faith, acceptance, and mental health: Working with religiously and culturally diverse families of LGBTQ youth. *Journal of the American Academy of Child & Adolescent Psychiatry, 59*(10), S348. https://doi.org/10.1016/j.jaac.2020.07.855

Gibbs, J. J., & Goldbach, J. (2015). Religious conflict, sexual identity, and suicidal behaviors among LGBT young adults. *Archives of Suicide Behavior, 19*(4), 472–488. https://doi.org/10.1080/13811118.2015.1004476

Hatzenbuehler, M. L., & Pachankis, J. E. (2016). Stigma and minority stress as social determinants of health among lesbian, gay, bisexual, and transgender youth: Research evidence and clinical implications. *Pediatric Clinics of North America, 63*(6), 985–997. https://doi.org/10.1016/j.pcl.2016.07.003

Hatzenbuehler, M. L., Pachankis, J. E., & Wolff, J. (2012). Religious climate and health risk behaviors in sexual minority youths: A population-based study. *American Journal of Public Health, 102*(4), 657–663. https://doi.org/10.2105/AJPH.2011.300517

Kennedy, S., & Cianciotto, J. (2006). *Homophobia at "hell house": Literally demonizing lesbian, gay, bisexual, and transgender youth*. National Gay and Lesbian Task Force Policy Institute.

Keo-Meier, C., & Ehrensaft, D. (Eds.). (2018). *The gender affirmative model: An interdisciplinary approach to supporting transgender and gender expansive children*. American Psychological Association. https://doi.org/10.1037/0000095-000

Kleiman, V. (Director), & Ryan, C. (Executive Producer). (2009). *Always my son* [Film]. Family Acceptance Project, San Francisco State University.

Kleiman, V. (Director), & Ryan, C. (Executive Producer). (2013). *Families are forever* [Film]. Family Acceptance Project, San Francisco State University. (Best Practices Registry for Suicide Prevention).

Mallory, C., Brown, C. N. T., & Conron, K. J. (2018, January). *Conversion therapy and LGBT youth*. The Williams Institute, UCLA School of Law. https://williamsinstitute. law.ucla.edu/demographics/conversion-therapy-and-lgbt-youth/

Maslowe, K. E., & Yarhouse, M. A. (2015). Christian parental reactions when a child comes out. *The American Journal of Family Therapy, 43*(4), 352–363. https:// doi.org/10.1080/01926187.2015.1051901

Movement Advancement Project. (2021). *Conversion "therapy" laws*. https://www. lgbtmap.org/equality-maps/conversion_therapy

Page, M. J. L., Lindahl, K. M., & Malik, N. M. (2013). The role of religion and stress in sexual identity and mental health among lesbian, gay, and bisexual youth. *Journal of Research on Adolescence, 23*(4), 665–677. https://doi.org/10.1111/jora.12025

Raifman, J., Moscoe, E., Austin, S. B., & McConnell, M. (2017). Difference-in-differences analysis of the association between state same-sex marriage policies and adolescent suicide attempts. *JAMA Pediatrics, 171*(4), 350–356. https://doi.org/ 10.1001/jamapediatrics.2016.4529

Russell, S. T., & Fish, J. N. (2016). Mental health in lesbian, gay, bisexual, and transgender (LGBT) youth. *Annual Review of Clinical Psychology, 12*(1), 465–487. https:// doi.org/10.1146/annurev-clinpsy-021815-093153

Ryan, C. (2009). *Supportive families, healthy children: Helping families with lesbian, gay, bisexual, and transgender children*. Family Acceptance Project, Marian Wright Edelman Institute, San Francisco State University.

Ryan, C. (2014). Generating a revolution in prevention, wellness, and care for LGBT children and youth. *Temple Political & Civil Rights Law Review, 23*(2), 331–344.

Ryan, C. (2015, January 7). Parents don't have to choose between their faith and their LGBT kids. *The Washington Post*. https://www.washingtonpost.com/national/ religion/parents-dont-have-to-choose-between-their-faith-and-their-lgbt-kids-commentary/2015/01/07/e3ec4a9c-96bc-11e4-8385-866293322c2f_story.html? utm_term=.104c709be171

Ryan, C. (2019a). The Family Acceptance Project's model for LGBTQ youth. *Journal of the American Academy of Child & Adolescent Psychiatry, 58*(10), S28–S29. https:// doi.org/10.1016/j.jaac.2019.07.123

Ryan, C. (2019b). *Family behaviors that increase your LGBTQ child's health & well-being* [Educational Poster]. Family Acceptance Project, Marian Wright Edelman Institute, San Francisco State University.

Ryan, C. (2019c). *Family behaviors that increase your LGBTQ child's health & well-being—Version for conservative settings* [Educational Poster]. Family Acceptance Project, Marian Wright Edelman Institute, San Francisco State University.

Ryan, C. (2019d). *Family behaviors that increase your LGBTQ child's risk for serious health & mental health problems* [Educational Poster]. Family Acceptance Project, Marian Wright Edelman Institute, San Francisco State University.

Ryan, C. (2019e). *Poster guidance for Healthy Futures posters.* Family Acceptance Project, Marian Wright Edelman Institute, San Francisco State University.

Ryan, C. (2020). Family rejection is a health hazard for LGBTQ children and youth. *Journal of the American Academy of Child & Adolescent Psychiatry, 59*(10), S336. https://doi.org/10.1016/j.jaac.2020.07.817

Ryan, C. (in press). *Implementing the Family Acceptance Project's family support model: Practice guidance.* Family Acceptance Project, Marian Wright Edelman Institute. San Francisco State University.

Ryan, C., & Chen-Hayes, S. (2013). Educating and empowering families of LGBTQ K-12 students. In E. S. Fisher & K. Komosa-Hawkins (Eds.), *Creating school environments to support lesbian, gay, bisexual, transgender, and questioning students and families: A handbook for school professionals* (pp. 209–229). Routledge.

Ryan, C., Huebner, D., Diaz, R. M., & Sanchez, J. (2009). Family rejection as a predictor of negative health outcomes in White and Latino lesbian, gay, and bisexual young adults. *Pediatrics, 123*(1), 346–352. https://doi.org/10.1542/peds.2007-3524

Ryan, C., & Rees, R. A. (2012). *Supportive families, healthy children: Helping Latter-day Saint families with lesbian, gay, bisexual & transgender children.* Family Acceptance Project, Marian Wright Edelman Institute, San Francisco State University.

Ryan, C., Russell, S. T., Huebner, D., Diaz, R., & Sanchez, J. (2010). Family acceptance in adolescence and the health of LGBT young adults. *Journal of Child and Adolescent Psychiatric Nursing, 23*(4), 205–213. https://doi.org/10.1111/j.1744-6171.2010.00246.x

Ryan, C., Sampson, M., Fullenkamp, J., & Peterson, J. (2018, January). *Integrating the Family Acceptance Project's family support model into family group decision-making to increase family support for LGBTQ children and youth to prevent placement in foster care* [Paper presentation]. Twenty-Second Annual Meeting of the Society for Social Work and Research, Washington, DC, United States.

Ryan, C., Toomey, R. B., Diaz, R. M., & Russell, S. T. (2018). Parent-initiated sexual orientation change efforts with LGBT adolescents: Implications for young adult mental health and adjustment. *Journal of Homosexuality, 67*(2), 159–173. https://doi.org/10.1080/00918369.2018.1538407

Salerno, J. P., Williams, N. D., & Gattamorta, K. A. (2020). LGBTQ populations: Psychologically vulnerable communities in the COVID-19 pandemic. *Psychological Trauma: Theory, Research, Practice, and Policy, 12*(S1), S239–S242. https://doi.org/10.1037/tra0000837

Substance Abuse and Mental Health Services Administration. (2014). *A practitioner's resource guide: Helping families to support their LGBT children* (HHS Publication No. PEP14-LGBTKIDS).

Substance Abuse and Mental Health Services Administration. (2015). *Ending conversion therapy: Supporting and protecting LGBTQ youth.* https://store.samhsa.gov/product/Ending-Conversion-Therapy-Supporting-and-Affirming-LGBTQ-Youth/SMA15-4928

Substance Abuse and Mental Health Services Administration. (2017). *Family, parent, and caregiver peer support in behavioral health.* https://www.samhsa.gov/sites/default/files/programs_campaigns/brss_tacs/family-parent-caregiver-support-behavioral-health-2017.pdf

Toomey, R. B., Syvertsen, A. K., & Shramko, M. (2018). Transgender adolescent suicide behavior. *Pediatrics, 142*(4), e20174218. https://doi.org/10.1542/peds.2017-4218

Turban, J. L., Beckwith, N., Reisner, S. L., & Keuroghlian, A. S. (2020). Association between recalled exposure to gender identity conversion efforts and psychological distress and suicide attempts among transgender adults. *JAMA Psychiatry, 77*(1), 68–76. https://doi.org/10.1001/jamapsychiatry.2019.2285

Yarhouse, M. A., & Tan, E. S. N. (2005). Addressing religious conflicts in adolescents who experience sexual identity confusion. *Professional Psychology, Research and Practice, 36*(5), 530–536. https://doi.org/10.1037/0735-7028.36.5.530

5 THE ROLE OF RELIGION IN SEXUAL ORIENTATION CHANGE EFFORTS AND GENDER IDENTITY CHANGE EFFORTS

THOMAS G. PLANTE

If a person is gay and seeks out the Lord and is willing, who am I to judge that person?

–Pope Francis

And what does the Lord require of you? To act justly and to love mercy and to walk humbly with your God.

–Micah 6:8

The various religious and spiritual traditions have provided thoughtful reflection and guidance regarding the biggest questions and concerns of life since perhaps the dawn of humans on the planet and the formation of group identities. These great wisdom traditions that we are familiar with today (e.g., Christianity, Islam, Judaism, Hinduism, Buddhism) developed and became established during the Axial Age (i.e., the pivotal age of religious development of the major religious traditions between the eighth and third centuries

https://doi.org/10.1037/0000266-006
The Case Against Conversion "Therapy": Evidence, Ethics, and Alternatives,
D. C. Haldeman (Editor)

B.C.E.; Armstrong, 2006), and they have had millennia to fine-tune their views and perspectives about eternal questions of life, death, and human behavior. These religious traditions and their leaders have been highly influential in community and personal life for thousands of years. Religion, religious organizations, and clerics continue to be extremely influential in the 21st century, not only for people of faith but also for everyone, because they often are deeply involved with and try to influence secular politics, laws, public policy, and expectations for behavior throughout the land (Fox, 2018). Additionally, services that are provided by religious institutions, such as hospitals, schools, universities, clinics, shelters, and charities, impact people of faith as well as those unaffiliated with any religion or religious institutions (Armstrong, 2006; Chaves, 2017).

When it comes to topics related to sex, religious traditions and clerics have a lot to say. Sexual ethics and expected behavior are highlighted within most religious traditions that include guidance and rules about how people should manage their sexual desires, behavior, and commitments (Grabowski, 2012; May et al., 2011; Pruss, 2012). Religious traditions and leaders may determine whom you can partner with, and they often speak to issues related to procreation, abortion, masturbation, homosexuality, premarital sex, marriage, and divorce. Conservative religious communities tend to be more prescriptive and restrictive about sexual ethics and behavior, and they typically frown upon or prohibit masturbation, premarital sex, homosexuality, abortion, contraception, and divorce (Edger, 2012). Although the press often highlights the beliefs of certain religious traditions, such as the Roman Catholic Church and evangelical Christian churches, most conservative religious traditions—including Orthodox Judaism and Mormonism—are similar with respect to sexual ethics and expected sexual behavior (Balkin et al., 2014). The religious traditions that tend to lean toward liberalism (e.g., Unitarianism) typically are more open, tolerant, and embracing of diverse sexual behaviors and identity. Nonetheless, many religious traditions that are well known for their conservative and restrictive sexual views (e.g., Roman Catholicism, Orthodox Judaism, and evangelical Christianity) also have more open, tolerant, and left-leaning elements (e.g., Reform Judaism; Salzman & Lawler, 2012).

This chapter focuses on the role of religion in sexual orientation and gender identity change efforts (SOCE and GICE, respectively). It provides a general overview of the most common religious perspectives on sexual orientation and gender identity. It also examines some of the diverse religious perspectives on this topic from a variety of religious traditions, with a focus on the Abrahamic traditions. Finally, it discusses ways that mental health professionals may be able to work productively and collaboratively with religious institutions and leaders to best serve their clients and patients.

It is important to mention that religious traditions tend to use sacred scripture (e.g., the Bible), historical traditions, and moral philosophy to determine their views and prescriptions on sexual behavior and ethics rather than contemporary social science research. Therefore, to better understand where their views, perspectives, and prescriptions come from, one must examine critical elements of these influences and most especially sacred scripture (Countryman, 2013). Additionally, to further complicate the matter, little quality empirical social science research has been conducted in this area as of this date. Much more research is clearly needed in the psychology and sociology of religion as it relates to lesbian, gay, bisexual, transgender, queer, and intersex (LGBTQI+) populations and engagement with SOCE and GICE.

WHY THE TENSION BETWEEN SOME RELIGIOUS TRADITIONS AND SEXUAL ORIENTATION AND GENDER IDENTITY?

Many people assume that traditional religious institutions tend to be completely against any deviance from heterosexual marital relationships and that homosexuality and LGBTQI+ identities and behavior are always sinful and bad and should be changed. Certainly, numerous news reports highlight the tensions that sometimes arise between religious communities and LGBTQI+ communities. For example, the well-known and media-savvy Westboro Baptist Church often receives national press attention as its members picket military funerals and other high-profile events with signs stating that LGBTQI+ people are sinful and will burn in hell for who they are and how they behave with others. (Full disclosure: My wife's cousin, Rabbi Mychal Copeland, a high-profile lesbian rabbi who was a chaplain at Stanford University several years ago, was the target of a Westboro Baptist Church protest.) Other examples include several national stories about bakeries refusing to make wedding cakes for gay and lesbian couples and town clerks refusing (for religious reasons) to issue marriage licenses to gay and lesbian couples even when it is legal for them to do so and illegal not to.

These and many other examples that receive a great deal of national press attention do not adequately reflect the complex and nuanced relationship between various religious institutions and LGBTQI+ communities. Although it is impossible to fully unpack these complicated relationships here, this chapter presents some of the factors that have contributed to these tensions in some, but not all, religious communities.

The Bible and LGBTQI+ Issues: The Influence of the Abrahamic Religious Traditions

Many people cite biblical references (as well as moral philosophy using natural law theory, which suggests that morally correct behavior follows the dictates of nature; d'Entrèves, 2017; Finnis, 2011) for their condemnation of LGBTQI+ orientations and behavior. Those from the Abrahamic religious traditions who embrace the Hebrew Bible—called the Tanakh by Jews, the Old Testament by Christians, and the Tawrat by Muslims—cite key passages to support their views, most particularly in the Book of Leviticus (18:22 and 20:13) and Genesis (1:27–28 and 2:24). Additionally, those who focus on natural law theory from moral philosophy (Finnis, 2011) suggest that sexual behavior is meant for reproduction only, and thus any deviance from heterosexual intercourse violates natural, or God-designed, law (Budziszewski, 2014). Relevant biblical passages often cited by those from the Abrahamic traditions include the following:

- "You shall not lie with a male as with a woman; it is an abomination." (*English Standard Version*, 2001, Leviticus 18:22)

- "If a man lies with a male as with a woman, both of them have committed an abomination; they shall surely be put to death; their blood is upon them." (*English Standard Version*, 2001, Leviticus 20:13)

- "So God created mankind in His own image, in the image of God he created them; male and female he created them. God blessed them and said to them, 'Be fruitful and increase in number; fill the earth and subdue it.'" (*New International Version*, 2011, Genesis 1:27–28)

- "That is why a man leaves his father and mother and is united to his wife, and they become one flesh." (*New International Version*, 2011, Genesis 2:24)

In the New Testament, Christians often use several letters attributed to Saint Paul to defend their views about the wrongfulness of LGBTQI+ behaviors. The relevant passages include the following:

- "Because of this, God gave them over to shameful lusts. Even their women exchanged natural sexual relations for unnatural ones. In the same way the men also abandoned natural relations with women and were inflamed with lust for one another. Men committed shameful acts with other men, and received in themselves the due penalty for their error." (*New International Version*, 2011, Romans 1:26–27)

- "Or do you not know that wrongdoers will not inherit the kingdom of God? Do not be deceived: Neither the sexually immoral nor idolaters nor adulterers nor men who have sex with men nor thieves nor the greedy nor drunkards nor slanderers nor swindlers will inherit the kingdom of God." (*New International Version*, 2011, I Corinthians 6:9–10)

- ". . . for the sexually immoral, for those practicing homosexuality, for slave traders and liars and perjurers—and for whatever else is contrary to the sound doctrine." (*New International Version*, 2011, I Timothy 1:10)

In Islam, the Qur'an has very few references about homosexuality, with only one passage that directly addresses the issue, but it does so in a way that forbids adultery and fornication for everyone regardless of sexual orientation:

> And as for those who are guilty of an indecency from among your women, call to witnesses against them four (witnesses) from among you; then if they bear witness confine them to the houses until death takes them away or Allah opens some way for them. And as for the two who are guilty of indecency from among you, give them both a punishment; then if they repent and amend, turn aside from them; surely Allah is Oft-returning (to mercy), the Merciful. (4:15–16)

Homoerotic relationships and desires were integrated into the premodern Arab cultures, while women's same-sex sexual relationships were very rarely commented on because they didn't involve penetration or affect their roles in the family and society. However, in more modern times, extreme homophobic beliefs and practices are common, with executions of gay and lesbian Muslims occurring in Iran, Saudi Arabia, and elsewhere as an example (Habib, 2010; Wilson, 2015).

It is important to mention that biblical scripture is often misused by those who quote it but ignore the contexts of these sacred texts, including details about the author and intended audience, what the text meant at the time of the writing, and how intended audience members at the time likely received it. Indeed, cherry-picking or proof-texting parts of sacred scripture to justify including discrimination and biases in one's particular point of view is very common, perhaps because these texts are part of the official canon of the religious traditions they represent. For example, the New Testament states,

> Slaves, obey your earthly masters with respect and fear and sincerity of heart, just as you would show to Christ. And do this not only to please them while they are watching, but as servants of Christ, doing the will of God from your heart. (*Berean Study Bible*, 2020, Ephesians 6:5–6)

Similar instructions seemingly support slavery elsewhere (e.g., Colossians 3:22, I Peter 2:18–20). These passages were used to justify slavery from before the founding of the United States through the U.S. Civil War.

Similar passages require wives to be obedient and subservient to their husbands. For example, the New Testament states,

> Wives, obey your husbands as you obey the Lord. The husband is the head of the wife, just as Christ is the head of the church people. The church is His body and he saved it. Wives should obey their husbands in everything, just as the church people obey Christ. (*Worldwide English (New Testament)*, 1996, Ephesians 5:22–24)

Similar quotes can be found elsewhere as well (e.g., I Peter 3). Other dramatic quotes include those that likely were not intended to be taken literally, such as the prescription to pluck out your eyes if they cause you to sin: "And if your eye causes you to stumble, gouge it out and throw it away. It is better for you to enter life with one eye than to have two eyes and be thrown into the fire of hell" (*New International Version*, 2011, Matthew 18:9).

Typically, and sadly, those who are most adamant about their judgmental, discriminatory biases on the basis of biblical texts are not thoughtful theologians, scholars, or experts on these sacred texts. Zealots tend to ignore texts that contradict their claims. Intolerant Christians, for example, fail to recognize that Jesus never directly mentioned, commented on, or gave any instructions about homosexuality or any LGBTQI+ behaviors. Additionally, they tend to ignore biblical instructions about not judging others, such as "Do not judge, and you will not be judged. Do not condemn, and you will not be condemned. Forgive, and you will be forgiven" (*Berean Study Bible*, 2020, Luke 6:37). Remarkably, there are many more biblical statements about not judging or condemning others than the very few that address homosexuality or LGBTQI+ behavior (for additional examples about not judging others, see Matthew 7:1–3, Luke 6:41, John 8:7, Romans 2:1, Romans 14:10, Romans 14:13, I Corinthians 4:5, James 4:11, and Ezekiel 16:52–56).

Non-Abrahamic Religious Traditions and LGBTQI+ Issues

Thus far I have focused on the Abrahamic religious traditions (i.e., Judaism, Christianity, and Islam), but what do other religious traditions say about LGBTQI+ issues and behavior? Briefly, the sacred texts of Hinduism (i.e., the Upanishads) include many examples of miraculous sex changes (e.g., Shikhandini, King Ila) as well as examples of nonvaginal sex or *ayoni* (Vanita, 2015). Historically, Hinduism didn't judge or persecute LGBTQI+ people, but over time and after the influence of British colonizers, Hindus have often incorporated Western views on sexuality. Hindu priests perform same-sex weddings, but there are more conservative and militant Hindu groups (e.g., Sangh Parivar) who tend to borrow from right-leaning Christian rhetoric on issues related to sexuality and sexual expression (Vanita, 2015).

Buddhism tends to value monastic celibacy. However, some variants of Buddhism practice sexual yoga. In the West, Buddhism tends to be accepting of LGBTQI+ orientations and behavior, focusing on consensual relationships rather than sexual orientation and preferences (Gross, 2015).

Native Americans throughout North America also have a history of being more accepting of sexual diversity, but, as with some variants of Hinduism, the influence of Western Abrahamic traditions and colonization has impacted native cultural practices and beliefs, resulting in more homophobia and transphobia (Wilson, 2015).

Overall, the Abrahamic traditions tend to have more difficulty with LGBTQI+ orientations and behavior than do Eastern and non-Abrahamic religious traditions (Copeland & Rose, 2015) and thus are the focus of this chapter. However, more conservative and fundamentalist religious traditions, from the West or East, tend to be less tolerant of LGBTQI+ orientations and behavior than are those that are more liberal.

RELIGION-BASED EFFORTS TO CHANGE LGBTQI+ ORIENTATIONS AND BEHAVIOR

Mental health communities and professional mental health organizations have universally condemned so-called "conversion therapy," better labeled *SOCE*—that is, therapy aimed at changing homosexual or other LGBTQI+ persons into heterosexuals (see Adelson & American Academy of Child and Adolescent Psychiatry Committee on Quality Issues, 2012; American Psychiatric Association Commission on Psychotherapy by Psychiatrists, 2000; American Psychological Association Task Force on Appropriate Therapeutic Responses to Sexual Orientation, 2009; Substance Abuse and Mental Health Services Administration, 2015). These organizations include language in their ethics codes to respect sexual identity and diversity and to do so without pathologizing member of the LGBTQI+ community or their sexual behaviors and preferences.

However, some religious communities can and do discriminate against LGBTQI+ persons. For example, the Vatican issued an instruction in 2005 (Congregation for Catholic Education, 2005) stating clearly that those men with "deep-seated homosexuality" were forbidden to be ordained as priests in the Roman Catholic Church. Church deacons, who can marry, also cannot be homosexual. Yet research suggests that a large number of Roman Catholic priests (up to almost 50% according to some estimates) would privately describe themselves as homosexual (Kappler et al., 2013; Plante, 2007). Thus, although the Roman Catholic Church forbids those with deep-seated homosexual tendencies from being ordained clerics, it has many more homosexually identified clerics than found in the general population by a wide margin. Additionally, the Roman Catholic Church, like many generally conservative churches, refuses to marry or bless same-sex couples as well and thus does not acknowledge or accept their marital unions.

Some churches sponsor and support SOCE and related programming for their members. A homosexual patient of mine, "Jeff," who was raised as an Episcopalian and converted to Roman Catholicism, was greatly influenced by a very conservative religious order within the Roman Catholic Church (Opus Dei) and chose, against my professional advice, to attend a weeklong treatment program in Texas that tried to convert him to heterosexuality. He reported that he wasn't "converted" by his participation in the program but enjoyed the company of men with similar concerns and mentioned that he encountered mostly Mormon clients while there (see Dehlin et al., 2015).

Research has failed to show any evidence for the efficacy of SOCE (e.g., Flentje et al., 2013; Maccio, 2010, 2011), and many professional groups, including the American Psychological Association and the American Psychiatric Association, require their members not to participate or encourage participation in SOCE. Additionally, laws now exist in many jurisdictions prohibiting SOCE (see Chapter 9, this volume). Nonetheless, some professionals and paraprofessionals continue to provide these treatments (see Nicolosi, 1992, 1994, 2009).

WHY DO SOME RELIGIOUS GROUPS ENCOURAGE SOCE WITHOUT EVIDENCE OR SUPPORT FROM THE PROFESSIONAL HEALTH AND MENTAL HEALTH COMMUNITY?

There are likely two reasons why some religious groups continue to support SOCE after its rejection by most professional health care and mental health groups. First, many maintain a strong and perhaps unshakable belief that homosexuality and any LGBTQI+ desire or behavior is wrong, sinful, and against God's will (Edger, 2012; Grabowski, 2012; May et al., 2011). Typically, they turn to selected biblical passages or natural law theory to defend their positions and feel that these sources of support and evidence will always trump whatever professional organizations, local laws, or social science research might offer, suggest, or demand. They cannot accept nonheterosexual orientations and behavior under any circumstances. Second, many believe that prayer and religion-based efforts to change sexual orientation and behavior (including the use of exorcism) can work miracles. In defense of their point of view, many refer to the New Testament and reported words of Jesus himself: "Truly I tell you, if you have faith as small as a mustard seed, you can say to this mountain, 'Move from here to there,' and it will move. Nothing will be impossible for you" (*New International Version*, 2011, Matthew 17:20). Many also refer to another quote from Jesus from the same Gospel:

> Again I tell you, it is easier for a camel to go through the eye of a needle than for someone who is rich to enter the kingdom of God. When the disciples heard this, they were greatly astonished and asked, "Who then can be saved?" Jesus looked at them and said, "With man this is impossible, but with God all things are possible." (*New International Version*, 2011, Matthew 19:24–26)

The parables of the mustard seed and the camel through the eye of the needle are often mentioned when people suggest that prayer can work miracles even when situations and concerns appear completely impossible to resolve. Additionally, Roman Catholics even have a patron saint (St. Jude) to whom they pray for "lost causes." In short, some people of faith believe that if their faith is strong enough, and if they pray hard enough, then miracles can happen, including a change in sexual identity and orientation. With this mindset, no empirical research or policies from well-informed and highly respected professional organizations or legal codes will change their perspectives and beliefs (Sacks, 2011; Subhi & Geelan, 2012).

HOW CAN MENTAL HEALTH PROFESSIONALS SUPPORT PATIENTS WHO HAVE CONFLICTS ABOUT THEIR SEXUAL ORIENTATION AND THEIR RELIGIOUS BELIEFS AND IDENTITY?

Many secular mental health professionals may find it very difficult to understand or believe that clients who come from religious traditions, affiliations, and groups that reject their sexual orientation and behavior may not want to leave these communities. Therapists may suggest that their clients can resolve these conflicts and challenges simply by finding a more accepting and accommodating religious community and tradition. For example, a Roman Catholic might turn to the Episcopal or Lutheran Church, an Orthodox Jew might join a Reform synagogue, and a Mormon might join a nondenominational church.

The truth is that religious identity and affiliation are often experienced as a core part of who clients are and what they are about (e.g., Ellison et al., 2013; Hood et al., 2018), as closely woven into the fabric of someone's being as are race, ethnicity, and gender. Additionally, their faith, rituals, and traditions may also be parts of their identity, so leaving a religious community and tradition may not be an option (Ganzevoort et al., 2011). However, most religious communities do have subbranches that include congregants and clerics who are fully supportive of LGBTQI+ patients. Some are informal networks, while others include systematic programs (e.g., the Dignity program within the Roman Catholic Church; Whitehead, 2013). Therapists can support patients by encouraging them to reflect thoughtfully about their options, the basis for their conflict with their sexual orientation, and the possibility of seeking consultation and connection with parts of their religious organizations that might help, support, and accept them (Barnes & Meyer, 2012). For those patients who do decide to leave their religious communities, therapists can help support their efforts to find new communities that will fully support them and nurture their spiritual and religious needs in affirming ways (Whitehead, 2013; Wood & Conley, 2014).

HOW CAN MENTAL HEALTH PROFESSIONALS WORK COLLABORATIVELY WITH RELIGIOUS GROUPS THAT ENGAGE IN AND SUPPORT SOCE FOR LGBTQI+ PERSONS?

Evidence-based, secular-minded, and ethical mental health and health care professionals can easily become frustrated with what they may perceive as religion-based behavior that is discriminatory, homophobic, intolerant, and narrow-minded among those supporting and offering SOCE. I suggest that professionals can find ways to counter these feelings and behaviors and try to work productively with the religious communities who engage in and support conversion therapy (Whitman & Bidell, 2014). Here are four principles for doing so.

Always Engage in Evidence-Based Treatment Services

It is critically important for mental health and health care professionals to engage in high-quality and evidence-based diagnostic and treatment services. In fact, we are mandated to do so by professional guidelines, ethics codes, and state licensing laws. Because quality research evidence doesn't support the use of SOCE, competent licensed mental health and health care professionals shouldn't engage in or support such efforts. We need to be attentive to best practices and clinical guidelines within our respective professions, and we must not deviate from these approaches for the sake of accommodating someone's religion-based biases. In short, professionals need to be mindful of and practice within their professional limits and guidelines at all times. If necessary, professionals can secure consultation from peers or experts in the field when situations call for help and peer guidance.

Always Be Mindful of Ethical Principles

Each of the mental health and health care professions has its own ethics codes to guide their professional work. Typically, these codes highlight being respectful and responsible, maintaining integrity, behaving competently, and practicing with concern for those with whom they work. The ethical principles typically highlighted in all of the major professional organizations' ethics codes can be easily remembered with the acronym RRICC: respect, responsibility, integrity, competence, and concern (Plante, 2004). Ethics codes also underscore efforts to be nondiscriminatory toward others and to respect diversity, most especially diversity based on race, ethnicity, gender, sexual orientation and identity, and religion. Thus, it is important for us to treat everyone in a similar manner and not to deny or discriminate against those from LGBTQI+ communities. Respect for religion and religious diversity is important also, but we cannot discriminate or violate the rights of sexually diverse clients based on our or their religious beliefs, practices, or identifications.

Approach Religious Groups With Accommodation, Humility, and the Expectation of Goodness in Mind

In working with those from religious organizations with whom we may have little experience or perhaps have difficulties, it is important to be respectful. We don't need to agree with those who hold strong views different from our own, but it is important to try to understand them and their perspective. Approaching others with humility is helpful in avoiding arrogant, all-knowing behavior or perspectives. We must behave in professional and nondiscriminatory ways with those who hold views that we might find offensive or at least very hard to understand and appreciate. In addition, trying to see the goodness in others, even when we strongly disagree with them, can help to create and maintain a dialogue that will be more productive for everyone involved.

Consult With Clerics

Health care and mental health care professionals typically feel comfortable consulting and working with each other. They often have shared experiences, language, and goals that make working together comfortable and easy. Many professionals feel much less comfortable working with and consulting with clerics, especially those with whom they have little or no experience and who hold beliefs, practices, and perspectives very different from their own. It is critically important to develop working relationships with clerics and those who represent religious traditions when we are working with clients and patients from these traditions. Having respectful, collaborative, and welcoming conversations can go a long way toward finding common ground in treatment and ultimately serves our clients and patients better (Plante, 2013). Below are a couple examples of positive collaborations with clerics.

Fr. James Martin is a Jesuit priest, a popular author, and an editor of *America* magazine and was the official chaplain of the popular late night show *The Colbert Report*. A large part of his work and ministry is to support the LGBTQI+ community, including a popular 2017 book (*Building a Bridge: How the Catholic Church and the LGBT Community Can Enter Into a Relationship of Respect, Compassion, and Sensitivity*) as well as a variety of lectures and support efforts. Because he is high profile and generally well liked in the more moderate to liberal branches of the Catholic Church, he has become a loud and outspoken voice working toward reconciliation between LGBTQI+ Catholics and the Church. By all accounts, his efforts have been an important contribution to a more positive relationship between the LGBTQI+ community and the Catholic Church, and his efforts have been encouraged by Pope Francis as well.

Rabbi Mychal Copeland (see Copeland & Rose, 2015) acts as the head rabbi of the only LGBTQI+ Jewish synagogue in San Francisco, California (Congregation Sha'ar Zahav). Her ministry focuses on serving the LGBTQI+ community within the structures of the Jewish tradition as well as within interfaith families. LGBTQI+ congregants are welcomed and celebrated in this unique synagogue.

Both Fr. Martin and Rabbi Copeland work closely with mental health professionals and refer to them as needed to help work with those who they minister to. A close working relationship between these spiritual leaders and popular clerics with the mental health community offers a more affirming and seamless effort to integrate religion, mental health, and LGBTQI+ concerns among those who seek help with this integration. They provide role models for others to emulate.

CONCLUSION

Religious traditions and organizations often have different points of view regarding LGBTQI+ orientations and behavior. In general, those from more Western and conservative groups tend to have less sympathy for LGBTQI+ issues than do those from more Eastern and liberal traditions. The Abrahamic religious traditions from conservative branches of Judaism, Christianity, and

Islam tend to have the strongest aversion to LGBTQI+ orientations and behaviors and are thus most likely to support conversion therapies.

Mental health and health care professionals cannot provide or support conversion therapies for LGBTQI+ clients when their professional organizations, ethics codes, and local laws prohibit such therapies. For this reason, religious groups that wish to offer and encourage these treatments typically rely on paraprofessionals from their own religious institutions to offer these services to their members. Research thus far has failed to offer support for the efficacy of these treatments, which are still provided.

It behooves health and mental health professionals to provide evidence-based best practices in their work and to be respectful of their clients' dignity without discrimination. They need to respect and avoid discrimination against LGBTQI+ clients, but they must also respect and avoid discrimination against people from religious traditions and groups that they may not agree with, relate to, or like.

APPENDIX: HELPFUL RESOURCES

Books:
- Copeland, M., & Rose, D. (2015). *Struggling in good faith: LGBTQI inclusion from 13 American religious perspectives*. Skylight Paths Publishing.

- Martin, J. (2017). *Building a bridge: How the Catholic Church and the LGBT community can enter into a relationship of respect, compassion, and sensitivity*. HarperOne.

Nonreligious organizations:
- Human Rights Campaign, faith resources, https://www.hrc.org/resources/religion-faith

- National LGBTQ Task Force, Video: Faith leaders analyze Fulton v. City of Philadelphia Oral Arguments, http://www.thetaskforce.org/issues/faith

- GLAAD Religion, Faith and Values Program, http://www.glaad.org/programs/faith

Christian-focused organizations:
- DignityUSA, http://www.dignityusa.org
- New Ways Ministry, http://www.newwaysministry.org
- Call to Action, http://www.cta-usa.org
- Affirmation: LGBTQ Mormons, Families, & Friends, http://www.affirmation.org
- Soulforce, http://www.soulforce.org

- Gay, Lesbian and Affirming Disciples Alliance, Inc., http://www.gladalliance.org
- Q Christian Fellowship, http://www.qchristian.org
- Metropolitan Community Churches, http://www.mccchurch.org
- Believe Out Loud, http://www.believeoutloud.com
- The Evangelical Network, https://www.ten.lgbt

Other religion-focused organizations:
- Muslim Alliance for Sexual and Gender Diversity, http://www.muslimalliance.org
- Keshet, https://www.keshetonline.org
- The Gay and Lesbian Vaishnava Association, Inc., http://www.galva108.org

REFERENCES

Adelson, S. L., & American Academy of Child and Adolescent Psychiatry Committee on Quality Issues. (2012). Practice parameter on gay, lesbian, or bisexual sexual orientation, gender nonconformity, and gender discordance in children and adolescents. *Journal of the American Academy of Child & Adolescent Psychiatry, 51*(9), 957–974. https://doi.org/10.1016/j.jaac.2012.07.004

American Psychiatric Association Commission on Psychotherapy by Psychiatrists. (2000). Position statement on therapies focused on attempts to change sexual orientation (reparative or conversion therapies). *The American Journal of Psychiatry, 157*(10), 1719–1721.

American Psychological Association Task Force on Appropriate Therapeutic Responses to Sexual Orientation. (2009). *Report of the Task Force on Appropriate Therapeutic Responses to Sexual Orientation.* American Psychological Association.

Armstrong, K. (2006). *The great transformation: The beginning of our religious traditions.* Anchor.

Balkin, R. S., Watts, R. E., & Ali, S. R. (2014). A conversation about the intersection of faith, sexual orientation, and gender: Jewish, Christian, and Muslim perspectives. *Journal of Counseling and Development, 92*(2), 187–193. https://doi.org/10.1002/j.1556-6676.2014.00147.x

Barnes, D. M., & Meyer, I. H. (2012). Religious affiliation, internalized homophobia, and mental health in lesbians, gay men, and bisexuals. *American Journal of Orthopsychiatry, 82*(4), 505–515. https://doi.org/10.1111/j.1939-0025.2012.01185.x

Berean Study Bible. (2020). Bible Hub. https://biblehub.com

Budziszewski, J. (2014). *The line through the heart: Natural law as fact, theory, and sign of contradiction.* Open Road Media.

Chaves, M. A. (2017). *American religion: Contemporary trends.* Princeton University Press.

Congregation for Catholic Education. (2005, November 29). *Concerning the criteria for the discernment of vocations with regard to persons with homosexual tendencies in view of their admission to the seminary and to holy orders.*

Copeland, M., & Rose, D. (2015). *Struggling in good faith: LGBTQI inclusion from 13 American religious perspectives.* Skylight Paths Publishing.

Countryman, W. (2013). *Dirt, greed and sex: Sexual ethics in the New Testament and their implications for today*. SCM Press.

Dehlin, J. P., Galliher, R. V., Bradshaw, W. S., Hyde, D. C., & Crowell, K. A. (2015). Sexual orientation change efforts among current or former LDS church members. *Journal of Counseling Psychology, 62*(2), 95–105. https://doi.org/10.1037/cou0000011

d'Entrèves, A. P. (2017). *Natural law: An introduction to legal philosophy*. Routledge. https://doi.org/10.4324/9781315125138

Edger, K. (2012). Evangelicalism, sexual morality, and sexual addiction: Opposing views and continued conflicts. *Journal of Religion and Health, 51*(1), 162–178. https://doi.org/10.1007/s10943-010-9338-7

Ellison, C. G., Fang, Q., Flannelly, K. J., & Steckler, R. A. (2013). Spiritual struggles and mental health: Exploring the moderating effects of religious identity. *The International Journal for the Psychology of Religion, 23*(3), 214–229. https://doi.org/10.1080/10508619.2012.759868

English Standard Version Bible. (2001). Crossway Bibles. https://biblehub.com

Finnis, J. (2011). *Natural law and natural rights*. Oxford University Press.

Flentje, A., Heck, N. C., & Cochran, B. N. (2013). Sexual reorientation therapy interventions: Perspectives of ex-ex-gay individuals. *Journal of Gay & Lesbian Mental Health, 17*(3), 256–277. https://doi.org/10.1080/19359705.2013.773268

Fox, J. (2018). *An introduction to religion and politics: Theory and practice*. Routledge. https://doi.org/10.4324/9781315183787

Ganzevoort, R. R., Van der Laan, M., & Olsman, E. (2011). Growing up gay and religious. Conflict, dialogue, and religious identity strategies. *Mental Health, Religion & Culture, 14*(3), 209–222. https://doi.org/10.1080/13674670903452132

Grabowski, J. S. (2012). *Sex and virtue: An introduction to sexual ethics* (Vol. 2). Catholic University of America Press.

Gross, R. M. (2015). Buddhism. In M. Copeland & D. Rose (Eds.), *Struggling in good faith: LGBTQI inclusion from 13 American religious perspectives* (pp. 11–26). Skylight Paths Publishing.

Habib, S. (2010). *Islam and homosexuality*. Praeger.

Hood, R. W., Jr., Hill, P. C., & Spilka, B. (2018). *The psychology of religion: An empirical approach*. Guilford Publications.

Kappler, S., Hancock, A., & Plante, T. G. (2013). Roman Catholic gay priests: Internalized homophobia, sexual identity, and psychological well-being. *Pastoral Psychology, 62*(6), 805–826. https://doi.org/10.1007/s11089-012-0505-5

Maccio, E. M. (2010). Influence of family, religion, and social conformity on client participation in sexual reorientation therapy. *Journal of Homosexuality, 57*(3), 441–458. https://doi.org/10.1080/00918360903543196

Maccio, E. M. (2011). Self-reported sexual orientation and identity before and after sexual reorientation therapy. *Journal of Gay & Lesbian Mental Health, 15*(3), 242–259. https://doi.org/10.1080/19359705.2010.544186

May, W., Lawler, R., & Boyle, J. (2011). *Catholic sexual ethics: A summary, explanation, & defense*. Our Sunday Visitor.

New International Version Bible. (2011). Biblica, Inc. https://biblehub.com

Nicolosi, J. (1992). *Reparative therapy of male homosexuality*. Jason Aronson.

Nicolosi, J. (1994). *Healing homosexuality*. Jason Aronson.

Nicolosi, J. (2009). *Shame and attachment loss: The practical work of reparative therapy.* InterVarsity Press.

Plante, T. G. (2004). *Do the right thing: Living ethically in an unethical world.* New Harbinger.

Plante, T. G. (2007). Homosexual applicants to the priesthood: How many and are they psychologically healthy? *Pastoral Psychology, 55*(4), 495–498. https://doi.org/10.1007/s11089-006-0051-0

Plante, T. G. (2013). Consultation with religious institutions. In K. I. Pargament, A. Mahoney, & E. P. Shafranske (Eds.), *APA handbook of psychology, religion, and spirituality* (Vol. 2, pp. 511–526). American Psychological Association. https://doi.org/10.1037/14046-026

Pruss, A. R. (2012). *One body: An essay in Christian sexual ethics.* University of Notre Dame Press. https://doi.org/10.2307/j.ctvpj7d0g

The Qu'ran. (M.A.S. Abdul Haleem, Trans.). (2004). Oxford University Press.

Sacks, J. (2011). Pray away the gay: An analysis of the legality of conversion therapy by homophobic religious organizations. *Rutgers Journal of Law & Religion, 13,* 67–86.

Salzman, T. A., & Lawler, M. G. (2012). *Sexual ethics: A theological introduction.* Georgetown University Press.

Subhi, N., & Geelan, D. (2012). When Christianity and homosexuality collide: Understanding the potential intrapersonal conflict. *Journal of Homosexuality, 59*(10), 1382–1402. https://doi.org/10.1080/00918369.2012.724638

Substance Abuse and Mental Health Services Administration. (2015). *Ending conversion therapy: Supporting and affirming LGBTQ youth* (HHS Publication No. SMA15-4928). U.S. Department of Health and Human Services.

Vanita, R. (2015). Hinduism. In M. Copeland & D. Rose (Eds.), *Struggling in good faith: LGBTQI inclusion from 13 American religious perspectives* (pp. 61–75). Skylight Paths Publishing.

Whitehead, A. L. (2013). Religious organizations and homosexuality: The acceptance of gays and lesbians in American congregations. *Review of Religious Research, 55*(2), 297–317. https://doi.org/10.1007/s13644-012-0066-1

Whitman, J. S., & Bidell, M. P. (2014). Affirmative lesbian, gay, and bisexual counselor education and religious beliefs: How do we bridge the gap? *Journal of Counseling and Development, 92*(2), 162–169. https://doi.org/10.1002/j.1556-6676.2014.00144.x

Wilson, A. (2015). First Nations (Native Americans). In M. Copeland & D. Rose (Eds.), *Struggling in good faith: LGBTQI inclusion from 13 American religious perspectives* (pp. 51–60). Skylight Paths Publishing.

Wood, A. W., & Conley, A. H. (2014). Loss of religious or spiritual identities among the LGBT population. *Counseling and Values, 59*(1), 95–111. https://doi.org/10.1002/j.2161-007X.2014.00044.x

Worldwide English Bible (New Testament). (1996). SOON Educational Publications. https://biblegateway.com

PART III

AFFIRMATIVE APPROACHES: GUIDELINES AND ETHICS

6

APA'S GUIDELINES FOR PSYCHOLOGICAL PRACTICE WITH LESBIAN, GAY, AND BISEXUAL CLIENTS AND SEXUAL ORIENTATION CHANGE EFFORTS

A Brief History

KRISTIN A. HANCOCK AND DOUGLAS C. HALDEMAN

It is important for psychologists—particularly those who provide mental health services in the areas of sexual orientation and gender diversity—to understand the role that professional practice guidelines have played in the field of psychology. Knowledge of these guidelines—what they are and what they are not—is vital to their appropriate use. The American Psychological Association (APA) has developed a number of professional practice guidelines, adopted them as association policy, and made them available for professional and public use. The APA (2000) *Guidelines for Psychotherapy With Lesbian, Gay, and Bisexual Clients* played a pivotal role in the development of and criteria for the association's practice guidelines. These guidelines also provided a foundation for the education and training of professional psychologists in lesbian, gay, and bisexual (LGB) issues in psychotherapy. This set of guidelines—and those that followed, including the *Guidelines for Psychological Practice With Lesbian, Gay, and Bisexual Clients* (APA, 2012) and the *Guidelines for Psychological Practice With Transgender and Gender Nonconforming People* (APA, 2015a)—have advanced our knowledge of what constitutes competent and affirmative practice with lesbian, gay,

https://doi.org/10.1037/0000266-007
The Case Against Conversion "Therapy": Evidence, Ethics, and Alternatives,
D. C. Haldeman (Editor)

bisexual, transgender, and gender nonconforming clients. This chapter provides important information about the history of professional practice guidelines (see Table 6.1 for a summary) and the history of the original *Guidelines for Psychotherapy With Lesbian, Gay, and Bisexual Clients* (APA, 2000). The chapter then discusses implications for the further development of APA policy with regard to sexual orientation change efforts (SOCE).

TABLE 6.1. The Development of Professional Practice Guidelines

Year	Who	What
1957	Hooker	First study to challenge homosexuality as mental illness
1962	Bieber	Psychoanalytic study of clinical patients in conversion treatment
1973	American Psychiatric Association	Removed homosexuality from the *Diagnostic and Statistical Manual of Mental Disorders* (Drescher, 2015)
1975	American Psychological Association (APA) Council of Representatives	"Remove the Stigma" Resolution on Homosexuality (Conger, 1975)
1981	American Psychiatric Association	*Ego-Dystonic Homosexuality* removed from the *Diagnostic and Statistical Manual of Mental Disorders* (Drescher, 2015)
1985	American Psychological Association Council of Representatives	Establishment of Division 44 (APA, 2013)
1991	Garnets et al.	Bias in Psychotherapy with LGB Study published
1991	Nicolosi	*Reparative Therapy of Male Homosexuality* published
1994	Haldeman	First major lit review of CT
1998	American Psychological Association	First resolution on CT adopted
2000	American Psychological Association (Hancock, Haldeman)	First set of LGB practice guidelines adopted by the American Psychological Association
2000	National Association of Social Workers, American Psychiatric Association, American Psychoanalytic Association, American Counseling Association	Policies opposing CT published (Human Rights Campaign, 2018)
2001	Drescher, Shidlo, and Schroeder	First compendium of CT studies
2009	American Psychological Association Task Force Appropriate Therapeutic Responses to Sexual Orientation (Chair, Glassgold)	Report on CT (major literature review) and second CT resolution (APA, 2009a, 2009b)

TABLE 6.1. The Development of Professional Practice Guidelines *(Continued)*

Year	Who	What
2012	American Psychological Association Guidelines Task Force (Hancock & Haldeman, Cochairs)	Second version of LGB guidelines adopted and refined due to more and better psychological research (APA, 2012)
2012	California	First law passed prohibiting CT by licensed mental health professionals with minors (Mohammadi, 2021)
2013	Exodus International	Long-time paraprofessional CT organization folded; founders claimed fraud (Lovett, 2013)
2015	New Jersey Supreme Court	CT declared a form of consumer fraud (Mohammadi, 2021)
2018	Ryan et al.	Population-based study showing increased risk of suicidality
2020	Blosnich et al.	First population-based study showing significant increased risk of harm from CT
2021	American Psychological Association Task Force on Psychological Practice With Sexual Minority Persons	Third set of LGB guidelines adopted
2021	American Psychological Association	Third resolution on CT adopted in clear opposition to CT

Note. CT = conversion therapy; LGB = lesbian, gay, and bisexual.

PROFESSIONAL PRACTICE GUIDELINES: INCLUSIONS AND EXCLUSIONS

All psychologists are required to familiarize themselves with the *Ethical Principles of Psychologists and Code of Conduct* (Ethics Code; APA, 2017). Psychology has employed various iterations of the Ethics Code since 1953. The Ethics Code contains fundamental principles that serve as the foundation for the more specific ethical standards that follow. The standards described in the Ethics Code are enforceable rules regarding psychologists' conduct. Although violations of these standards do not necessarily determine legal liability or any other legal consequences and do not necessarily constitute a barrier to licensure, association sanctions may result when a psychologist violates any of these standards (APA Policy and Planning Board, 2014). Thus, standards may be viewed as mandatory.

Guidelines are not standards. Guidelines are "aspirational in intent" and "include pronouncements, statements, or declarations that suggest or recommend specific professional behavior, endeavor, or conduct for psychologists or for individuals or organizations that work with psychologists" (APA Policy and Planning Board, 2014, p. 517). While guidelines represent the profession's position on what constitutes good practice, they are not accompanied by a legal enforcement mechanism. That said, they are nevertheless powerful tools for the education and training of psychologists.

Generally, guidelines were developed in response to a growing emphasis on evidence-based medicine in the 1990s and the rising costs of health care. In their history of the rise of guidelines for professional practice, Reed et al. (2002) described research in the 1980s (Wennberg, 1984) that found "unexplained" variations in costs for specific procedures in the treatment of specific conditions. Reed et al. also noted that the managed care industry then began to portray health care professionals as wasteful and inefficient and as a cause of higher medical costs. Soon afterward, health care systems and plans "pursued goals of reducing practice variation and standardizing care, developing increasingly specific rules (standards, guidelines, practice parameters, critical pathways, best practices, etc.) for the provision of care" (Reed et al., 2002, p. 1041). APA began developing guidelines in an effort to "facilitate the continued systematic development of the profession and assure a high level of professional practice by psychologists" (APA, 1995, p. 2). Taking a leadership role in the development of guidelines also ensured that the association would exercise authority regarding the guidance that psychologists were to receive. Guidelines were thus taken up originally with the intention of standardizing treatment and containing costs across practitioners as well as to make sure that psychology, not some managed care organization, created these guidelines.

The nomenclature on guidelines has been refined over the past decade. There are now two types of practice guidelines: clinical practice guidelines and professional practice guidelines (APA, 2015b). Clinical practice guidelines focus on specific disorders and interventions. In contrast, the *Guidelines for Psychological Practice With Lesbian, Gay, and Bisexual Clients* (APA, 2012) and the *Guidelines for Psychological Practice With Transgender and Gender Nonconforming People* (APA, 2015a) are both professional practice guidelines. Professional practice guidelines are developed to promote the competence of practitioners and to "assist the practitioner in the provision of high-quality psychological services by providing well-supported practical guidance and education in a particular practice area" (APA, 2015b, p. 824). These guidelines are supported by methodologically sound empirical evidence and by "professional consensus"—that is, agreement among experts in the particular field, practitioner surveys, literature reviews, and so on (APA, 1995, 2015b).

Keeping professional practice guidelines up to date is essential. Psychological research and professional literature continue to evolve and refine and sometimes change our understanding of areas of professional practice. For this reason, professional practice guidelines are revised regularly, at intervals not to exceed a period of 10 years (APA, 2015b).

Professional practice guidelines are developed for a variety of reasons. For example, there may be legal or regulatory issues that impact psychologists' practice (e.g., court decisions, case law, legislation). These guidelines may benefit the public (e.g., by avoiding harm, improving service delivery, or providing assistance in working with an emerging, underserved, or vulnerable population). Professional practice guidelines can also be developed to provide professional guidance to practitioners as psychology grows and expands to create new areas of practice, techniques, and approaches. The *Guidelines for Psychotherapy With Lesbian, Gay, and Bisexual Clients* (Division 44/Committee on Lesbian, Gay, and Bisexual Concerns Task Force on Guidelines for Psychotherapy With Lesbian, Gay, and Bisexual Clients, 2000) and the *Guidelines for Psychological Practice With Lesbian, Gay, and Bisexual Clients* (APA, 2012) were developed to address the biased, inappropriate, and inadequate care of LGB clients in psychotherapy. A third version of these guidelines, *Guidelines for Psychological Practice With Sexual Minority Persons*, was adopted by APA in 2021.

HISTORY OF THE LESBIAN, GAY, AND BISEXUAL GUIDELINES

The presumption that homosexuality was a mental disorder coincided with advances in medicine toward the end of the 19th century and prevailed for at least half of the 20th century (Hancock & Greenspan, 2010). Thus, during this period, the task for medicine was to discover the etiology of homosexuality and then develop a treatment for it. Then, in 1957, a pivotal study by Evelyn Hooker found that there was no difference between non-clinical samples of homosexual men and heterosexual men on projective test responses. Her findings challenged the notion that homosexuality per se was a mental illness and that projective testing could be used to reveal this.[1] In light of these results, and because of the enormous stigma that accompanied mental illness, the American Psychiatric Association removed

---

[1]Prior to the 1980s, in most studies, participants were not asked about a bisexual orientation. It therefore could be assumed that many of the studies on gay and lesbian people also included people who would now be regarded as bisexual.

homosexuality from its nomenclature in 1973 (Lyons, 1973). Soon afterward, in 1974, the American Psychological Association adopted its strong position regarding homosexuality, stating that "homosexuality per se implies no impairment in judgment, reliability, or general social and vocational abilities" (Conger, 1975).

An entire generation of research regarding the psychological adjustment of gay men and lesbians followed these momentous actions on the part of organized psychiatry and psychology. Studies revealed no significant differences between heterosexual and homosexual individuals on a range of mental health variables that included general psychological functioning (Pillard, 1988; Rothblum, 1994; Weinberg & Williams, 1974), cognitive abilities (Tuttle & Pillard, 1991), and self-esteem (Savin-Williams, 1990). The decision to remove homosexuality from the official diagnostic nomenclature paved the way for psychological research that found gay men and lesbians to be no more psychologically impaired than their heterosexual counterparts.[2] A review of research that supported the notion of homosexuality as psychopathology found these studies to have a wide range of methodological flaws, including inappropriate comparison groups, faulty sampling, and questionable outcome measures (Gonsiorek, 1991). In the first challenges to SOCE, Davison (1976) and Haldeman (1991) challenged the existence of these "treatment approaches":

> Perhaps conversion therapy seemed viable when homosexuality was still thought to be an illness; at this point, it is an idea whose time has come and gone. At no point has there been empirical support for the idea of conversion; indeed, the methodological flaws in these studies are enormous. It now makes sense to discontinue focusing on conversion attempts and focus instead on healing and educating an intolerant social context. Some will say that an individual has the "right to choose" conversion treatment. Such a choice, however, is almost always based on the internalized effects of a hostile family and an intolerant society. As long as we focus on homosexuality itself as the problem, we miss the point. (Haldeman, 1991, pp. 159–160)

Following the adoption of APA's 1974 resolution on homosexuality (Conger, 1975), APA's Committee on Lesbian and Gay Concerns was interested in exploring whether the practice of psychologists had evolved. In 1984, 10 years after the APA passed its resolution, a task force was formed to investigate the practice of psychologists with lesbian and gay clients. Garnets et al. (1991) conducted a survey of psychologists now referred to as the "Bias Study." This study documented a wide range of biased, inadequate,

---

[2]Similar findings were noted pertaining to bisexual women and men by Fox (1996).

and inappropriate care in the provision of mental health services to lesbian and gay clients. Some of the practices described in this survey of more than 2,500 psychologists were addressed by the standards of APA's Ethics Code (e.g., Competence, Client Welfare). Other practices were not. Garnets et al. noted the following examples:

- A lesbian struggling with her sexual identity was challenged by her therapist, "If you have a uterus, don't you think you should use it?" (p. 967)

- The therapist continued to focus upon [patients] being "gay" as "the problem" rather than what the person sought help for such as relationship problems, trouble handling guilt about it with family or work, general social anxiety, or other problems totally unrelated to being gay. (p. 967)

- A lesbian dropped her male therapist because, when she told him that she was "into women," he responded by telling her that he didn't care because he had a client who was "into dogs." (p. 967)

The authors concluded that psychologists needed additional assistance in avoiding bias in their service provision to lesbian and gay clients.

Fortunately, the Bias Study also collected information from participants on what was considered to be beneficial or exemplary care. Data were organized into categories of assessment, intervention, identity, relationships, and therapist expertise and education (Garnets et al., 1991). These data provided a foundation for building psychotherapy guidelines with LGB clients.

SEXUAL ORIENTATION CHANGE EFFORTS IN PROFESSIONAL PRACTICE GUIDELINES

Given the aforementioned history, it was inevitable that conversion therapy would be mentioned in the first set of LGB guidelines (Division 44/Committee on Lesbian, Gay, and Bisexual Concerns Task Force on Guidelines for Psychotherapy With Lesbian, Gay, and Bisexual Clients, 2000) as an example of biased and inappropriate care, rooted in a disproven notion that LGB people were pathological simply as a function of same-sex attraction and behavior. However, the authors of these guidelines were also sensitive to the concerns raised by practitioners in the development of the APA (1998) "Resolution on Appropriate Therapeutic Responses to Sexual Orientation." These concerns were primarily based on the "slippery slope" argument (i.e., that once one form of therapy was prohibited due to lack of scientific validity, other forms of therapy might be jeopardized). The potential banning of conversion therapy, even with verbiage as mild as "discourages," was viewed by the powerful practice groups within the organization as an assault on practitioner autonomy. As a result, the 1998 resolution (APA, 1998) was primarily a recitation of the elements of the APA Ethics Code that could be implicated in conversion therapy (see Chapter 9, this volume). As is the case with most "first efforts" in the domain of policy, this resolution did not enjoin psychologists from practicing conversion therapy. However, it did put the therapy world on notice that there were potentially some serious ethical pitfalls associated with the concept.

Because APA policies (including practice guidelines) are passed in a political environment, the authors of the first set of LGB guidelines, having participated in the crafting and adoption of the 1998 policy, were careful not to evoke opposition from the practice community. So, in the first set of guidelines (Division 44/Committee on Lesbian, Gay, and Bisexual Concerns Task Force on Guidelines for Psychotherapy With Lesbian, Gay, and Bisexual Clients, 2000), the authors approached the issue of so-called "conversion therapy" with caution. Practitioners were advised to consider elements of stigma and internalized self-devaluation as significant in LGB persons' discomfort with, and possible attempt to change, their sexual orientation. Additionally, these first guidelines admonished the practitioner that antigay or homophobic attitudes on the part of the therapist can exacerbate the distress about same-sex attraction internalized by the client as a result of societal stigma (Division 44/Committee on Lesbian, Gay, and Bisexual Concerns Task Force on Guidelines for Psychotherapy With Lesbian, Gay, and Bisexual Clients, 2000).

At this time, many in the LGB psychological community asked why a stronger statement could not be adopted—one that would identify "conversion therapy" as a discredited form of potentially harmful treatment that had no empirical support and should be banned. APA governance created a complex policymaking structure that turns slowly. Consensus among mainstream psychologists seemed to be that because the APA is a professional organization and not an advocacy organization, it was unlikely to prohibit conversion therapy in the absence of controlled studies indicating harm (Haldeman, 2002a). There were anecdotal reports of harm; however, there were also anecdotal reports of "cures." Both pro- and anti-conversion-therapy groups claimed the mantle of science, although the weakness of the pro-conversion-therapy studies' methodologies led many LGB psychologists to label them "science in drag" (Haldeman, 1994).

The task force that developed the next APA (2009a) report, entitled *Appropriate Affirmative Responses to Sexual Orientation Distress and Change*

Efforts, recommended that use of the terms *conversion therapy* and *reparative therapy* be discontinued because they inaccurately suggest that these interventions constitute a legitimate form of treatment. Instead, this task force coined the term *sexual orientation change efforts*, or *SOCE*. Admittedly, this acronym is more cumbersome and less recognizable than *conversion therapy*, but a short explanation was seen as well worth the improvement in accuracy. This change proved pivotal in advocating for legislative initiatives to oppose SOCE (see Chapter 9).

Furthermore, the 2009 report (APA, 2009a) provided a significant breakthrough in the case against SOCE. The task force included a content-naïve methodologist whose task was to review the extant literature on SOCE for quality. In her review of nearly 100 studies going back decades, Miller (APA, 2009a) found no evidence to support the claims of SOCE practitioners that their methods were successful in changing sexual orientation or even in assisting people with unwanted same-sex attractions in managing their behavior. These studies were found to be rife with methodological flaws, as mentioned previously.

The results of one high-profile study (Spitzer, 2003) purporting to demonstrate that sexual orientation can be changed in therapy were touted as proof to contradict the conclusions of the aforementioned review of the literature. Its publication sent shock waves through the lesbian, gay, bisexual, and transgender (LGBT) community, given the disparity between the study's results and conventional wisdom, as well as the fact that the study's author, Robert Spitzer, had previously been considered an ally to the LGBT community given his role in the declassification of homosexuality from the *Diagnostic and Statistical Manual of Mental Disorders* many years earlier. Closer examination, however, revealed significant flaws in his research, calling into question its conclusions on a number of fronts (Drescher & Zucker, 2006). Ultimately, Spitzer himself recanted his findings as fraudulent (Spitzer, 2012) and apologized to the LGBT community for the damage done.

Additionally, the 2009 APA report (APA, 2009b) found evidence of harm to individuals, relying heavily on a study conducted by Shidlo and Schroeder (2002). The results of this study revealed various forms of harm accrued by SOCE participants, including suicidality and other depressive symptoms, high-risk sexual behaviors in the wake of unsuccessful SOCE, and anger at therapists for having been lied to and wasting time and resources on SOCE (Shidlo & Schroeder, 2002). These findings and other forms of harm among SOCE participants have since been replicated (Dehlin et al., 2015; Fjelstrom, 2013). In the context of inadequate empirical support and evidence of potential for serious harm, the 2009 APA report (APA, 2009b) advocated instead for client-centered approaches that enable individuals to explore their sexual orientation freely without the specter of a preconceived unrealistic therapeutic outcome such as SOCE (APA, 2009a).

The second set of LGB guidelines (*Guidelines for Psychological Practice With Lesbian, Gay, and Bisexual Clients*; APA, 2012) provided a much stronger statement opposing SOCE. Guideline No. 3 states, in part, "efforts to change sexual orientation have not been shown to be effective or safe" (APA, 2012, p. 14). Although stopping short of recommending outright prohibition of SOCE, Guideline No. 3 illustrates the lack of efficacy and the potential for psychoemotional damage to those who undergo SOCE. A variety of negative treatment outcomes, along with a treatment protocol for helping clients recover from SOCE, had been identified (Haldeman, 2002b).

Complicating matters for the profession, to say nothing of the challenges faced by most SOCE clients, was the conflict between sexual orientation and religious identification/affiliation. Tozer and Hayes (2004) found that the overwhelming majority of those who seek SOCE do so out of a conviction that same-sex attraction is incompatible with their religious beliefs. For such individuals, lack of access to SOCE was seen by conservative religious persons, as well as by some psychologists, as unfairly limiting therapeutic options for conflicted same-sex-attracted individuals. A number of options have been developed to address the concerns of such individuals. One study (Lefevor et al., 2019) identified four options for a convenience sample of 1,782 same-sex-attracted individuals with respect to gender of partner and relationship structure. The research team found that the subjects in the "same-sex relationship" group had the least incidence of depression and anxiety along with the greatest amount of life satisfaction and physical health. These results suggest that there are a number of ways for conflicted same-sex-attracted individuals to deal with their discomfort: entering into a same-sex partnership, engaging in sexual abstinence (celibacy), affiliating with a more gay-friendly religious denomination, and other pathways. Caution is advised, however, for those who decide to ignore their primary same-sex attractions and engage in undesired and potentially fraudulent and unsustainable but socially/culturally sanctioned opposite-sex relationships (Moore, 2015).

Guidelines on SOCE, in the generic sense, have been developed by entities other than APA, if we count advisory statements that are intended to guide practice. For example, a recent statement by a Substance Abuse and Mental Health Services Administration (SAMHSA) advisory panel of research and practice experts who reviewed professional statements, research, and clinical practice guidelines (SAMHSA, 2015) declared that "SOCE are coercive, can be harmful, and should not be part of behavioral health treatment" (p. 1). This statement is echoed by a number of national and international health organizations. Scientific advice, however, only goes so far to counteract the effects of what is essentially a religious perspective: that same-sex attraction and behavior are immoral because they contravene a particular, idiosyncratic interpretation of scripture.

CONTINUING THE WORK: A STATUS REPORT ON RESEARCH AND THE POLITICAL CLIMATE

In the time that has passed since the 2009 APA resolution and task force report (APA, 2009b), changes on a variety of fronts—scientific and legislative— have affected the ways in which SOCE is viewed. This section assesses some of those changes and makes recommendations for future work in this area.

Several factors have led to SOCE's prominence in the public eye. First and foremost, public opinion has grown far more accepting of nonheterosexual orientations and nonbinary gender identities (Flores, 2014). Against this backdrop of increased social tolerance, national and international organizations have publicly opposed SOCE. In 2011, challenges to SOCE took a new turn with the adoption of the first legislation in the country to ban licensed mental health providers from engaging in SOCE with minors. Moreover, in addition to the aforementioned opposition from SAMHSA (2015), the United Nations classified SOCE as a human rights violation in 2013, stating that SOCE constitutes "abuses in health-care settings that may cross a threshold of mistreatment that is tantamount to torture or cruel, inhuman, or degrading treatment or punishment" (United Nations Human Rights Council, 2013). At this writing, anti-SOCE laws have been adopted in a number of jurisdictions, and legislation aimed at prohibiting or limiting SOCE has been introduced in every state, as well as on the federal level (see Chapter 9, this volume).

It should be noted that, ideally, empirical research guides public policy, not the other way around. In the past 10 years, research on SOCE has accelerated. Many of these newer studies reflect a significant methodological improvement over their predecessors in that their subjects are derived from population-based samples as opposed to convenience samples. Population-based samples create more robust data sets that are ultimately more generalizable to the world of a difficult-to-study population such as SOCE participants. One such study found that SOCE was associated with sexual identity distress (Dehlin et al., 2015). Another found dissociation and emotional numbness, characterized by compulsive behaviors and/or depression and anxiety (Jacobsen & Wright, 2014). Yet another study revealed disconnection to parts of the self (Fjelstrom, 2013). A large population-based study found that SOCE participants did not report sexual orientation or even sexual behavior change; in fact, participants endorsed elevated levels of distress due to self-blame for the "treatment" failure (Flentje et al., 2014). One study purporting to show enduring change in sexual orientation as a result of SOCE featured a sample limited to White cisgender men in conservative religious communities who experience strong support for entering into a mixed-gender marriage, along with the threat of excommunication if they do not (Jones & Yarhouse, 2011). Nevertheless, even with this limited sample demographic, the authors report that many cases of change were reversed or retracted (Jones & Yarhouse, 2011). Another study found more mental health problems (including depression) and lower levels of life satisfaction, social support, and socioeconomic status among young adults whose parents attempted to change their sexual orientation during adolescence; an even greater intensity of these negative outcomes was associated with using religious or mental health interventions in the attempts to change their sexual orientation (Ryan et al., 2018). The same study found that lesbian, gay, bisexual, transgender, and questioning or queer (LGBTQ) youth who had been obliged to undergo SOCE by their parents were two to three times more likely to attempt suicide than was a control group of LGBTQ adolescents.

Other recent studies of LGBTQ adolescents and young adults paint a similar picture. An examination of data from a 2011 survey of 21,247 college-age adults found that religiosity was strongly correlated with sexual minority suicide ideation and attempts (Lytle et al., 2018). The authors concluded that attachment to antigay religious organizations and communities significantly increases the likelihood of emotional distress and suicidality, particularly for those youth who are questioning their sexual orientation. These findings are consistent with the long-held view that attachment to an antigay religious institution is a significant motivator for an individual to seek SOCE, placing the individual at risk for any number of negative social or spiritual outcomes in the event that the individual fails to change sexual orientation.

However, empirical findings go only so far to counteract the proliferation of what is essentially a religious perspective: that same-sex attraction and behavior are immoral because they contravene a particular, idiosyncratic interpretation of scripture. To identify conservative religious doctrine as the main issue to be addressed in future guideline and policy statements may be both reductionistic as well as politically impractical. It is inaccurate to suggest that policy or guideline statements have any influence on religious dogma, as noted in APA's (2008) "Resolution on Religious, Religion-Related, and/or Religion-Derived Prejudice." This policy statement draws a line between the provinces of social science and religion, defending against the incursion of religious dogma into social-science-based policy while disavowing any attempt on the part of psychology to influence religion (APA, 2008).

Attachment to a conservative antigay religious organization is, for most conflicted same-sex-attracted persons, a complex proposition. The doctrines of such groups may bind their followers with fear. At the same time, the followers themselves derive social (including familial) support and validation as well as ready-made answers to the fundamental existential questions of meaning and purpose in life (Haldeman, 2018). Excommunication from this world into the orbits of an unfamiliar LGBT community seem unthinkable to many—hence, the continued popularity of SOCE.

On a political level, religious freedom is currently sacrosanct. In fact, free exercise of religious belief is used as the primary argument against legislation that would limit or prohibit SOCE (Haldeman, 2018). SOCE proponents, defending their practices against proposed legislation that would curtail or eliminate their industry, argue that SOCE should be protected as a matter of religious freedom so that those whose same-sex attractions are incompatible with their religious beliefs have treatment options—however dangerous and poorly supported those treatments are. Related issues include the ability of psychology training programs to determine their own curricula (as in the "conscience clause" issue), women's reproductive rights, and other concerns in which personal freedoms based on diversity may collide with religion-sanctioned actions (e.g., Hancock, 2014; Russell & Bohan, 2014). The courts have upheld bans on SOCE and have even labeled SOCE a form of consumer fraud (see Chapter 9, this volume). However, the courts have also shown an appetite for valuing religious freedom over sexual orientation, as in the Masterpiece Cakeshop case (U.S. Supreme Court, 2017). In this case, the U.S. Supreme Court found the Colorado Civil Rights Commission in violation of the U.S. Constitution's free exercise clause when it sanctioned a bakery for refusing to provide a wedding cake for a same-sex couple on the grounds of religious objection.

The message here is clear to anyone who would limit what is regarded as religion-based discrimination. As long as a business owner couches discriminatory practice or behavior in terms of religious objection, such discrimination is permissible against anyone viewed as contravening that person's religious beliefs. The question becomes the extent to which religion-based discrimination may be supported. A wedding cake may be one thing, but housing and employment is quite another. This bakery decision could well be seen as precedent to withhold medical care from same-sex individuals.

These matters remain unresolved. One thing is clear, however: Guidelines may serve to inform future policy development and legislative initiatives regarding SOCE.

MOVING FORWARD

The value of professional practice guidelines is significant—not only for practice but also for education and training, consultation, and the development of social policy. Many organizations have developed and promulgated advisory statements around SOCE and will continue to do so. However, the exacting architecture of an actual guideline statement allows for an understanding of the statement's scientific foundation and application. Statements are rendered stronger by this required structure. Historically, each iteration of APA's professional practice guidelines addressing psychological practice with LGB clients has offered greater clarity with respect to both empirical basis and recommended application. With respect to SOCE, the most recent version of the professional practice guidelines that cover psychological practice with LGB clients (APA Task Force on Psychological Practice With Sexual Minority Persons, 2021) provides further assistance to practitioners and can rely on a stronger scientific foundation.

This most recent set of guidelines, *Guidelines for Psychological Practice With Sexual Minority Persons*, provides a summary of the substantial research in LGBT psychology from 2011 to 2021. In this decade, studies with robust data sets establish empirically what has been reported anecdotally for decades: that conversion therapies are harmful. The harms associated with conversion therapies are numerous but include increased risk of suicidality, depression, substance abuse, and other mental health sequelae. These data permit a much stronger statement opposing the use of conversion therapies (Guideline No. 4, "Psychologists understand that sexual orientations are not mental illnesses, and that efforts to change sexual orientation cause harm"; APA Task Force on Psychological Practice With Sexual Minority Persons, 2021).

Several factors have contributed to the heightened visibility of SOCE in recent years. The potential for SOCE to cause long-lasting harm, particularly among youth, has been well documented. A number of serious mental health consequences resulting from SOCE have been examined in this chapter (Dehlin et al., 2015; Ryan et al., 2018), and some researchers have identified SOCE's reinforcement of minority stress and societal stigma as a significant causal element in the potential for SOCE to cause harm (Herek & McLemore, 2013). Given the suicidality data alone, one might consider whether SOCE constitutes a public health hazard. Additionally, SOCE is in the news more frequently than ever before. This media coverage results, in part, from the consideration of anti-SOCE legislation in nearly every state of the union, but also from other factors. For example, it is deemed newsworthy when ex-ex-gay leaders come out as gay or when they publicly disparage the SOCE programs they founded (National Center for Lesbian Rights, 2019). SOCE is reflected in entertainment media as well, with a feature-length film, *Boy Erased*, having been nominated for two Academy Awards. SOCE is an issue that is not going away anytime soon.

In light of the above, it seems clear that professional health care and humanitarian organizations and agencies have a responsibility to use the most current, methodologically sound data in developing professional practice guidelines and policies on SOCE. APA, for example, has what is likely the most comprehensive and sophisticated approach to the development of guidelines and policies. To strengthen its position on SOCE, it would need more durable evidence, including more population-based studies, which is critical in the study of a difficult population to research. Fortunately, a cadre of new researchers may well be in a position to provide such data.

Historically, APA and other major mental health and medical organizations have provided guidance to health care providers in the form of some degree of criticism or outright prohibition of SOCE. It is likely that further research will allow for stronger admonitions of this harmful practice. Opposing SOCE, however, will not resolve the conflict that many people feel regarding their sexual orientation—the conflict that causes them to seek SOCE in the first place. In a world without SOCE, what legitimate therapeutic options need to be developed for the sexually conflicted?

The APA SOCE Task Force (APA, 2009b) answered this question by recommending the following for those conflicted about same-sex attraction: acceptance and support, comprehensive assessment, active coping, social support, identity exploration and development, and reduction of internalized stigma. This is a good start, but further development of these terms in this particular therapeutic context is required. Pachankis (2018), for example, advocated for LGBT-specific treatment protocols across a spectrum of modalities. Furthermore, it has recently been observed that there are evidence-based treatments for individuals in conflict about their sexual orientation that are effective and do not risk harming the individual (Chaudoir et al., 2017).

Developing professional practice guidelines to address SOCE has always been a very sensitive endeavor, given its overlap with conservative organized religion. It is time, however, to recognize the potential health risks posed by SOCE and to develop policies and guidelines that serve to avoid harm, protect the vulnerable, and inform the public. This undertaking will require evidence—and courage.

REFERENCES

American Psychological Association. (1995). *Criteria for guideline development and review*.

American Psychological Association. (1998). Resolution on appropriate therapeutic responses to sexual orientation. *American Psychologist, 53*(8), 934–935. https://doi.org/10.1037/0003-066X.53.8.882

American Psychological Association. (2000). Guidelines for psychotherapy with lesbian, gay, and bisexual clients. *American Psychologist, 55*, 1440–1451. https://doi.org/10.1037/0003-066X.55.12.1440

American Psychological Association. (2008). Resolution on religious, religion-related, and/or religion-derived prejudice. *American Psychologist, 63*(5), 431–434. https://doi.org/10.1037/0003-066X.63.5.360

American Psychological Association. (2009a). Appropriate affirmative responses to sexual orientation distress and change efforts. *American Psychologist, 65*(5), 385–475. https://doi.org/10.1037/a0019553

American Psychological Association. (2009b). *Report of the American Psychological Association Task Force on Appropriate Therapeutic Responses to Sexual Orientation.* https://www.apa.org/pi/lgbt/resources/therapeutic-response.pdf

American Psychological Association. (2012). Guidelines for psychological practice with lesbian, gay, and bisexual clients. *American Psychologist, 67*(1), 10–42. https://doi.org/10.1037/a0024659

American Psychological Association. (2013). *About Division 44.* Retrieved May 19, 2021, from https://www.apadivisions.org/division-44/about

American Psychological Association. (2015a). Guidelines for psychological practice with transgender and gender non-conforming people. *American Psychologist, 70*(9), 832–864. https://doi.org/10.1037/a0039906

American Psychological Association. (2015b). Professional practice guidelines: Guidance for developers and users. *American Psychologist, 70*(9), 823–831. https://doi.org/10.1037/a0039644

American Psychological Association. (2017). *Ethical principles of psychologists and code of conduct* (2002, Amended June 1, 2010, and January 1, 2017). http://www.apa.org/ethics/code/index.aspx

American Psychological Association. (2021, February). *APA resolution on sexual orientation change efforts.* https://www.apa.org/about/policy/resolution-sexual-orientation-change-efforts.pdf

American Psychological Association Policy and Planning Board. (2014). APA guidelines: Their importance and a plan to keep them current: 2013 annual report of the Policy and Planning Board. *American Psychologist, 69*(5), 511–519. https://doi.org/10.1037/a0036643

American Psychological Association Task Force on Psychological Practice With Sexual Minority Persons. (2021). *Guidelines for psychological practice with sexual minority persons.* https://www.apa.org/about/policy/psychological-sexual-minority-persons.pdf

Bieber, I. (1962). *Male homosexuality: A psychoanalytic study.* Basic Books.

Blosnich, J. R., Henderson, E. R., Coulter, R. W. S., Goldbach, J. T., & Meyer, I. H. (2020). Sexual orientation change efforts, adverse childhood experiences, and suicide ideation and attempt among sexual minority adults, United States, 2016–2018. *American Journal of Public Health, 110,* 1024–1030. https://doi.org/10.2105/AJPH.2020.305637

Chaudoir, S. R., Wang, K., & Pachankis, J. E. (2017). What reduces sexual minority stress? A review of the intervention "toolkit." *Journal of Social Issues, 73*(3), 586–617. https://doi.org/10.1111/josi.12233

Conger, J. (1975). Proceedings of the American Psychological Association, for the year 1974: Minutes of the annual meeting of Council of Representatives. *American Psychologist, 30,* 620–651.

Davison, G. C. (1976). Homosexuality: The ethical challenge. *Journal of Consulting and Clinical Psychology, 44*(2), 157–162. https://doi.org/10.1037/0022-006X.44.2.157

Dehlin, J. P., Galliher, R. V., Bradshaw, W. S., Hyde, D. C., & Crowell, K. A. (2015). Sexual orientation change efforts among current or former LDS church members. *Journal of Counseling Psychology, 62*(2), 95–105. https://doi.org/10.1037/cou0000011

Division 44/Committee on Lesbian, Gay, and Bisexual Concerns Task Force on Guidelines for Psychotherapy With Lesbian, Gay, and Bisexual Clients. (2000). Guidelines for psychotherapy with lesbian, gay, and bisexual clients. *American Psychologist, 55*(12), 1440–1451. https://doi.org/10.1037/0003-066X.55.12.1440

Drescher, J. (2015). Out of *DSM*: Depathologizing homosexuality. *Behavioral Sciences, 5*(4), 565–575. https://doi.org/10.3390/bs5040565

Drescher, J., Shidlo, A., & Schroeder, M. (2001). *Sexual conversion therapy: Ethical, clinical and research perspectives.* CRC Press.

Drescher, J., & Zucker, K. (2006). *Ex-gay research: Analyzing the Spitzer study and its relation to science, religion, politics, and culture.* Harrington Park Press.

Fjelstrom, J. (2013). Sexual orientation change efforts and the search for authenticity. *Journal of Homosexuality, 60*(6), 801–827. https://doi.org/10.1080/00918369.2013.774830

Flentje, A., Heck, N. C., & Cochran, B. N. (2014). Experiences of ex-ex-gay individuals in sexual reorientation therapy: Reasons for seeking treatment, perceived helpfulness and harmfulness of treatment, and post-treatment identification. *Journal of Homosexuality, 61*(9), 1242–1268. https://doi.org/10.1080/00918369.2014.926763

Flores, A. R. (2014). *National trends in public opinion on LGBT rights in the United States.* The Williams Institute. https://williamsinstitute.law.ucla.edu/publications/trends-pub-opinion-lgbt-rights-us/

Fox, R. (1996). Bisexuality in perspective: A review of theory and research. In B. Firestein (Ed.), *Bisexuality: The psychology and politics of an invisible minority* (pp. 263–291). Sage.

Garnets, L., Hancock, K. A., Cochran, S. D., Goodchilds, J., & Peplau, L. A. (1991, September). Issues in psychotherapy with lesbians and gay men. A survey of psychologists. *American Psychologist, 46*(9), 964–972. https://doi.org/10.1037/0003-066X.46.9.964

Gonsiorek, J. (1991). The empirical basis for the demise of the illness model of homosexuality. In J. Gonsiorek & J. Weinrich (Eds.), *Homosexuality: Research implications for public policy* (pp. 115–136). Sage. https://doi.org/10.4135/9781483325422.n8

Haldeman, D. C. (1991). Sexual orientation conversion therapy for gay men and lesbians: A scientific examination. In J. Gonsiorek & J. Weinrich (Eds.), *Homosexuality: Research implications for public policy* (pp. 149–160). Sage. https://doi.org/10.4135/9781483325422.n10

Haldeman, D. C. (1994). The practice and ethics of sexual orientation conversion therapy. *Journal of Consulting and Clinical Psychology, 62*(2), 221–227. https://doi.org/10.1037/0022-006X.62.2.221

Haldeman, D. C. (2002a). Gay rights, patient rights: The implications of sexual orientation conversion therapy. *Professional Psychology, Research and Practice, 33*(3), 260–264. https://doi.org/10.1037/0735-7028.33.3.260

Haldeman, D. C. (2002b). Therapeutic antidotes: Helping gay and bisexual men recover from conversion therapies. *Journal of Gay and Lesbian Psychology, 5*(3–4), 117–130. https://doi.org/10.1300/J236v05n03_08

Haldeman, D. C. (2018). Appropriate therapeutic responses to questioning sexual orientation. *Journal of Health Service Psychology, 44,* 62–67. https://doi.org/10.1007/BF03544664

Hancock, K. A. (2014). Student beliefs, multiculturalism, and client welfare. *Psychology of Sexual Orientation and Gender Diversity, 1*(1), 4–9. https://doi.org/10.1037/sgd0000021

Hancock, K. A., & Greenspan, K. (2010). Emergence and development of the psychological study of lesbian, gay, bisexual, and transgender issues. In J. C. Chrisler & D. R. McCreary (Eds.), *Handbook of gender research in psychology* (Vol. 1, pp. 59–78). Springer Press. https://doi.org/10.1007/978-1-4419-1465-1_4

Herek, G. M., & McLemore, K. A. (2013). Sexual prejudice. *Annual Review of Psychology, 64*(1), 309–333. https://doi.org/10.1146/annurev-psych-113011-143826

Hooker, E. (1957). Male homosexuality in the Rorschach. *Journal of Projective Techniques, 21,* 18.

Human Rights Campaign. (2018). *Policy and position statements on conversion therapy.* https://www.hrc.org/resources/policy-and-position-statements-on-conversion-therapy

Jacobsen, J., & Wright, R. (2014). Mental health implications in Mormon women's experiences with same-sex attraction: A qualitative study. *The Counseling Psychologist, 42*(5), 664–696. https://doi.org/10.1177/0011000014533204

Jones, S. L., & Yarhouse, M. A. (2011). A longitudinal study of attempted religiously mediated sexual orientation change. *Journal of Sex & Marital Therapy, 37*(5), 404–427. https://doi.org/10.1080/0092623X.2011.607052

Lefevor, G. T., Beckstead, A. L., Schow, R. L., Raynes, M., Mansfield, T. R., & Rosik, C. H. (2019). Satisfaction and health within four sexual identity relationship options. *Journal of Sex & Marital Therapy, 45*(5), 355–369. https://doi.org/10.1080/0092623X.2018.1531333

Lovett, I. (2013, June 23). After 37 years of trying to change people's sexual orientation, group is to disband. *The New York Times.* https://www.nytimes.com/2013/06/21/us/group-that-promoted-curing-gays-ceases-operations.html

Lyons, R. D. (1973, December 16). Psychiatrists, in a shift, declare homosexuality no mental illness. *The New York Times,* 1.

Lytle, M. C., Blosnich, J. R., De Luca, S. M., & Brownson, C. (2018). Association of religiosity with sexual minority suicide ideation and attempt. *American Journal of Preventive Medicine, 54*(5), 644–651. https://doi.org/10.1016/j.amepre.2018.01.019

Mohammadi, F. (2021, January 11). *Protecting the most vulnerable among us: Why the United States should criminalize conversion therapy on minors*. American Bar Association. https://www.americanbar.org/groups/criminal_justice/publications/criminal-justice-magazine/2021/winter/protecting-most-vulnerable-among-us-why-united-states-should-criminalize-conversion-therapy-minors

Moore, C. (2015). Meet the women who pick up the pieces after their husbands come out. *Out Magazine*. https://www.out.com/news-opinion/2015/8/13/meet-women-who-pick-pieces-after-their-husbands-come-out

National Center for Lesbian Rights. (2019). *Former ex-gay leaders unite in opposition to conversion therapy*. https://bornperfect.org/former-ex-gay-leaders

Nicolosi, J. (1991). *Reparative therapy of male homosexuality*. Jason Aronson.

Pachankis, J. E. (2018). The scientific pursuit of sexual and gender minority mental health treatments: Toward evidence-based affirmative practice. *American Psychologist, 73*(9), 1207–1219. https://doi.org/10.1037/amp0000357

Pillard, R. (1988). Sexual orientation and mental disorder. *Psychiatric Annals, 18*(1), 52–56. https://doi.org/10.3928/0048-5713-19880101-15

Reed, G. M., McLaughlin, C. J., & Newman, R. (2002). American Psychological Association policy in context. The development and evaluation of guidelines for professional practice. *American Psychologist, 57*(12), 1041–1047. https://doi.org/10.1037/0003-066X.57.12.1041

Rothblum, E. D. (1994). "I only read about myself on bathroom walls": The need for research on the mental health of lesbians and gay men. *Journal of Consulting and Clinical Psychology, 62*(2), 213–220. https://doi.org/10.1037/0022-006X.62.2.213

Russell, G. M., & Bohan, J. S. (2014). Towards a contextual understanding of psychology trainees' religious conflicts. *Psychology of Sexual Orientation and Gender Diversity, 1*(4), 293–301. https://doi.org/10.1037/sgd0000072

Ryan, C., Toomey, R. B., Diaz, R. M., & Russell, S. T. (2018). Parent-initiated sexual orientation change efforts with LGBT adolescents: Implications for young adult mental health and adjustment. *Journal of Homosexuality, 7*, 1–15. https://doi.org/10.1080/00918369.2018.1538407

Savin-Williams, R. (1990). *Gay and lesbian youth: Expressions of identity*. Hemisphere.

Shidlo, A., & Schroeder, M. (2002). Changing sexual orientation: A consumer's report. *Professional Psychology, Research and Practice, 33*(3), 249–259. https://doi.org/10.1037/0735-7028.33.3.249

Spitzer, R. L. (2003). Can some gay men and lesbians change their sexual orientation? 200 participants reporting a change from homosexual to heterosexual orientation. *Archives of Sexual Behavior, 32*(5), 403–417. https://doi.org/10.1023/A:1025647527010

Spitzer, R. L. (2012). Spitzer reassesses his 2003 study of reparative therapy of homosexuality. [Letter to the Editor]. *Archives of Sexual Behavior, 41*(4), 757. https://doi.org/10.1007/s10508-012-9966-y

Substance Abuse and Mental Health Services Administration. (2015). *Ending conversion therapy: Supporting LGBTQ youth*. https://store.samhsa.gov/product/Ending-Conversion-Therapy-Supporting-and-Affirming-LGBTQ-Youth/SMA15-4928

Tozer, E. E., & Hayes, J. A. (2004). Why do individuals seek conversion therapy? The role of religiosity, internalized homonegativity, and identity development. *The Counseling Psychologist, 32*(5), 716–740. https://doi.org/10.1177/0011000004267563

Tuttle, G. E., & Pillard, R. C. (1991). Sexual orientation and cognitive abilities. *Archives of Sexual Behavior, 20*(3), 307–318. https://doi.org/10.1007/BF01541849

United Nations Human Rights Council. (2013, February). Report of the Special Rapporteur on torture and other cruel, inhuman, or degrading treatment or punishment, Juan E. Mendez (A/HRC/22/53). https://www.ohchr.org/documents/hrbodies/hrcouncil/regularsession/session22/a.hrc.22.53_english.pdf

U.S. Supreme Court. (2017). *Masterpiece Cakeshop, LTD, et al. v. Colorado Civil Rights Commission et al.* https://www.supremecourt.gov/opinions/17pdf/16-111_j4el.pdf

Weinberg, M., & Williams, C. (1974). *Male homosexuals: Their problems and adaptations.* Oxford University Press.

Wennberg, J. E. (1984). Dealing with medical practice variations: A proposal for action. *Health Affairs, 3*(2), 6–32. https://doi.org/10.1377/hlthaff.3.2.6

7

USING THE APA GUIDELINES FOR PSYCHOLOGICAL PRACTICE TO DEVELOP TRANS-AFFIRMING COUNSELING FOR TRANS AND GENDER NONCONFORMING CLIENTS

ANNELIESE A. SINGH, RAVEN K. COKLEY, AND FRANK B. GORRITZ

This chapter describes how helping professions may use the American Psychological Association (APA; 2015) *Guidelines for Psychological Practice With Transgender and Gender Nonconforming Clients* (hereinafter, TGNC Guidelines) to develop practices that affirm transgender and gender nonconforming (TGNC) clients. The first section of the chapter reviews the four major theoretical frameworks that are embedded within the guidelines to describe the key importance of these theoretical frameworks in TGNC-affirming practice. Then, we describe the 16 TGNC-affirming guidelines, with a special focus on how each of these guidelines counters gender identity change efforts (GICE). In doing so, we also review how the guidelines may be applied in everyday practice. In the final section of this chapter, we describe other TGNC-affirming documents, such as the World Professional Association for Transgender Health Standards of Care (Coleman et al., 2012) and the American Counseling Association (2010) Competencies for Counseling With Transgender Clients, that inform TGNC-affirming practice and challenge any GICE or sexual orientation change efforts (SOCE).

https://doi.org/10.1037/0000266-008
The Case Against Conversion "Therapy": Evidence, Ethics, and Alternatives,
D. C. Haldeman (Editor)

DEFINITION OF TRANS-AFFIRMING COUNSELING AND PSYCHOLOGICAL PRACTICE

Trans counseling and psychological practice within western[1] contexts is certainly not new; however, approaches that address power, privilege, and oppression within the therapeutic relationship to develop specific affirming approaches certainly are more recent (dickey & Singh, 2017). Although a substantial literature base had existed calling for and articulating major components of affirming counseling and psychological practice with lesbian, gay, and bisexual (LGB) individuals, little attention was paid to developing affirming approaches with TGNC people until Arlene Lev's (2004) ground-breaking text, *Transgender Emergence: Therapeutic Guidelines for Working With Gender-Variant People and Their Families*. Lev challenged the field of TGNC mental health to consider not only how to best support TGNC clients and their unique needs but also the disempowering counseling and psychological practices TGNC clients regularly faced when accessing services.

The history of TGNC mental health care that Lev was challenging was one in which TGNC clients experienced strict gatekeeping from helping professionals (Richmond et al., 2017). TGNC clients seeking a medical and social transition were expected to dissolve preexisting marriages if their current gender identity would result in a "homosexual union" (Denny, 2002). Clients also experienced extensive psychological testing to "prove" their gender identity was "stable." Therapeutic interventions often took place in university hospital settings, which contributed to a medicalized approach to TGNC health, focusing on body modifications as one of the defining features of TGNC identity. Furthermore, the *Harry Benjamin International Gender Dysphoria Association's Standards of Care for Gender Identity Disorders*, Sixth Version (W. Meyer et al., 2001), included a criterion that TGNC clients undergo a "real-life experience" of living in their identified gender prior to receiving approval to proceed with medical transitions. This requirement regularly placed TGNC clients who did want medical interventions in great danger because they did not "pass" for their identified gender due to extensive societal antitrans bias.

Over time, TGNC activists and community organizers called for change in these types of disaffirming treatments (Chang et al., 2019; Lev, 2004). In addition, mental health professionals began to call for models of informed

---

[1]We are intentionally electing to not capitalize "western" to continuously acknowledge and remember the impact of white and western colonization on the lives of TGNC people.

consent with regard to TGNC medical care so TGNC people could access their physicians directly for hormones without a letter of approval. As the movement for more affirming practices with TGNC clients grew, a cohesive definition of trans-affirming care was developed:

> practice that [is] culturally-relevant for TGNC clients and their multiple social identities, addresses the influence of social inequities on the lives of TGNC clients, enhances TGNC client resilience and coping, advocates to reduce systemic barriers to TGNC mental and physical health, and leverages TGNC client strengths. (Singh & dickey, 2017, p. 4)

The *APA Guidelines for Psychological Practice With Transgender and Gender Nonconforming Clients* (2015), which are a major part of the movement toward TGNC-affirming care, describe five domains of practice: (a) foundational knowledge; (b) stigma, discrimination, and barriers; (c) lifespan development; (d) assessment, therapy, and intervention; and (e) research, education, and training.

TGNC-AFFIRMING THEORETICAL FRAMEWORKS

Four theoretical frameworks are embedded throughout the APA TGNC Guidelines that are foundations for TGNC-affirming practice: (a) multicultural counseling competency, (b) social justice and advocacy, (c) TGNC minority stress, and (d) resilience and trauma. Each of these theoretical frameworks, described next, specifically guides clinicians toward engaging in TGNC-affirming practice, which is antithetical to GICE.

Multicultural Competency

Multiculturalism is a guiding perspective within the TGNC Guidelines that helps clinicians ensure they have the self-awareness of attitudes and beliefs about TGNC people, knowledge about TGNC-affirming approaches, and the skills to work in an affirming manner with TGNC clients. The guidelines also draw from the revision of the multicultural counseling competencies to bring attention to the role of action and advocacy within TGNC mental health (Ratts et al., 2016). In addition, the guidelines integrate attention to the important intersecting identities and experiences (e.g., race/ethnicity, sexual orientation, ability, social class, and immigration status) that TGNC clients hold. This approach to intersectionality does not merely include the listing of the multiple identities TGNC clients have but rather examines the interlocking oppressions that influence TGNC people's identities and experiences (e.g., racism, sexism, classism, heterosexism, ableism; Budge et al., 2016; Crenshaw, 1991). For instance, older TGNC adults experience interlocking oppressions, such as heterosexism and ageism (dickey & Bower, 2017). A TGNC Indigenous older adult living with mental health, cognitive, and/or physical health disabilities may also experience oppressive systems of racism and ableism. Therefore, TGNC-affirming practice takes a holistic view of the intersectional power structures that influence mental and physical well-being.

Social Justice and Advocacy

The TGNC Guidelines integrate social justice and advocacy as key roles of helping professionals. Whereas developing multicultural counseling competencies in psychological practice with TGNC clients facilitates rapport-building and ensures ethical care, social justice and advocacy approaches acknowledge the ways that privilege and oppression identities and experiences of both the client and clinician influence the therapeutic relationship (Ratts et al., 2016). Because of extensive societal anti-TGNC bias and discrimination, clinicians providing affirming care identify the ways their practice settings replicate societal inequities (Chang, Singh, & Rossman, 2017; Chang et al., 2018; dickey et al., 2017). In doing so, clinicians identify as social change agents who do not limit their advocacy to their clinical settings but rather extend their advocacy to larger systems of change (e.g., lobbying, policy change).

TGNC Minority Stress

As discussed in Chapter 3 of this book, the minority stress model (I. H. Meyer, 2003) was initially developed to articulate the additive, continuous, and persistent mental health stressors and disparities that LGB clients face that are embedded within interpersonal interactions, institutions, and cultures, making minority stress a given in everyday life. Shipherd et al. (2019) applied the minority stress model to TGNC people, who may experience external forms of stress related to difficulties in obtaining medical care and safe access to restrooms. Exposure to these external forms of stress leads to internal stressors among TGNC people such as internalized stigma, identity concealment, and fear of rejection (Barr et al., 2018; Shipherd et al., 2019). Furthermore, struggles with these internal stressors among TGNC people cause further difficulties in being able to cope with trauma related to stigma (Shipherd et al., 2019).

Resilience and Trauma

Although the minority stress model (I. H. Meyer, 2003, 2010, 2015) acknowledged that people who experience minority stress can also be resilient to this stress, the TGNC Guidelines included resilience and trauma theoretical frameworks due to the extensive hate crimes, violence, and other discrimination that TGNC people face. Many of these experiences of trauma then create physical and mental health vulnerabilities (e.g., suicidality, substance abuse, depression, anxiety) for TGNC people (James et al., 2016; Richmond et al., 2017). Researchers have studied not only the pervasive structural violence that TGNC people experience but also the resilience strategies that TGNC people develop to navigate multiple and intersecting oppressions (e.g., anti-TGNC bias and racism, classism, heterosexism, ableism; Singh et al., 2011). This is not the everyday resilience studies that were grounded in western and white[2] frameworks that defined *resilience* as hardiness and individual when understanding why some children were more resilient than others (while not looking at other factors related to oppression such as racism and classism). These TGNC resilience strategies are grounded in the resistance and navigation of TGNC societal oppression (including GICE) and can include ability to self-define one's own TGNC identity, access to a TGNC-affirming community, ability to identify intersecting oppressions when they are occurring, accessing and sharing financial and legal resources, engaging in collective advocacy, and cultivating hope—and, for some—spirituality (Hudson & Romanelli, 2020; Singh, 2013; Singh & McKleroy, 2011; Singh et al., 2011, 2013, 2014). Clinicians can continuously explore resilience to oppression to counter minority stress (Singh, 2018).

DOMAINS OF TRANS-AFFIRMING PRACTICE: EXPLORING APPLICATION OF THE TGNC GUIDELINES

There are 16 guidelines within the five domains of the TGNC Guidelines. These guidelines can specifically guide TGNC-affirming mental health care because they are grounded in professional consensus regarding the components of TGNC-affirming care. Because of the scholarly base and the professional consensus, helping professionals can refer to these guidelines not only to guide their own psychological practice but also to challenge the use

---

[2]We are intentionally electing to not capitalize "white" to continuously acknowledge and remember the impact of white and western colonization on the lives of TGNC people.

of change efforts with regard to gender identity and gender expression. We describe the guidelines within the domains next.

Foundational Knowledge and Awareness

The first domain of the TGNC Guidelines sets the stage for TGNC-affirming practice through focusing on clinicians' awareness, knowledge, and skills. There are four guidelines in this domain: (1) understanding that gender is a nonbinary construct, (2) knowing that gender identity and sexual orientation are interrelated but not synonymous social constructs, (3) understanding how gender identities intersect and influence various other sociocultural identities, and (4) developing an awareness of how clinicians' attitudes toward gender identity and expressions can both directly and indirectly influence the care that they offer to TGNC people and their families (APA, 2015). Without foundational knowledge and awareness, clinicians can misunderstand gender identities outside of the gender binary. The lack of foundational knowledge and awareness can lead to GICE such as pressuring TGNC people to transition to a binary gender identity, which enacts nonbinary erasure (J. Bradford et al., 2013). Each of these guidelines shifts clinicians' work away from GICE by underscoring the need for them to have an in-depth understanding of gender and to affirm TGNC people and the positive influence that affirming care can have on TGNC health outcomes.

Guideline 1: Psychologists understand that gender is a nonbinary construct that allows for a range of gender identities and that a person's gender identity may not align with sex assigned at birth.

This guideline refers to mental health clinician understanding that TGNC gender identities may shift and fluctuate at any given place or time. Specifically, TGNC people have described shifts in their gender identities as part of self-exploration, as well as part of encompassing broad spectrums of gender in its fluidity (N. J. Bradford et al., 2019). Furthermore, TGNC people have described themselves as experiencing distress due to expectations that one's gender identity has to remain fixed or unambiguous due to *cisnormative*[3] perceptions of gender (Diamond & Butterworth, 2008; Johnson, 2016). Therefore, clinicians can better support TGNC clients by assisting them in exploring their unique gender expression through affirming their TGNC identity, exploring identity descriptors (e.g., trans, nonbinary, genderqueer,

---

[3]*Cisnormative* refers to the embedded default in society to assumptions and privileging of cisgender identities. Cisnormativity creates oppressive environments and experiences for TGNC people.

agender) that are congruent with their gender identity, and exploring pronouns that feel affirming to them (e.g., she/her/hers, he/him/his, gender-neutral pronouns such as they/them/theirs, zem/zir/zirself, and hir/hir/hirself; APA, 2015).

Guideline 2: Psychologists understand that gender identity and sexual orientation are distinct but interrelated constructs.

Clinicians are urged to understand the complex and necessary understanding that gender identity and sexual orientation should not be conflated, although there may be overlaps (APA, 2015). Clinicians can offer support to TGNC clients by using language and offering resources specific to gender identity and sexual orientation, affirming these identities as valuable ones to explore while addressing some of the discord that TGNC people may experience as a result of internalizing negative messages about these identities. This guideline also encourages clinicians to develop awareness about GICE and SOCE, as well as how these unethical practices can present themselves in clinical work with TGNC clients (Fish & Russell, 2020). Although both types of efforts are harmful, they can impact TGNC people in uniquely harmful ways, which further urges clinicians to understand the harm associated with conflating gender identity and sexual orientation (Fish & Russell, 2020). Clinicians can ask exploration questions, such as "How do your gender and sexual orientation identities intersect with one another—and how might they be different?" to affirm the ways they may be still coming to know about their gender and sexual orientation identity development and also help TGNC clients find the language of advocacy that is often needed when they experience questioning and other forms of bias about their gender and sexual orientation identities. For those clients who have experienced GICE or SOCE, it is especially important to affirm that it may take some time for them to gain clarity about the overlaps and distinctions in their gender and sexual orientation identity development due to discrimination and trauma they have experienced from others who might have wanted or still do want them to adhere to a gender and/or sexual orientation identity that does not fit who they truly are.

Guideline 3: Psychologists seek to understand how gender identity intersects with the other cultural identities of TGNC people.

Clinicians seek to understand how other sociocultural identities (e.g., race/ethnicity, social class, age, educational status, employment status, immigration status, country of origin, religion) also intersect with gender identity and gender expression (APA, 2015). It is important for clinicians to remember not to overemphasize gender identity and gender expression, especially if the client has not stated that these topics are areas of concern. For instance, TGNC people who are BIPOC (Black, Indigenous, People of Color) experience interlocking oppressions of anti-TGNC bias and racism. In another example, TGNC people who live with cognitive, physical health, and/or mental health disabilities experience ableism in addition to anti-TGNC bias and other societal oppressions related to a targeted identity (e.g., LGBTQ+, immigrant). Clinicians can specifically explore these multiple and intersecting identities in affirming ways by asking, "What other lived identities and experiences are important to you along with your gender identity?" and exploring any negative stereotypes or messages that TGNC clients may have internalized due to other interlocking oppressions (e.g., racism, sexism, heterosexism, classism, ableism, xenophobia).

Guideline 4: Psychologists are aware of how their attitudes about and knowledge of gender identity and gender expression may affect the quality of care they provide to TGNC people and their families.
This guideline articulates ways that clinicians can identify how their attitudes and beliefs about TGNC identities and experiences have direct and indirect influences on the experiences of TGNC clients when accessing care. Evidence-based practices and client collaboration are recommendations for clinicians (APA, 2015). A lack of knowledge, skills, and awareness further perpetuates TGNC client maltreatment. Therefore, clinicians must continuously ask themselves three important questions to ensure ethical and affirming practice with TGNC clients: (a) What negative and disaffirming messages have I learned and internalized about TGNC clients? (b) What is my current knowledge base about TGNC-affirming practice? and (c) What changes do I need to make in my practice to ensure I am creating TGNC-affirming clinical environments?

Stigma, Discrimination, and Barriers

The second domain of TGNC-affirming practice includes three guidelines: (5) identifying how the discrimination experienced by TGNC people influences health/wellness outcomes, (6) addressing the influence of institutional barriers to treatment for TGNC people, and (7) emphasizing the need to foster and create societal change that leads to more affirming environments, systems, and practices for TGNC clients and communities (APA, 2015). These guidelines are essential to affirmative care with TGNC clients, given that 27% of TGNC people reported discrimination in health care, 22% of TGNC people reported discrimination in employment, and 9% of TGNC people reported discrimination in housing per J. Bradford et al.'s (2013) health initiative study. Furthermore, TGNC people experience difficulties when encountering gatekeeping from medical providers in regard to gender-affirming medical interventions (H. M. Meyer et al., 2020; Saad et al., 2019). These three guidelines encourage clinicians to be aware of societal trans prejudice not only to help TGNC clients increase their well-being and self-advocacy but also to explicitly seek to develop environments that are affirming of TGNC identities and experiences, which are inconsistent with GICE.

Guideline 5: Psychologists recognize how stigma, prejudice, discrimination, and violence affect the health and well-being of TGNC people.

This guideline encourages clinicians to develop awareness, knowledge, and skills related to the various forms of oppression and discrimination that TGNC people experience in order to better assist, assess, and advocate on behalf of their TGNC clients and their communities (APA, 2015). Providing more affirming services may include referring TGNC people to housing systems and health care clinicians who are affirming to TGNC people; affirming services may also include clinicians seeking information about resources to assist TGNC people in fighting against other institutional forms of oppression, such as workplace discrimination. To do so, clinicians must continuously collect TGNC-affirming resources to share with clients.

Guideline 6: Psychologists strive to recognize the influence of institutional barriers on the lives of TGNC people and to assist in developing TGNC-affirmative environments.

In following this guideline, clinicians aspire to self-assess and examine the accessibility of their office spaces and service locations, which includes acknowledging how cisgender privilege may show up in these spaces (e.g., an awareness of overt and covert cues related to the physical and psychological safety of TGNC people in the office, such as signage and use of language; APA, 2015). Clinicians can do a TGNC audit of every part of their practice. For example, what would TGNC clients encounter that would indicate TGNC-affirming messages when they first enter your office, interact with your website, complete intake paperwork, or use the restroom? It is important to take an intersectional approach here and note if these facets of your practice are largely affirming of white TGNC people, or is a range of TGNC BIPOC images included? Another question to ask is, "Could a TGNC person using a wheelchair easily access my office?" Affirming TGNC clinical practice should elevate the excellence in your practice for serving and affirming people of all identities.

Guideline 7: Psychologists understand the need to promote social change that reduces the negative effects of stigma on the health and well-being of TGNC people.

Clinicians interrupt systems of oppression against TGNC people, including housing affordability, discrimination, education, employment, health care, physical and emotional violence, and other forms of social inequity (APA, 2015). A major component of this guideline is the call for civic and political engagement by clinicians, as it relates to addressing the systemic barriers that TGNC people encounter in society. This work may occur at the local, state, or national level, in a manner that is both affirming of and collaborative with TGNC people. As a clinician it is important to continuously ask, "How am I advocating for policy change in my clinical setting to create TGNC-affirming environments?" and "Where can I advocate for TGNC-affirming lobbying and legislation to reduce the harm of anti-TGNC societal bias?"

Lifespan Development

In this third domain, two guidelines describe particular needs related to lifespan development and TGNC-affirming care: (8) children and adolescents and (9) older adulthood.

Guideline 8: Psychologists working with gender-questioning and TGNC youth understand the different developmental needs of children and adolescents and that not all youth will persist in a TGNC identity into adulthood.

Clinicians provide TGNC-affirming care to children and adolescents by understanding the inherent fluidity of gender as they experience it. For instance, clinicians can have awareness, knowledge, and skills related to supporting and affirming children and adolescents in exploring their identities without presuming a cisgender or TGNC identity (Edwards-Leeper, 2017; Ehrensaft, 2012; Jost & Janicka, 2020). These two developmental guidelines outline the barriers that TGNC children, adolescents, and older adults face due to the intersections of anti-TGNC bias with adultism (the oppression of TGNC children and adolescents) or ageism (the oppression of TGNC older adults). These guidelines also describe the components of gender-affirming care across the lifespan, which explicitly excludes GICE and SOCE.

Learning to support families of children and adolescents exploring gender is also crucial, as there has been much misinformation about this developmental stage (Chang, Cohen, & Singh, 2017). For example, much of the earlier research suggested that the majority of gender creative children and adolescents in a TGNC clinic sample did not persist in a TGNC identity into adulthood. However, this research has been widely critiqued, as attention was called to those gender creative children and adolescents who may have left the clinic and/or dropped out of the study because of a lack of TGNC-affirming care yet were counted as desisters (Tishelman et al., 2015). Clinicians should be aware that anti-TGNC organizations have capitalized on this research as a way to endorse GICE, given previous skepticism about whether adolescents could be trusted to make their own decisions about their gender identity (Edwards-Leeper, 2017). The guidelines explain that GICE is considered unethical in the field because it does not affirm the gender of children and adolescents however their gender may evolve (Edwards-Leeper, 2017; Hidalgo et al., 2013).

Specific attention to interdisciplinary care that clinicians coordinate when providing TGNC-affirming practice with TGNC children and adolescents is described in Guideline 8. Clinicians must work not only with the family and loved ones of the child or adolescent but also with stakeholders in school and community settings to ensure TGNC children and adolescents have affirming awareness, knowledge, and skills that they can use to take action in affirming their gender identity and gender expression (Chang, Cohen, & Singh, 2017). Some of these interdisciplinary care relationships may include working with TGNC-affirming endocrinologists during puberty (or providing education and resources to physicians who have not worked with TGNC children and adolescents previously to ensure affirming care) and coordinating meetings with families and school educators and administrators to establish affirming bathroom use and classroom experiences.

Guideline 9: Psychologists strive to understand both the particular challenges that TGNC elders experience and the resilience they can develop.

This guideline articulates how clinicians can provide TGNC-affirming care to older adults, especially as they interact with institutions and healthcare providers that often are unaware or—worse—biased against TGNC identities. Furthermore, TGNC adults may be less likely to seek out health care services due to fears of discrimination from service providers, which enhances clinicians' responsibility to provide affirmative care (Warren & Steffen, 2020). Because TGNC people of all ages can also experience high rates of housing and food insecurity due to family rejection, employment discrimination, and losing their homes, TGNC adults can experience extremely challenging minority stress. For instance, TGNC older adults may need to move back home and live with people from whom they experience gender identity rejection and invalidation. Specifically, 57% of TGNC people reported experiencing significant rejection from family members (Grant et al., 2011). In addition, as they access assisted living and hospice care, their generational cohort may not have knowledge of TGNC people in general. Clinicians can serve as strong advocates in working with these institutions to ensure TGNC-affirming care. TGNC older adults who come to understand their gender identities and gender expressions later in life may also experience many "firsts" during a medical and/or social transition (should they want this) that intersect with their other multiple identities, which makes support and advocacy important roles during this developmental stage.

Assessment, Therapy, and Intervention

In this fourth domain of TGNC-affirming practice, there are five guidelines: (10) identifying the relationship between mental health concerns and gender minority stress, (11) knowing that TGNC-affirming care and experiences increase client well-being, (12) understanding romantic and sexual relationships, (13) supporting a diversity of parenting and family formation, and (14) collaborating and working effectively with interdisciplinary providers. These five guidelines, which shift clinicians away from GICE, help them understand how to engage in assessment, therapy, and intervention efforts that enhance TGNC client well-being and to remind clients of the expectations of affirming care they should be receiving from other interdisciplinary providers.

Guideline 10: Psychologists strive to understand how mental health concerns may or may not be related to a TGNC person's gender identity and the psychological effects of minority stress.

This guideline helps clinicians providing TGNC-affirming care to consider how clients' gender identity needs intersect with other mental health concerns. For instance, TGNC people often present with suicidality, depression, anxiety, and other mood disorders. Many times, as TGNC clients receive affirming care, these mood disturbances remit as they (if desired) access resources and support for medical and/or social transition (Ducheny et al., 2017). It is important for clinicians to manage multiple presenting diagnoses when they occur but also to be very careful not to institute gatekeeping practices. For instance, clinicians are asked to write letters for TGNC clients seeking medical and surgical intervention. Only rarely should clinicians institute barriers to TGNC clients experiencing other mental health concerns (e.g., not providing a referral letter for medical treatment). Consultation and collaboration with TGNC-affirming colleagues is crucial to determine the best course if there is any concern.

Guideline 11: Psychologists recognize that TGNC people are more likely to experience positive life outcomes when they receive social support or trans-affirmative care.

This guideline reminds clinicians that TGNC-affirming care is the standard practice as TGNC client well-being increases in relationship to social support. These positive mental health outcomes are important to discuss with not only clients but also their loved ones and other providers they may interact with during, for instance, a medical and/or social transition. This guideline is especially helpful in guiding difficult conversations with people who are not affirming of TGNC identities and experiences. Clinicians can share the increased rates of depression, anxiety, suicidality, substance abuse, housing and food insecurity, legal and financial stressors, health care stressors, and other negative health and well-being outcomes that exist for TGNC people that could be decreased by social support of family and friends and other important social support structures for TGNC clients (Singh & Burnes, 2010).

Guideline 12: Psychologists strive to understand the effects that changes in gender identity and gender expression have on the romantic and sexual relationships of TGNC people.

Guideline 13: Psychologists seek to understand how parenting and family formation among TGNC people takes a variety of forms.

These two guidelines recognize that TGNC clients may want to build families and (unless identifying as asexual) have sexual/romantic relationships. With regard to family-building, this guideline describes the variety of family constitutions that can occur. TGNC clients who identify their gender identity early in life may have secured reproductive material for later family-building prior to hormone treatment, which is a discussion that occurs developmentally earlier than it occurs with their age peers. In addition, across the lifespan, some TGNC people on hormone treatment may need to pause this treatment to become pregnant. In these instances, clinicians should be prepared to provide resources (e.g., in-person and online support groups) that help clients through what can be a difficult time emotionally and physically as their body changes. Some TGNC clients may experience divorce or loss of custody as a result of affirming their gender identity and need access to TGNC-affirming legal resources. Also, clients in preexisting relationships may experience different sexual attractions as they come to know and experience their identified gender, which can affect current and future relationships. In each of these instances, discussions of sex, sexuality, and sexual orientation are important areas of TGNC-affirming care for clinicians to engage in with clients.

Guideline 14: Psychologists recognize the potential benefits of an interdisciplinary approach when providing care to TGNC people and strive to work collaboratively with other providers.

This guideline urges clinicians to become familiar with and knowledgeable about the various providers with whom TGNC clients will interact and be prepared to work collaboratively with them. Previous guidelines, especially Lifespan Development Guidelines 8 and 9, introduced this idea (Ducheny et al., 2017). A specific guideline of interdisciplinary collaboration and consultation is provided here because many of the providers with whom TGNC clients interact with may not be TGNC-affirming due to lack of knowledge or explicit anti-TGNC bias. In each of these instances, clinician advocacy is important in determining the best TGNC-affirming referrals (e.g., medical, legal, support groups) in a geographic location as well as in becoming aware of TGNC-affirming resources that may be out of the local or state area (e.g., access to TGNC-affirming surgeons). It is important to note that these collaborations do not always involve specific TGNC care. For instance, TGNC adolescents may be applying to college and not see their gender represented on an application form, or a TGNC person in middle adulthood may be experiencing misgendering in a spiritual setting. To provide TGNC-affirming care, clinicians build an ongoing directory of wide-ranging resources that are supportive of clients.

Research, Education, and Training

The fifth domain of the TGNC Guidelines urges clinicians who engage in research, education, and training to integrate TGNC-affirming practices into their activities. There are two guidelines in this domain: (15) using ethical practices in research that examines gender in general and/or TGNC identities and (16) providing TGNC-affirming environments in education and training contexts. These final two guidelines provide clear direction for explicitly affirming TGNC research, education, and training approaches and moving away from a focus on change efforts.

Guideline 15: Psychologists respect the welfare and rights of TGNC participants in research and strive to represent results accurately and avoid misuse or misrepresentation of findings.

This guideline encourages researchers to know the historical influence of research and assessment on the lives of TGNC people. For instance, research historically examined TGNC identities from a binary perspective using gate-keeping procedures in study designs and other research activities. In addition, general studies examining gender identity more broadly or other research topics often do not include TGNC identities in demographic questions, and/or they include TGNC identities in nonaffirming ways. This guideline also invites researchers to consider how TGNC-specific research may influence TGNC mental health. For instance, correct pronoun and name use and an awareness of the wide range of TGNC gender identities are important for the rapport-building necessary to working affirmatively in research activities and settings with this community. Because TGNC communities are often over-studied and underserved, TGNC participants may have a significant distrust of researchers (Sevelius et al., 2017). However, TGNC people have also illus-trated the need to have increased representation of their narratives within social science research (de Vries, 2012). Therefore, having a TGNC com-munity advisory board is important not only to ensure that research topics, questions, design, implementation, and findings are TGNC-affirming but also to help distribute findings that can support TGNC communities in need of research on a wide variety of topics (e.g., housing, discrimination, resilience, health care, education).

Guideline 16: Psychologists seek to prepare trainees in psychology to work competently with TGNC people.
In following this guideline, those in mental health education and training settings identify ways to develop education and training environments where trainees gain TGNC competencies. Clinicians must become familiar not only with these current guidelines but also with the common presenting issues TGNC people have regarding their gender identity and gender expression. In addition, trainees must learn that their role is not gatekeeping (Singh & Burnes, 2010) but rather providing quality care and facilitating access to necessary TGNC client resources (e.g., letters of referral, informed consent medical care, in-person and online support groups and resources). Trainers and supervisors are also urged to consider how their education training envi-ronments replicate cisgenderism and make changes to education processes (e.g., admissions paperwork, correct name and pronoun usage, inclusion of TGNC content in coursework, work with alumni) to integrate TGNC-affirming perspectives throughout the curriculum and training.

OTHER USES OF THE TGNC GUIDELINES

The APA (2015) TGNC Guidelines are not simply 16 specific ways to aspire to develop TGNC-affirming practice. They are also clear articulations that GICE and SOCE are not a part of affirming or ethical counseling and psychological practice. Clinicians should also be aware of other important professional documents as well that they can use in tandem with the APA TGNC Guidelines to ensure ethical and TGNC-affirming practice.

World Professional Association for Transgender Health Standards of Care

The *World Professional Association for Transgender Health Standards of Care* (Version 7[4]; SOC-7; Coleman et al., 2012) provides standards for several disciplines (e.g., mental health, medicine) working with TGNC clients in medical and/or social transitions. These standards explicitly describe GICE as unethical. The SOC-7 also outlines four major tasks of mental health clinicians: (a) assess gender dysphoria; (b) provide needed resources for potential medical and/or social transition; (c) assess, diagnose, and discuss the possible mental health concerns that may accompany gender dysphoria; and (d) assess eligibility, explore, and refer to medical interventions (if desired). The current SOC-7 is clear that there is not a required length of counseling for a letter of referral. It also recognizes informed consent models as important components of TGNC-affirming care as clinicians present clients with options if those clients want medical transition care. The SOC-7 is also clear that GICE are antithetical to TGNC-affirming care.

American Counseling Association *Counseling Competencies for Working With Transgender Clients*

The American Counseling Association (ACA; 2010) *Counseling Competencies for Working With Transgender Clients* articulates eight areas of competency that guide counselor training with regard to TGNC clients: (a) professional orientation and ethical practice, (b) social and cultural diversity, (c) human growth and development, (d) career development, (e) helping relationships, (f) group work, (g) assessment, and (h) research and program evaluation. Within these eight domains are specific competencies describing TGNC-affirming practice. The ACA is clear that GICE is antithetical to TGNC-affirming care.

LIMITATIONS OF THE AMERICAN PSYCHOLOGICAL ASSOCIATION TGNC GUIDELINES AND CLINICIAN ADVOCACY

Although the APA TGNC Guidelines (APA, 2015) describe 16 key components of TGNC-affirming practice that counter GICE and SOCE, the document has limitations. The first limitation is the evolving nature of TGNC

---

[4]The SOC are currently under revision.

identities and necessary care. The writing of the guidelines began in 2011, and the guidelines were endorsed in 2015. For instance, Guideline 8, which addresses care for children and adolescents, was written prior to several U.S. states passing laws to firmly articulate GICE and SOCE as illegal mental health practice. Although this guideline states that GICE with children and adolescents is unethical, if written more recently, it may have taken an even stronger stance. In addition, although clinician advocacy is discussed throughout the document and words such as "inequities" are used, the document is limited with regard to contexts of justice and equity in TGNC clients' lives. With the pervasive and unrelenting nature of anti-TGNC societal biases embedded in interpersonal interactions, institutions, and cultures, further describing clinicians' role in social justice and advocacy is very important (DeBlaere et al., 2019; dickey et al., 2017). Finally, the guidelines were grounded in the TGNC scholarship existing at the time, and much recent scholarship has focused on new areas in TGNC-affirming health (e.g., acute stress, biomarkers, cardiovascular health) that clinicians can seek to stay informed of through professional development (e.g., journals, conferences, workshops).

CONCLUSION

One of the hallmark accomplishments of the APA (2015) TGNC Guidelines was to clearly delineate the major theoretical grounding and components of TGNC-affirming practice grounded in the abundance of existing literature with TGNC people and communities. The guidelines contain more than 300 references that describe and point to the clear need for clinicians to provide TGNC-affirming practice to counter societal health disparities, and this scholarship has continued to grow in its scope and urgency. The guidelines not only steer clinicians away from GICE and SOCE but also identify them as unethical. The APA has been clear in its February 2021 resolutions against GICE and SOCE that TGNC-affirming practice is ethical and that clinicians have a responsibility to create clinical environments that help clients who have experienced GICE and SOCE heal and learn not only that their gender and sexual orientation identities are their own to define but also that harm they have experienced in unethical practice is not a standard of our mental health professions (APA, 2021a, 2021b). Therefore, clinicians can use these APA TGNC Guidelines not only to frame their own professional development with TGNC clients but also to use as an advocacy tool when working with TGNC clients.

REFERENCES

American Counseling Association. (2010). American Counseling Association competencies for counseling with transgender clients. *Journal of LGBT Issues in Counseling*, *4*(3–4), 135–159. https://doi.org/10.1080/15538605.2010.524839

American Psychological Association. (2015). Guidelines for psychological practice with transgender and gender nonconforming people. *American Psychologist, 70*(9), 832–864. https://doi.org/10.1037/a0039906

American Psychological Association. (2021a, February). *APA resolution on gender identity change efforts.* https://www.apa.org/about/policy/resolution-gender-identity-change-efforts.pdf

American Psychological Association. (2021b, February). *APA resolution on sexual orientation change efforts.* https://www.apa.org/about/policy/resolution-sexual-orientation-change-efforts.pdf

Barr, S., Budge, S., & Adelson, J. (2018). Transgender community belongingness as a mediator between strengths of transgender identity and well-being. *Journal of Counseling Psychology, 63*(1), 87–97. https://doi.org/10.1037/cou0000127

Bradford, J., Reisner, S. L., Honnold, J. A., & Xavier, J. (2013). Experiences of transgender-related discrimination and implications for health: Results from the Virginia Transgender Health Initiative Study. *American Journal of Public Health, 103*(10), 1820–1829. https://doi.org/10.2105/AJPH.2012.300796

Bradford, N. J., Rider, G. N., Catalpa, J. M., Morrow, Q. J., Berg, D. R., Spencer, K. G., & McGuire, J. K. (2019). Creating gender: A thematic analysis of genderqueer narratives. *International Journal of Transgenderism, 20*(2–3), 155–168. https://doi.org/10.1080/15532739.2018.1474516

Budge, S. L., Thai, J. L., Tebbe, E. A., & Howard, K. A. S. (2016). The intersection of race, sexual orientation, socioeconomic status, trans identity, and mental health outcomes. *The Counseling Psychologist, 44*(7), 1025–1049. https://doi.org/10.1177/0011000015609046

Chang, S. C., Cohen, J. R., & Singh, A. A. (2017). Working with TGNC primary caregivers and family concerns across the lifespan. In A. A. Singh & l. m. dickey (Eds.), *Affirmative counseling and psychological practice with transgender and gender nonconforming clients* (pp. 143–159). American Psychological Association. https://doi.org/10.1037/14957-007

Chang, S. C., Singh, A. A., & Rossman, K. (2017). Gender and sexual orientation diversity within the TGNC community. In A. A. Singh & l. m. dickey (Eds.), *Affirmative counseling and psychological practice with transgender and gender nonconforming clients* (pp. 19–40). American Psychological Association.

Chang, S. C., Singh, A. A., & dickey, l. m. (2018). *A clinician's guide to gender-affirming care: Working with transgender and gender nonconforming clients.* New Harbinger.

Chang, S. C., Singh, A. A., & dickey, l. m. (2019). *Affirming mental health practice and treatment with gender diverse clients.* New Harbinger.

Coleman, E., Bockting, W., Botzer, M., Cohen-Kettenis, P., DeCuypere, G., Feldman, J., Fraser, L., Green, J., Knudson, G., Meyer, W. J., Monstrey, S., Adler, R. K., Brown, G. R., Devor, A. H., Ehrbar, R., Ettner, R., Eyler, E., Garofalo, R., Karasic, D. H., . . . Zucker, K. (2012). Standards of care for the health of transsexual, transgender, and gender-nonconforming people, version 7. *International Journal of Transgenderism, 13*(4), 165–232. https://doi.org/10.1080/15532739.2011.700873

Crenshaw, K. (1991). Mapping the margins: Intersectionality, identity politics, and violence against women of color. *Stanford Law Review*, *43*(6), 1241–1299. https://doi.org/10.2307/1229039

DeBlaere, C., Singh, A. A., Wilcox, M. M., Cokley, K. O., Delgado-Romero, E. A., Scalise, D. A., & Shawahin, L. (2019). Social justice in counseling psychology: Then, now, and looking forward. *The Counseling Psychologist*, *47*(6), 938–962. https://doi.org/10.1177/0011000019893283

Denny, D. (2002). The politics of diagnosis and a diagnosis of politics: How the university-affiliated gender clinics failed to meet the needs of transsexual people. *Transgender Tapestry*, *98*, 17–27.

de Vries, K. M. (2012). Intersectional identities and conceptions of the self: The experience of transgender people. *Symbolic Interaction*, *35*(1), 49–67. https://doi.org/10.1002/symb.2

Diamond, L. M., & Butterworth, M. (2008). Questioning gender and sexual identity: Dynamic links over time. *Sex Roles*, *59*(5–6), 365–376. https://doi.org/10.1007/s11199-008-9425-3

dickey, l. m., & Bower, K. (2017). Aging and TGNC identities: Working with older adults. In A. A. Singh & l. m. dickey (Eds.), *Affirmative counseling and psychological practice with transgender and gender nonconforming clients* (pp. 161–174). American Psychological Association.

dickey, l. m., & Singh, A. A. (2017). Social justice and advocacy for transgender and gender-diverse clients. *Psychiatric Clinics of North America*, *40*(1), 1–13. https://doi.org/10.1016/j.psc.2016.10.009

dickey, l. m., Singh, A. A., Chang, S. C., & Rehrig, M. (2017). Advocacy and social justice: The next generation of counseling and psychological practice with transgender and gender nonconforming clients. In A. A. Singh & l. m. dickey (Eds.), *Affirmative counseling and psychological practice with transgender and gender nonconforming clients* (pp. 247–262). American Psychological Association. https://doi.org/10.1037/14957-013

Ducheny, K., Hendricks, M. L., & Keo-Meier, C. L. (2017). TGNC-affirmative interdisciplinary care. In A. A. Singh & l. m. dickey (Eds.), *Affirmative counseling and psychological practice with transgender and gender nonconforming clients*. American Psychological Association.

Edwards-Leeper, L. (2017). Affirmative care of TGNC children and adolescents. In A. A. Singh & l. m. dickey (Eds.), *Affirmative counseling and psychological practice with Transgender and Gender Nonconforming clients* (pp. 119–142). American Psychological Association. https://doi.org/10.1037/14957-006

Ehrensaft, D. (2012). From gender identity disorder to gender identity creativity: True gender self child therapy. *Journal of Homosexuality*, *59*(3), 337–356. https://doi.org/10.1080/00918369.2012.653303

Fish, J. N., & Russell, S. T. (2020). Sexual orientation and gender identity change efforts are unethical and harmful [Editorial]. *American Journal of Public Health*, *110*(8), 1113–1114. https://doi.org/10.2105/AJPH.2020.305765

Grant, J. M., Mottet, L., Tanis, J. E., Harrison, J., Herman, J., & Keisling, M. (2011). *Injustice at every turn: A report of the National Transgender Discrimination Survey*.

Hidalgo, M. A., Ehrensaft, D., Tishelman, A. C., Clark, L. F., Garofalo, R., Rosenthal, S. M., Spack, N. P., & Olson, J. (2013). The gender affirmative model: What we know and what we aim to learn. *Human Development, 56*(5), 285–290. https://doi.org/10.1159/000355235

Hudson, K. D., & Romanelli, M. (2020). "We are powerful people": Health-promoting strategies of LGBTQ Communities of Color. *Qualitative Health Research, 30*(8), 1156–1170. https://doi.org/10.1177/1049732319837572

James, S. E., Herman, L. L., Rankin, S., Keisling, M., Mottet, L., & Anafi, M. (2016). *The report of the 2015 U.S. Transgender Survey.* National Center for Transgender Equality and National Gay and Lesbian Task Force.

Johnson, A. H. (2016). Transnormativity: A new concept and its validation through documentary film about transgender men. *Sociological Inquiry, 86*(4), 465–491. https://doi.org/10.1111/soin.12127

Jost, A. M., & Janicka, A. (2020). Patient-centered care: Providing safe spaces in behavioral health settings. In M. Forcier, G. Van Schalkwyk, & J. L. Turban (Eds.), *Pediatric gender identity: Gender-affirming care for transgender and gender diverse youth* (pp. 101–109). Springer. https://doi.org/10.1007/978-3-030-38909-3_7

Lev, A. I. (2004). *Transgender emergence: Therapeutic guidelines for working with gender-variant people and their families.* Haworth Clinical Practice.

Meyer, H. M., Mocarski, R., Holt, N. R., Hope, D. A., King, R. E., & Woodruff, N. (2020). Unmet expectations in health care settings: Experiences of transgender and gender diverse adults in the Central Great Plains. *Qualitative Health Research, 30*(3), 409–422. https://doi.org/10.1177/1049732319860265

Meyer, I. H. (2003). Prejudice, social stress, and mental health in lesbian, gay, and bisexual populations: Conceptual issues and research evidence. *Psychological Bulletin, 129*(5), 674–697. https://doi.org/10.1037/0033-2909.129.5.674

Meyer, I. H. (2010). Identity, stress, and resilience in lesbians, gay men, and bisexuals of color. *The Counseling Psychologist, 38*(3), 442–454.

Meyer, I. H. (2015). Resilience in the study of minority stress and health of sexual and gender minorities. *Psychology of Sexual Orientation and Gender Diversity, 2*(3), 209.

Meyer, W., Bockting, W., Cohen-Kettenis, P., Coleman, E., Diceglie, D., Devor, H., Gooren, L., Hage, J., Kirk, S., Kuiper, B., Laub, D., Lawrence, A., Menard, Y., Patton, J. F., Schaefer, L. C., Webb, A., & Wheeler, C. C. (2001). The Harry Benjamin International Gender Dysphoria Association's standards of care for gender identity disorders, sixth version. *Journal of Psychology & Human Sexuality, 13*, 1–30. https://doi.org/10.1300/J056v13n01_01

Ratts, M. J., Singh, A. A., Nassar-McMillan, S., Butler, S. K., & McCullough, J. R. (2016). Multicultural and social justice counseling competencies: Guidelines for the counseling profession. *Journal of Multicultural Counseling and Development, 44*(1), 28–48. https://doi.org/10.1002/jmcd.12035

Richmond, K., Burnes, T. R., Singh, A. A., & Ferrara, M. (2017). Assessment and treatment of trauma with TGNC clients: A feminist approach. In A. A. Singh & l. m. dickey (Eds.), *Affirmative counseling and psychological practice with transgender and gender nonconforming clients* (pp. 191–212). American Psychological Association. https://doi.org/10.1037/14957-010

Saad, T. C., Rodger, D., & Blackshaw, B. P. (2019). Responding to objections to gatekeeping for hormone replacement therapy. *Journal of Medical Ethics, 45*(12), 828–829. https://doi.org/10.1136/medethics-2019-105813

Sevelius, J., dickey, l. m., & Singh, A. A. (2017). Engaging in TGNC-affirmative research. In A. A. Singh & l. m. dickey (Eds.), *Affirmative counseling and psychological practice with transgender and gender nonconforming clients* (pp. 231–246). American Psychological Association.

Shipherd, J. C., Berke, D., & Livingston, N. A. (2019). Trauma recovery in the transgender and gender diverse community: Extensions of the minority stress model for treatment planning. *Cognitive and Behavioral Practice, 26*(4), 629–646. https://doi.org/10.1016/j.cbpra.2019.06.001

Singh, A. A. (2013). Transgender youth of color and resilience: Negotiating oppression and finding support. *Sex Roles, 68*(11–12), 690–702. https://doi.org/10.1007/s11199-012-0149-z

Singh, A. A. (2018). *Queer and trans resilience workbook: Skills for navigating sexual orientation and gender identity.* New Harbinger.

Singh, A. A., & Burnes, T. R. (2010). Shifting the counselor role from gatekeeping to advocacy: Ten strategies for using the ACA Competencies for Counseling Transgender Clients for individual and social change. *Journal for Lesbian, Gay, Bisexual, and Transgender Issues in Counseling, 4*(3–4), 241–255. https://doi.org/10.1080/15538605.2010.525455

Singh, A. A., & dickey, l. m. (2017). *Affirmative counseling and psychological practice with transgender and gender nonconforming clients.* American Psychological Association. https://doi.org/10.1037/15959-007

Singh, A. A., Hays, D. G., & Watson, L. S. (2011). Strength in the face of adversity: Resilience strategies of transgender individuals. *Journal of Counseling and Development, 89*(1), 20–27. https://doi.org/10.1002/j.1556-6678.2011.tb00057.x

Singh, A. A., & McKleroy, V. S. (2011). "Just getting out of bed is a revolutionary act": The resilience of transgender people of color who have survived traumatic life events. *Traumatology, 17*(2), 34–44. https://doi.org/10.1177/1534765610369261

Singh, A. A., Meng, S., & Hansen, A. (2013). "It's already hard enough being a student": Developing affirming college environments for trans youth. *Journal of LGBT Youth, 10*(3), 208–223. https://doi.org/10.1080/19361653.2013.800770

Singh, A. A., Meng, S. E., & Hansen, A. W. (2014). "I am my own gender": Resilience strategies of trans youth. *Journal of Counseling and Development, 92*(2), 208–218. https://doi.org/10.1002/j.1556-6676.2014.00150.x

Tishelman, A. C., Kaufman, R., Edwards-Leeper, L., Mandel, F. H., Shumer, D. E., & Spack, N. P. (2015). Serving transgender youth: Challenges, dilemmas, and clinical examples. *Professional Psychology, Research and Practice, 46*(1), 37–45. https://doi.org/10.1037/a0037490

Warren, A. R., & Steffen, A. M. (2020). Reactions and preferences for training among area agency on aging providers working with transgender and gender nonconforming older adults. *Journal of Applied Gerontology, 39*(5), 545–554. https://doi.org/10.1177/0733464819868057

8

THE APPLICATION OF ETHICAL PRINCIPLES, STANDARDS, AND PRACTICES TO SEXUAL ORIENTATION CHANGE EFFORTS AND GENDER IDENTITY CHANGE EFFORTS

LINDA F. CAMPBELL

Cultural diversity; legislative actions that are affirmative of lesbian, gay, bisexual, and transgender people; and societal awareness of nonhetero-sexual orientation and gender nonconforming identities have increased greatly in recent years. How is it, then, that discrimination, prejudice, and stigma still abound? Effective advocacy, antidiscriminatory policies and practices, accurate educative information, and persistent commitment by survivors of maltreatment and their allies have created a welcoming platform for the oppressed, victimized, and marginalized to seek affirming mental health services. Barriers to affirming treatment continue to be maintained by remaining forms of bigotry, prejudice, and efforts to stigmatize those who vary from heterosexual and cisgender identities. Life for sexual minorities (SM) and transgender/nonconforming (TG/NC) individuals means the endurance of a level of minority stress that can create the urgency to escape the intolerable social maltreatment even by implausible methods such as conversion "therapy."

Efforts to tap into the vulnerabilities of SM and TG/NC individuals have taken the form of sexual orientation change efforts (SOCE) and gender identity change efforts (GICE), which postulate a method of changing sexual

https://doi.org/10.1037/0000266-009
The Case Against Conversion "Therapy": Evidence, Ethics, and Alternatives,
D. C. Haldeman (Editor)

orientation or gender identity. Other chapters in this book discuss research, sources of minority stress, guidelines, public policy, and other aspects of the impact of SOCE and GICE on the health and welfare of SM and TG/NC individuals. In this chapter, ethical principles, standards, and practices across the mental health fields are identified, and ethical aspects for professionals providing health services are discussed. Ethical concepts that are applicable to working with SM and TG/NC individuals are presented here, along with separate sections for each given the importance of distinct recognition of treatment and other therapeutic variables.

The principal underpinnings of ethical practice with SM and TG/NC individuals are echoed throughout ethics documents and many mental health associations' standards of care (American Counseling Association [ACA], 2014; American Psychological Association [APA], 2009, 2012; Substance Abuse and Mental Health Services Administration [SAMHSA], 2015; World Professional Association for Transgender Health [WPATH], 2012):

- Lesbian, gay, and bisexual orientations are not mental illnesses and are normal variants of human sexuality. Diversity in gender identity and expression is normative, and transgender nonbinary identity is not pathological.

- Stigma, prejudice, and discrimination significantly impact the health and well-being of SM and TG/NC individuals. The effect of these complex factors is an essential focus of psychotherapists.

- Change efforts are categorized as "health hazards" by the APA, American Medical Association, American Academy of Nursing, Clinical Social Work Association, American Academy of Family Physicians, and many other professional associations. Change efforts exacerbate the experience of stigma and prejudice by further marginalizing and isolating individuals.

In light of the psychological, social, and physical barriers that fuel minority stress for SM and TG/NC individuals, specifically identified ethical principles and standards of primary significance drawn from various codes are highlighted below.

BENEFICENCE AND AVOIDING HARM

Avoiding harm and safeguarding the welfare of those with whom mental health professionals (MHPs) work are priorities in working with SM and TG/NC clients. The position of change efforts is that SM and TG/NC individuals have a disorder that needs to be treated (Shidlo & Gonsiorek, 2017). Health professionals do not treat nonconditions and normal states of functioning. Defining a normal state as a disorder can legitimize the change effort treatment. Substantial evidence supports the harmful effects of change efforts with little or no evidence of improvement in health conditions (APA, 2009; Bradshaw et al., 2015). Failed attempts at change exacerbate individuals' feelings of guilt, shame, depression, and anxiety, among other minority stressors. Reported harmful effects include dissociation, anxiety, self-harm behaviors, and substance abuse (Haldeman, 2004). Participation in or facilitation of SOCE/GICE contributes to harm and violates the trust that MHPs protect the client's welfare.

Informed consent is a foundational concept in ethics codes that is the means by which beneficence and avoidance of harm are conveyed. Informed consent carries an additional dimension in work with SM and TG/NC clients, such as advocacy in legal processes, collaboration with medical professionals for transition, and preparation for disclosures to family. Beneficence and avoidance of harm communicated through informed consent speak to the value of transparency and full disclosure of the purpose and course of treatment, involvement of third parties, limits of confidentiality, potential outcomes, and expectations that clients may reasonably have of MHPs (APA, 2017a). In the context of GICE and SOCE, MHPs need to be prepared for the request by clients for change treatments. In compliance with informed consent standards, MHPs need to outline the affirmative treatment options but are also ethically bound to provide the most current scientific evidence for the treatment being requested and exercise their professional judgment in providing psychoeducational information, engaging in decision making, and determining choices. MHPs are mindful of the ethical obligation to fully inform clients of the purpose and course of treatment, potential outcomes, and reasonable expectations of treatment. Practitioners who engage in change efforts are violating the informed consent requirements of all mental health ethics codes if they do not inform clients that change treatments lack empirical evidence, have been publicly discredited, and have been found to be potentially harmful (APA, 2009; Flentje et al., 2014; SAMHSA, 2015).

RESPECT FOR THE RIGHTS AND DIGNITY OF OTHERS

Ethical principles across health professions identify clients' autonomy and right to independent decision making as among the highest values. These values are rooted in the shameful history of those with minority status who were exploited, subjected to maltreatment, and controlled by those with greater power. Until recently, health care often followed the vertical model of the profession in not informing patients of their specific treatment options but rather giving instructions to take a course of action without explanation or collaboration. Mental health professions have incorporated into their ethics code the importance of shared information, collaboration, and respect for the clients/patients to make decisions about their health care. The companion standard to autonomy is informed consent in that MHPs are ethically obligated to explain the purpose of treatment, the likely outcomes, the negative effects, and the possible impact on the individuals' lives.

The term *self-determination*, often used synonymously with *autonomy*, has become quite controversial as a concept used to justify GICE and SOCE. The rationale is that clients should be able to access their treatment of choice. The cloaking of discredited treatments in the guise of freedom of choice is another ethical violation: deception without full disclosure of the medical and psychological effects. Ironically and sadly, this very concept catapults clients back into the exploitation and manipulation that autonomy is intended to combat. MHPs are ethically bound to use evidence-based practice based on empirically supported research regarding treatment modalities. Informed consent enables MHPs to fully explain their chosen treatment plans and to disavow those treatments that have no empirically demonstrated effectiveness.

BASES FOR SCIENTIFIC AND PROFESSIONAL JUDGMENTS

Scientific knowledge and professional judgment are among the linchpins of any sound ethical framework. Psychologists and other MHPs base diagnoses, treatment decisions, and clinical goals on known scientific findings (APA, 2017a). They do not misrepresent research, and they ensure that their own biases do not take precedence over standards of practice or scientific knowledge (APA, 2009). They promote accuracy and truthfulness in practice and do not recommend practices that are likely to be ineffective or harmful. Treatments aimed at gender identity and sexual orientation change are not ethical (APA, 2011). Studies of change efforts have been shown to use flawed methodology and inaccurate statistical approaches (APA, 2009; Panozzo, 2013); furthermore, reports indicate no change effect and increased distress (Flentje et al., 2014). Psychologists are ethically responsible to be aware of research findings, to determine their treatments accordingly, and to be advocates for scientifically based practice that protects their clients.

Professional knowledge is the companion to scientific knowledge and is the means by which MHPs tailor scientifically based treatments to individual clients. In 2006, the APA Presidential Task Force on Evidence-Based Practice released its report. The definition that has become APA's official policy and is practiced by other health professions (Institute of Medicine, 2011) is "Evidence-based practice in psychology (EBPP) is the integration of the best available research with clinical expertise in the context of patient characteristics, culture, and preferences" (p. 273). This definition underscores the ethical standard requiring adherence to scientific knowledge and professional expertise, but it also adds a critical component of practice that has been known and valued for some years but was not codified until the passage of EBPP—specifically, patient characteristics, culture, and preferences. This standard of practice not only supports affirmative practice with SM and TG/NC clients but also specifies that these three variables (i.e., research, clinical expertise, and patient characteristics) are equal in importance. Those who sponsor change efforts are, in fact, violating all three requirements of evidence-based practice. The assumption that the patient characteristics of SM or TG/NC identities are the manifestation of a disorder, and therefore treatable, violates professional standards, guidelines, and sometimes legislative statutes.

In addition, EBPP specifically cites clinical expertise, not clinical judgment. Clinical expertise is based on standards of practice in a profession, yet some practitioners present their clinical judgment as clinical expertise that would not stand the test of standards of care. Finally, as already noted, empirically supported research on change efforts has not been demonstrated as effective treatment. MHPs need to take ethically grounded positions on change efforts and to advocate for adherence to evidence-based practice.

COMPETENCE

Practicing within scope of practice while developing a range of competency in working with diverse identities is a challenge and a professional imperative (Campbell & Arkles, 2017). Unlike choosing a scope of practice with a population (e.g., children) or practice activity (e.g., neuropsychology), MHPs provide services to clients who have intersecting identities that can be fluid and cannot be discretely categorized. Specialty and proficiency areas of the mental health professions can be declared outside of one's scope of practice, but ethics and diversity are two integral components of professional competence. All human beings have multiple identities, and ethical treatment of those identities is a professional imperative.

Ethical aspects of competence in the context of sexual orientation and gender identity require a competency level that goes beyond clinical and cultural competence to the expectation that MHPs have mastered knowledge and skills that ensure a quality standard of care. The levels of competencies can be identified as clinical competency, cultural competency, and gender-identity- and sexual-orientation-specific competency.

Clinical Competence

Mental health specialists practice within their scope of practice with the theoretical, technical, and therapeutic knowledge and skills required by their professions' standards of care. Clinical competence encompasses knowledge of empirically supported research regarding psychotherapy practice, skills commensurate with the practice of this knowledge, and an awareness of disavowed and discredited means of practice. Evidence-based practice, as noted earlier, requires practitioners to use their clinical expertise (not judgment) to apply the best empirically based research when developing treatment plans and psychotherapy interventions based on client/patient characteristics, preferences, and culture. In application to SM and TG/NC clients, this means that bona fide treatments such as operant conditioning, classical conditioning, exposure with response prevention, and other cognitive behaviorally sound approaches that have shown impressive outcomes with phobias, anxiety, and other mood disorders are not appropriate for change efforts because the application of cognitive behavioral approaches has not demonstrated lasting effects for change purposes (Shidlo & Schroeder, 2002). Furthermore, psychotherapy practice addresses mental health disorders and conditions, not normal states (APA, 2012).

Cultural Competence

"Psychologists' worldviews are rooted in their professional knowledge, personal life experience, and interactions with others . . . and these world views influence their . . . clinical conceptualizations and approaches" (APA, 2017b, p. 26). Ethics codes of all mental health professions reflect the importance of professionals gaining the knowledge, skills, and attitude to respect the dignity, welfare, and rights of all people of diverse identities (ACA, 2014; APA, 2017b; National Association of Social Workers, 2017; WPATH, 2012). Psychologists recognize how their attitudes and knowledge about lesbian, gay, and bisexual (LGB) issues (APA, 2012) and gender identity and expression (APA, 2015) may affect treatment. MHPs do not discriminate or exercise bias based on their own beliefs about sexual orientation (APA, 2009), and they do not engage in biased practices toward transgender and gender diverse people (ACA, 2014; APA, 2017b). The ethical and professional standard of practice is clear.

What does cultural competency mean beyond respecting others with whom we work, and how should practitioners think about their scope of practice in the context of SM and TG/NC individuals? Cultural competence entails being aware of one's own cultural and worldview, gaining knowledge of different cultural views, and developing positive attitudes toward those with different identities and belief systems. Individuals embody multiple identities whose prominence depends on context. At times, ethnicity may be more salient than gender, yet in a different context, gender or language may be more prominent. Because of the fluid nature and multiplicity of identities, MHPs develop a cultural competency across diversities to ensure effective practice. SM and TG/NC individuals are not always in psychotherapy to primarily address their identities or their interest in change efforts (Singh, 2013); furthermore, psychotherapy may progress to a need for greater specialty in SM and TG/ND issues than the attending clinician can offer. Clients may ask about change efforts whether they initially came to therapy for that purpose or not. Culturally competent clinicians incorporate knowledge and awareness of these possible trajectories of psychotherapy into their working alliance and treatment planning in order to provide competent care even for short-term or referral purposes.

Culturally competent clinicians are mindful of several ethical principles derived from the *Guidelines for Psychological Practice With Lesbian, Gay, and Bisexual Clients* (APA, 2012) and the *Guidelines for Psychological Practice With Transgender and Nonconforming People* (APA, 2015). These guidelines, which are described in greater detail in Chapters 6 and 7 of this book, are as follows:

- Clinicians understand that gender is a nonbinary construct and that gender identity may not align with sex assignment at birth. Clinicians should make this assumption regardless of the client's presenting problems.

- Same-sex attractions, feelings, and behavior are normal states of sexuality, and change efforts are not effective. MHPs do not ethically engage in discredited or potentially harmful treatment plans.

- Gender identity and sexual orientation are separate and distinct constructs and should be recognized as such in treatment.

- Clinicians recognize how their attitudes and knowledge about LGB and gender identity issues are relevant to and may affect their treatment planning and quality of care. Implicit bias can affect their interaction and decision making even if they are not consciously aware of their biases.

- Sexual orientation or gender identity may or may not be related to presenting and continuing mental health concerns and should not be assumed to be central to therapy.

- Clinicians understand how gender identity and sexual orientation intersect with other cultural identities. Psychotherapists take all primary identities into consideration before development of a treatment plan.

- Stigma, prejudice, and discrimination can significantly impact the health and well-being of TG/NC and SM individuals. Often psychotherapy focuses on the client's thoughts, feelings, and behaviors without considering the external environment and the context in which the client lives. Marginalized populations can be more affected by the stress, discrimination, and prejudice of their external experience than by their own intrapersonal dynamics.

- Clinicians gain understanding and knowledge regarding the impact that religious beliefs can have on SM and TG/NC clients. Typically, religious beliefs have been instilled over the client's lifetime. Beliefs, therefore, can be an integration of internalized prescriptions from family of origin and continued external messages from others. These factors can be highly significant to the client's well-being.

- Sexual and gender diversity can negatively impact family-of-origin relationships. Encouragement to disclose to family of origin should be cautiously considered given the potential for negative consequences.

- Currently constructed family may include people who are not legally or biologically related but who are members of a chosen family. For clients whose family of origin is not accepting of their identity, a healthy choice is to construct a chosen family. This decision and action can be important parts of therapy.

Sexual-Orientation-Specific and Gender-Identity-Specific Competencies in the Context of Change Efforts

Concerted focus on development of competencies at this level of practice with SM and TG/NC clients prepares MHPs to effectively engage with the full range of identities, external stressors, interpersonal dynamics, change requests, and other variables in the psychotherapeutic process. These competencies and skills can be attained through formal training, consultation, continuing education, and supervision. The ability to demonstrate acquired competencies is necessary for ethical practice. The following are specific areas of competence and acquired knowledge base applicable to practice with both SM and TG/NC clients:

- SOCE and GICE contribute to reinforced bias and stigma in society against SM and TG/NC individuals. Even passive acknowledgment of change efforts is harmful and implies a maladaptive mental status at best.

- It is inappropriate for MHPs to support clients in expectation of change (APA, 2009). MHPs may be concerned that clients will terminate if their change requests are not met. Clinician interest in retaining clients or concern for the working alliance should not override the ethical responsibility to adhere to evidence-based practice. Reflective listening and empathic responding are indicative of caring for the client and serve as a transition to appropriate treatments.

- MHPs develop knowledge and skills to conduct other treatment plans consistent with evidence-based practice. MHPs assess the level of investment that clients have in a change effort, and they develop their treatment plans accordingly in terms of development of the working alliance, pacing of exploration, engagement of insight, and enactment of the treatment plan.

- Change efforts are often in response to religious beliefs and tenets. MHPs become knowledgeable about the psychology of religion and incorporate their understandings into their treatment plans. Reflective listening and empathic responding are important tools in establishing a level of understanding that will allow clients to consider movement on the continuum of religious beliefs. A sound knowledge base of the psychology of religion allows MHPs to more effectively guide the exploration of alternatives.

- Religion is a diversity variable, and as such MHPs respect religious tenets of clients in balancing religion and sexual orientation or gender identity (Haldeman, 2004). A sound knowledge base of the psychology of religion and respect for religion as a diversity variable can foster client trust that the MHP is not trying to deprive the client of religious beliefs but rather broadening the spectrum for a healthy role of religion in the client's life. (For more details, see Chapter 5 of this book.)

- Avoidance of harm is a foundational ethical standard (APA, 2017b). MHPs inform their clients of the potential for harm in change efforts and explain their stance against change efforts in light of the lack of supporting evidence and the root causes of desire to change (e.g., stigma, minority stress, perceived religion-based dissonance; SAMHSA, 2015).

- MHPs understand requests for change efforts in light of sexual and gender identity stigma and minority stress. MHPs acknowledge and name the source of the stress and the negative external impact that fuels internal dissonance. Clients can erroneously perceive that their sexual or gender identity is maladaptive and therefore is the source of internal distress that makes change efforts attractive. Clients often do not realize that external oppression, bias, and discrimination are the root cause of internal distress, depression, anxiety, and other reactions to harmful minority treatment.

- Self-awareness, self-care, and use of consultation are important for the ongoing health and welfare of MHPs, as is continued monitoring for countertransference and other impediments to competent treatment.

- MHPs reflect on their own potential for implicit bias and take steps to resolve their own conflicts (Worthington et al., 2005) through consultation, supervision, and/or their own psychotherapy.

- MHPs are aware of their own religious beliefs and how they may impact their interactions and treatment of SM and TG/NC clients.

- Engagement in social justice and advocacy initiatives are an integral part of competent treatment. Engagement in these important activities goes beyond traditional views of the psychotherapists' role.

- MHPs achieve competency in using language that is affirming to people of diverse sexual orientations and gender identities.

MHPs whose practice focuses on sexual orientation or gender identity and who may face change effort requests are at the forefront of the mental health profession's establishment of practice in these important areas. Practice in both areas involves the acquisition of knowledge, skills, and attitudes specific to the practice. Following are the primary areas of expertise necessary for effective, ethical practice.

MHPs working with SM and TG/NC individuals are particularly alert to the impact of multiple marginalized identities, the importance of an integrated sense of self, and the understanding of complex dynamics of power and oppression. The impact of intersectionality was first recognized within the Black feminist movement and served to shed light on the experiences of discrimination and stigmatization held by those with multiple marginalized identities (Crenshaw, 1991) and to correct the erroneous perception of unidimensional stigma (Dyar et al., 2020). In recent years researchers have begun to chronicle these experiences. Sexual and gender minority individuals report higher occurrences of chronic illness and disabilities than do heterosexual and cisgender persons (Dispenza et al., 2017). Black, Latinx, and transgender people are much more often targeted for identity-related violence and hate crimes (English et al., 2018). Adolescents of multiple minority identities have greater likelihood of being bullied into suicidal ideation, and Black LGB youths were found to be more likely than were White heterosexual same-gender peers to express suicidal ideation (Mueller et al., 2015). Gay Black men, for example, often must navigate dual minority status in relationship to their church and to the stigma within their religious communities (Heard Harvey & Ricard, 2018).

Competence and avoidance of harm are key ethical elements in providing services to these populations. All individuals have intersecting identities; however, clients of multiple marginalized identities are most vulnerable to levels of stress and types of stigma that require MHPs to obtain not only clinical competence and cultural competence but also an understanding of the complexity of challenges as well as knowledge of tailored evidence-based treatment plans. Ethical aspects of treatment include the following: (a) awareness of identity centrality (i.e., relative identification with each of one's multiple marginalized identities; Shramko et al., 2018), (b) understanding of institutional and other structural inequities and systems of oppression impacting clients, and (c) incorporation of not only discriminatory and stigmatizing experiences but also strengths and sources of resilience into treatment (Adames et al., 2018). The positive aspects of intersectionality can be overlooked in the urgency to treat environmental stressors and internalized negative dynamics; however, these factors can and should be incorporated into development of coping mechanisms and strength-based treatments.

Sexual-Orientation-Specific Competencies in the Context of Change Efforts

The characteristics of clients who seek SOCE through professional interventions often reflect the following characteristics: (a) They are from rural backgrounds in which very little diversity exists or is allowed. (b) Their family of origin espouses very narrow, dogmatic values related to parental control cloaked in a traditional moral stance. (c) The family of origin embraces a religious orthodoxy based on control and judgment (Dehlin et al., 2015). (d) They live in small to midsize communities that have not accepted minority diversity, implicitly practice a hierarchical power structure, and are invested in maintaining the status quo.

Proponents of SOCE can exploit these factors and instill fear based on distorted absolutes such as rejection by family, friends, and God; certain illness; inability to have a family; societal rejection; and long-term unfulfillment (Haldeman & Hancock, 2017). MHPs through clinical interviews and other assessment can determine the nature and origin of clients' change requests and incorporate the cognitive distortions, disinformation, and feared consequences experienced by clients into their psychotherapy.

Multiple Identities

Ethics codes of all major mental health professions include as enforceable standards the importance of acquiring knowledge and skills in working with diverse identities. Implicit in this expectation is the understanding of the multiplicity of identities and rejection of the perception of discrete identities. Minority status can include all of the diversity factors depending on context, but within the United States, ethnicity, race, sexual orientation, gender identity, culture, and socioeconomic status are minority identities that have withstood a history of oppression and current discrimination (Singh et al., 2017). Multiple identities compound the stigma, bias, and maltreatment of individuals, increasing the minority stress and negative effects on health and well-being. MHPs need to be aware of and responsive to this complexity and be responsive to the whole person.

Sexual Minority Youth

Minority children and adolescents are particularly vulnerable to maltreatment. They may have experienced bias, stigma, and discrimination through their development, or without expressing their sexual orientation they may have lived in fear that they are not normal and they will be found out. They often do not have access to information or education to counter distortions and stigma. MHPs may face parental expectations for SOCE and must be prepared through informed consent to educate parents on the potential harmful effects of SOCE.

Advocacy for Sexual Minorities

The conventional 50-minute therapy hour in the therapist's office is less tenable when working with sexual minority clients. Advocacy is a competency cited in the APA Benchmark Competencies (2011) and is defined as the awareness of social, political, economic, and cultural factors that impact individuals, institutions, and systems. Advocacy initiatives for public policy changes (Flores, 2014), legislative changes, and leadership in opposing prejudice, discrimination, and change efforts not supported by empirical evidence are integral to ethical practice (Haldeman & Hancock, 2017).

Gender-Identity-Specific Competencies in the Context of Change Efforts

As noted earlier, competencies for MHPs with SM and TG/NC clients and other ethical standards may apply similarly to both populations but also reflect separate competencies. Gender identity introduces specific variables that are less applicable for mental health services with other disenfranchised groups.

Advocacy for Transgender and Nonconforming Clients

Advocacy for TG/NC clients includes some elements of the advocacy role described earlier. Additionally, MHPs may be asked to assist clients in (a) providing documentation for public use that affirms gender identity (e.g., public accommodations; Lev, 2009), (b) exercising sensitivity to military clients or others whose employment is restrictive toward TG/NC individuals (APA, 2015), (c) balancing therapeutic relationship and endorsement letters of attestation for legal or medical purposes, (d) working with parents who are requesting change efforts, (e) consulting with medical or other professionals during transition, and (f) providing assistance for legal name or gender marker change (APA, 2015). Ethical, legal, and regulatory knowledge is essential for these purposes. Advocacy based on good intentions rather than competency and ethical standing represents an unacceptable risk of harm (Campbell & Arkles, 2017).

Informed Consent

MHPs promote transparency, authenticity, and respect for their clients' autonomy. The informed consent is emblematic of this stance and is the contract with clients that should reflect purpose of treatment, limits of confidentiality, other standard elements (e.g., fees, logistics), and any information that clients need to make informed decisions. MHPs engage in gender-affirming practices. Clients should be informed that GICE does not align with the goals of psychotherapy, is not supported by empirical evidence, and is potentially harmful. When working with minors who cannot engage in legal agreements or contracts, MHPs still explain the elements of informed consent and seek the minor's assent.

Multiple Roles

Advocacy, consultation with other health and legal professionals, attestations, and other roles not typically held inevitably result in multiple roles. MHPs may find themselves at the same political, community, or professional events as clients or even participating in the same activity. MHPs can navigate these waters by (a) being alert to the possibility of exploitation or loss of objectivity, (b) including in the informed consent the potential for multiple roles and how those situations will be resolved, and (c) engaging in ongoing discussions with clients and encouraging them to inform the MHP if they become uncomfortable with any given situation.

Confidentiality

The scope for limits of confidentiality is greater in working with TG/NC clients, and the inclusion of clients in these decisions can impact the working relationship and trust. The role of MHPs, as noted earlier, can include court interactions, creation and modification of documents, collaboration with school personnel, and advocacy roles that go beyond the typical statutory range of confidentiality waivers. Should transitioning be a consideration, the involvement of MHPs with parents and family, medical professionals, and legal representatives can be important to the client's welfare. MHPs should explain to clients and to parents of minors the implications for confidentiality if the MHP is fully participatory. As is expected with all minor clients, even though they do not have legal authority to make decisions, the MHPs should explain in terms understandable to the client and make every effort to gain assent (Campbell & Arkles, 2017).

Record Keeping

Clinical notes, official and unofficial records, and any documents created by MHPs require sensitivity, knowledge of legal and ethical standards in record keeping, and full awareness of the implications of recorded content on the client's treatment plan and the access that third parties will have to the MHP's and client's records. A difficult and sensitive balancing between risk management and client welfare exists and requires thoughtful consideration. MHPs need their records to accurately reflect their decision making in treatment of clients and yet be sensitive to disclosures that could have a negative impact on or unintended consequences for clients.

Gender-specific application of ethical standards is critical to the competent treatment of TG/NC clients. The principles and standards are not different than they are for other populations, yet the interpretation and application are specific to TG/NC clients, much as they are for other minority identities. MHPs are aware that they are practicing tailored and enhanced application of ethical practices in working with SM and TG/NC individuals.

AFFIRMATIVE TREATMENT IN THE CONTEXT OF SEXUAL ORIENTATION CHANGE EFFORTS

Upon investigation, change efforts that claimed to be successful have primarily reflected components of established therapeutic modalities. Participants in change efforts reported a sense of feeling accepted, belonging to and confiding in a group, and feeling commonality with others (Tozer & Hayes, 2004). These experiences are not inherent in change efforts but rather are core conditions of Rogerian principles essential to the therapeutic relationship (Rogers, 1957). Building on empirically supported studies of common factors and psychotherapy effectiveness, the APA Task Force on Appropriate

Therapeutic Responses to Sexual Orientation (2009; Anton, 2010) developed a framework for affirmative therapeutic treatments for those seeking sexual orientation change. Ethical aspects of affirmative treatments are noted below and reflect the importance of ethical decision making. These approaches affirming of SM are in keeping with ethical principles of respect for the welfare of others, beneficence, and trustworthiness.

Acceptance and Support

Empathic capacity is a core element in working with SM and a skill without which ethical practice would not be achievable. Clients coming to therapy with an initial goal of orientation change must gain the MHP's fundamental understanding of their request in terms of positive regard, openness to their concerns, and support for their distress. The categorical rejection of the request for change by MHPs could instill hopelessness, loss of trust, and disengagement. MHPs recognize clients' need to reduce suffering and normalize the conflicts while creating a therapeutic alliance (Haldeman, 2004). The ethical expectation of doing no harm reinforces the importance of the establishment of empathy and positive regard before treatment decision making.

Assessment

Sexual orientation is one of many aspects of the whole person. Understanding the role and meaning of sexual orientation in a person's life requires exploration of developmental history, past emotional life events, traumas, view of self and others, and the influence of family, culture, and norms (Haldeman, 2004). Anxiety, depression, interpersonal deficits, and other symptoms can seem to be perpetuated by dissatisfaction with sexual orientation, whereas negative and traumatic life experience may well be factors in maintaining distress, self-disappointment, and hopelessness. Ethical standards for assessment expect MHPs to "conduct an examination of individuals adequate to support their statements or conclusion" (APA, 2017a, p. 13). Multiple data points and thoroughness in assessment provide for more accurate treatment.

Religion

Conservative religious beliefs are often the motivating factor for interest in change efforts (Hathaway et al., 2004). Religious and spiritual beliefs often have deep roots in family and cultural prescription; individuals may not even embrace these prescriptions, which have been indoctrinated into their identity. A full understanding of the role, meaning, and contemporary influence of religion in the client's life enables MHPs to proceed with empathy and authenticity. Some of the elements of this exploration include (a) understanding the beliefs, (b) understanding the connection between the distress and the beliefs (Hathaway et al., 2004), (c) identifying religious goals and motivations (Emmons & Paloutzian, 2003), and (d) exploring the impact of religious beliefs on the client's self-stigma and prejudice (Hunsberger & Jackson, 2005). Clients' histories and lived experiences with trauma, sexuality, abuse, rejection, and abandonment need to be respected and incorporated into therapy before healing can take place.

Active Coping

Reduction of life distress by changing the source of stress, leaving the environment, or changing the perception of the situation involves active coping mechanisms. Cognitive strategies are employed to reduce cognitive dissonance, which often results from the conflict of dealing with social stigma and the desire to be accepted and supported. Effective cognitive strategies include (a) extinguishing all-or-nothing thinking of being a bad or self-distaining person because of sexual orientation, (b) rejecting stereotypical thinking, (c) engaging in dialectical behavioral therapy or acceptance and commitment to reduce anxiety and stress, (d) reframing cognitions about sexual attractions, (e) reducing self-judgments, and (f) reappraising events and making positive meanings (Pachankis et al., 2015).

Other methods of active coping include emotion-focused strategies of realizing and resolving disappointments with self and learning to tolerate ambiguity and uncertainty with a positive attitude (Bartoli & Gillem, 2008). Coping techniques extend to reduction of religious dissonance by redirecting clients to overarching values such as charity, forgiveness, gratitude, kindness, and compassion, thereby building self-acceptance (Ritter, 2018).

Social Support

Individuals who have undergone SOCE often report that one of the primary positive outcomes of the experience is social support, interaction with those who have similar concerns and identities, and being a part of a group in contrast with ongoing marginalization. Success in SOCE can be generalized to the positive effects of group belongingness rather than the effectiveness of the change efforts. Social support is a powerful treatment component in affirmative psychotherapy. Self-help groups, affirming communities, social groups, and welcoming religious groups provide an environment for healing and self-acceptance and serve as buffers for minority stress, marginalization, and isolation (APA, 2009). An important role of MHPs is to connect clients to resources that provide these support experiences.

Identity Exploration and Development

The multiple aspects of identity play a central role in identity distress and in affirmative treatment. The incongruence that SM feel between societal/family norms and their experienced identity can be overwhelming and can be the primary source of distress and hopelessness. Individuals can resort to SOCE because they think that religious beliefs, family culture, and societal expectations cannot change but that they may be able to change their sexual orientation, thereby decreasing the dissonance. Affirmative therapy creates the climate for identity exploration and acceptance of multiple identities that may not all be congruent, and it moves individuals away from the concept of fixed identities into integration and fluidity of identities. Formation of a collective identity is particularly important for the health and well-being of SM (Worthington et al., 2008).

MHPs lead clients into identity exploration without expectations of an outcome. Helping individuals understand and embrace their multiple identities prepares clients to synthesize and integrate identities rather than compartmentalize and think of some identities as winning and others as losing. In meeting competency expectations, MHPs encourage clients in determining (a) goals for identity, (b) behavioral expression of sexual orientation, (c) public and private social roles, (d) gender role identity, and (e) forms of relationships (APA, 2009). This affirming approach reduces the gender stereotyping associated with dissonance and introduces more complex aspects of gender that affirm diversity and set the stage for identity integration. This approach also meets the competency expectation for MHPs working with this population.

AFFIRMATIVE TREATMENT IN THE CONTEXT OF GENDER IDENTITY CHANGE EFFORTS

Gender nonconformity is not the same status as gender dysphoria, which is distress caused by incongruence between sex assigned at birth and gender identity (Institute of Medicine, 2011). Only some TG/NC individuals experience gender dysphoria, and these individuals can become the targets of GICE. Provision of services to those experiencing gender dysphoria requires awareness of the ethical standards of competence to understand the tailoring of interventions at this developmental stage of decision making and the ethical obligation to adhere to known evidence-based practice regarding unsubstantiated change efforts. MHPs must acquire the knowledge and skills to conduct psychotherapy that explores all options for tailored treatment:

> Some individuals integrate their trans- or cross-gender feelings into the gender role they were assigned at birth and do not feminize or masculinize their body. For others, changes in gender role and expression are sufficient to alleviate gender dysphoria. Some individuals may need hormonal treatment, a possible change in gender role, but not surgery; others may need a change in gender role along with surgery, but not hormonal treatment. In other words, treatment for gender dysphoria has become more individualized. (WPATH, 2012, p. 5)

MHPs should explore the client's reasons for seeking services and identify the role that stigma and marginalization, and the ensuing anxiety, depression, and stress, have played in the client's belief that SOCE is the route to relief from their psychological distress. MHPs become familiar with the research and knowledge-based information that SOCE is an unethical means of treatment and that psychotherapy oriented to affirmative treatments is the standard of care (APA, 2015; SAMHSA, 2015; WPATH, 2012).

MHPs should not dismiss change effort requests, however, but rather meet clients at their level of understanding knowing that their dysphoria will be strongly exacerbated by their external experience of rejection and discrimination from significant others (e.g., peer groups, family). The role of MHPs is a critical one in providing guidance through informational resources, educating clients on the impact of negative stereotyping and discrimination, and exploring the potential for coexisting mental health concerns that also affect clients' dissatisfaction with self. Competencies include the knowledge and skills to provide supportive and affirming psychotherapy during the exploration of identity and determination of clients' goals without leading clients to a predetermined decision. In working with adolescents and children, MHPs have additional responsibility to provide parents with the educational information, support, and affirmation of the normality of their children and adolescents.

Treatment goals in working with clients experiencing gender dysphoria are (a) maximizing overall psychological well-being and quality of life, (b) reducing or eliminating gender dysphoria, and (c) facilitating long-term satisfaction with gender identity (WPATH, 2012). WPATH (2012) identified affirmative psychotherapeutic interventions, which include the following:

- clarifying gender identity and role
- exploring the impact of stigma and minority stress

- if desired by clients, facilitating changes in gender role expression
- supporting and promoting interpersonal skills and coexisting mental health concerns
- assisting clients in consideration of social gender role transition, facilitating an individualized plan, and considering the implications of change
- collaborating with clients on decision making about communication with family and others

More evidence-based treatment plans incorporate these principles of psychotherapy with greater specificity in intervention models that meet ethical standards of care for TG/NC client affirmation. Transgender-affirming cognitive behavior therapy (TA-CBT) is built on psychoeducation, challenging negative self-beliefs, and encouraging trans-affirming social connectedness (Austin & Craig, 2015). AFFIRM is the youth model of TA-CBT aimed at decreasing depression and strengthening coping skills (Austin et al., 2018).

CONCLUSION

These elements of affirmative treatment for SM and TG/NC individuals in the context of change efforts are consistent with and emblematic of ethical standards of care for MHPs. Competence, both clinical and subject specific, is critical for effective treatment and a healthy working alliance. Avoidance of harm, adherence to evidence-based practice, and respect for the welfare of others are the building blocks of other ethical standards described in this chapter.

MHPs hold positions of great responsibility and privilege in advocating for and implementing affirmative treatment models for SM and TG/NC clients while vigorously opposing change efforts that broadly violate ethical standards of multiple mental health professions. MHPs' roles are complex, reach beyond the 50-minute hour, and move beyond the traditional boundaries of treatment. Ethical practice is an eyes-wide-open commitment to clients, to communities, and to societal change.

REFERENCES

Adames, H. Y., Chavez-Dueñas, N. Y., Sharma, S., & La Roche, M. J. (2018). Intersectionality in psychotherapy: The experiences of an AfroLatinx queer immigrant. *Psychotherapy, 55*(1), 73–79. https://doi.org/10.1037/pst0000152

American Counseling Association. (2014). *ALGBTIC competencies for counseling transgender clients.* https://www.counseling.org/resources/competencies/algbtic_competencies.pdf

American Psychological Association. (2011). *Benchmark competencies.* https://www.apa.org/ed/graduate/revised-competency-benchmarks.doc

American Psychological Association. (2012). Guidelines for psychological practice with lesbian, gay, and bisexual clients. *American Psychologist, 67*(1), 10–42. https://doi.org/10.1037/a0024659

American Psychological Association. (2015). Guidelines for psychological practice with transgender and gender non-conforming people. *American Psychologist, 70*(9), 832–864. https://doi.org/10.1037/a0039906

American Psychological Association. (2017a). *Ethical principles of psychologists and code of conduct* (2002, Amended June 1, 2010, and January 1, 2017). https://www.apa.org/ethics/code/ethics-code-2017.pdf

American Psychological Association. (2017b). *Multicultural guidelines: An ecological approach to context, identity, and intersectionality.* https://www.apa.org/about/policy/multicultural-guidelines.pdf

American Psychological Association Presidential Task Force on Evidence-Based Practice. (2006). Evidence-based practice in psychology. *American Psychologist, 61*(4), 271–285. https://www.apa.org/pubs/journals/features/evidence-based-statement.pdf

American Psychological Association Task Force on Appropriate Therapeutic Responses to Sexual Orientation. (2009). *Report of the APA task force on appropriate therapeutic responses to sexual orientation.* https://www.apa.org/pi/lgbt/resources/therapeutic-response.pdf

Anton, B. S. (2010). Proceedings of the American Psychological Association for the legislative year 2009: Minutes of the annual meeting of the Council of Representatives and minutes of the meetings of the Board of Directors. *American Psychologist, 65*(5), 385–475. https://doi.org/10.1037/a0019553

Austin, A., & Craig, S. L. (2015). Transgender affirmative cognitive behavioral therapy: Clinical considerations and applications. *Professional Psychology, Research and Practice, 46*(1), 21–29. https://doi.org/10.1037/a0038642

Austin, A., Craig, S. L., & D'Souza, S. A. (2018). An AFFIRMative cognitive behavioral intervention for transgender youth: Preliminary effectiveness. *Professional Psychology, Research and Practice, 49*(1), 1–8. https://doi.org/10.1037/pro0000154

Bartoli, E., & Gillem, A. R. (2008). Continuing to depolarize the debate on sexual orientation and religion: Identity and the therapeutic process. *Professional Psychology, Research and Practice, 39*(2), 202–209. https://doi.org/10.1037/0735-7028.39.2.202

Bradshaw, K., Dehlin, J. P., Crowell, K. A., Galliher, R. V., & Bradshaw, W. S. (2015). Sexual orientation change efforts through psychotherapy for LGBQ individuals affiliated with the Church of Jesus Christ of Latter-day Saints. *Journal of Sex & Marital Therapy, 41*(4), 391–412. https://doi.org/10.1080/0092623X.2014.915907

Campbell, L. F., & Arkles, G. (2017). Ethical and legal concerns for mental health professionals. In A. Singh & l. m. dickey (Eds.), *Affirmative counseling and psychological practice with transgender and gender nonconforming clients* (pp. 95–119). American Psychological Association. https://doi.org/10.1037/14957-005

Crenshaw, K. W. (1991). Mapping the margins: Intersectionality, identity, politics, and violence against women of color. *Stanford Law Review, 43*(6), 1241–1299. https://doi.org/10.2307/1229039

Dehlin, J. P., Galliher, R. V., Bradshaw, W. S., Hyde, D. C., & Crowell, K. A. (2015). Sexual orientation change efforts among current or former LDS church members. *Journal of Counseling Psychology, 62*(2), 95–105. https://doi.org/10.1037/cou0000011

Dispenza, F., Varney, M., & Golubovic, N. (2017). Counseling and psychological practices with sexual and gender minority persons living with chronic illnesses/ disabilities (CID). *Psychology of Sexual Orientation and Gender Diversity, 4*(1), 137–142. https://doi.org/10.1037/sgd0000212

Dyar, C., Feinstein, B. A., Stephens, J., Zimmerman, A., Newcomb, M. E., & Whitton, S. W. (2020). Nonmonosexual stress and dimensions of health: Within group variation by sexual, gender, and race/ethnic identities. *Psychology of Sexual Orientation and Gender Diversity, 7*(1), 12–25. https://doi.org/10.1037/sgd0000348

Emmons, R. A., & Paloutzian, R. F. (2003). The psychology of religion. *Annual Review of Psychology, 54*(1), 377–402. https://doi.org/10.1146/annurev.psych.54.101601. 145024

English, D., Rendina, J., & Parsons, J. (2018). The effects of intersecting stigma: A longitudinal examination of minority stress, mental health, and substance use among Black, Latino, and multiracial gay and bisexual men. *Psychology of Violence, 8*(6), 669–679. https://doi.org/10.1037/vio0000218

Flentje, A., Heck, N. C., & Cochran, B. N. (2014). Experiences of ex-ex-gay individuals in sexual reorientation therapy: Reasons for seeking treatment, perceived helpfulness and harmfulness of treatment, and post-treatment identification. *Journal of Homosexuality, 61*(9), 1242–1268. https://doi.org/10.1080/00918369.2014. 926763

Flores, A. R. (2014). *National trends in public opinion on LGBT rights in the United States.* The Williams Institute. https://williamsinstitute.law.ucla.edu/wp-content/ uploads/POP-natl-trends-nov-2014.pdf

Haldeman, D. (2004). When sexual and religious orientation collide: Considerations in working with conflicted same-sex attracted male clients. *The Counseling Psychologist, 32*(5), 691–715. https://doi.org/10.1177/0011000004267560

Haldeman, D., & Hancock, K. (2017). Lesbian, gay, and bisexual health issues: Policy and practice. In K. DeBord, A. Fischer, K. Bieschke, & R. Perez (Eds.), *Handbook of sexual orientation and gender diversity in counseling and psychotherapy* (pp. 387–415). APA Books. https://doi.org/10.1037/15959-016

Hathaway, W. L., Scott, S. Y., & Garver, S. A. (2004). Assessing religious/spiritual functioning: A neglected domain in clinical practice? *Professional Psychology, Research and Practice, 35*(1), 97–104. https://doi.org/10.1037/0735-7028.35.1.97

Heard Harvey, C., & Ricard, R. (2018). Contextualizing the concept of intersectionality: Layered identities of African American women and gay men in the Black church. *Journal of Multicultural Counseling and Development, 46*(3), 206–218. https://doi.org/10.1002/jmcd.12102

Hunsberger, B., & Jackson, L. M. (2005). Religion, meaning, and prejudice. *Journal of Social Issues, 61*(4), 807–826. https://doi.org/10.1111/j.1540-4560.2005.00433.x

Institute of Medicine. (2011). *The health of lesbian, gay, bisexual, and transgender people: Building a foundation for better understanding.* The National Academies Press.

Lev, A. I. (2009). The ten tasks of the mental health provider: Recommendations for revision of the World Professional Association for Transgender Health's Standards of Care. *International Journal of Transgenderism, 11*(2), 74–99. https:// doi.org/10.1080/15532730903008032

Mueller, A. S., James, W., Abrutyn, S., & Levin, M. L. (2015). Suicide ideation and bullying among US adolescents: Examining the intersections of sexual orientation, gender, and race/ethnicity. *American Journal of Public Health, 105*(5), 980–985. https://doi.org/10.2105/AJPH.2014.302391

National Association of Social Workers. (2017). *Sexual orientation change efforts (SOCE) and conversion therapy with lesbians, gay men, bisexuals, and transgender persons* [Position statement]. https://www.socialworkers.org/LinkClick.aspx?fileticket=IQYALknHU6s%3D&portalid=0

Pachankis, J. E., Hatzenbuehler, M. L., Rendina, H. J., Safren, S. A., & Parsons, J. T. (2015). LGB-affirmative cognitive-behavioral therapy for young adult gay and bisexual men: A randomized controlled trial of a transdiagnostic minority stress approach. *Journal of Consulting and Clinical Psychology, 83*(5), 875–889. https://doi.org/10.1037/ccp0000037

Panozzo, D. (2013). Advocating for an end to reparative therapy: Methodological grounding and blueprint for change. *Journal of Gay & Lesbian Social Services: The Quarterly Journal of Community & Clinical Practice, 25*(3), 362–377. https://doi.org/10.1080/10538720.2013.807214

Ritter, K. (2018, August 9–12). *Integration of religious, spiritual, sexual, and gender identities: A demonstration of synthesis* [Conference session]. American Psychological Association 126th Annual Convention, San Francisco, CA, United States.

Rogers, C. (1957). The necessary and sufficient conditions of personality change. *Journal of Consulting Psychology, 21*(2), 95–103.

Shidlo, A., & Gonsiorek, J. C. (2017). Psychotherapy with clients who have been through sexual orientation change interventions or request to change their sexual orientation. In K. A. DeBord, A. R. Fischer, K. J. Bieschke, & R. M. Perez (Eds.), *Handbook of sexual orientation and gender diversity in counseling and psychotherapy* (pp. 291–312). American Psychological Association. https://doi.org/10.1037/15959-012

Shidlo, A., & Schroeder, M. (2002). Changing sexual orientation: A consumer's report. *Professional Psychology, Research and Practice, 33*(3), 249–259. https://doi.org/10.1037/0735-7028.33.3.249

Shramko, M., Toomey, R. B., & Anhalt, K. (2018). Profiles of minority stressors and identity centrality among sexual minority Latinx youth. *American Journal of Orthopsychiatry, 88*(4), 471–482. https://doi.org/10.1037/ort0000298

Singh, A. A. (2013). Transgender youth of color and resilience: Negotiating oppression, finding support. *Sex Roles, 68*(11–12), 690–702. https://doi.org/10.1007/s11199-012-0149-z

Singh, A. A., Hwahng, S. J., Chang, S. C., & White, B. (2017). Affirmative counseling with trans/gender-variant people of color. In A. Singh and l. m. dickey (Eds.), *Affirmative counseling and psychological practice with transgender and gender nonconforming clients* (pp. 41–68). American Psychological Association.

Substance Abuse and Mental Health Services Administration. (2015). *Ending conversion therapy: Supporting and affirming LGBTQ youth* (HHS Publication No. SMA15-4928). U.S. Department of Health and Human Services.

Tozer, E. E., & Hayes, J. A. (2004). Why do individuals seek conversion therapy? The role of religiosity, internalized homonegativity, and identity development. *The Counseling Psychologist, 32*(5), 716–740. https://doi.org/10.1177/0011000004267563

World Professional Association for Transgender Health. (2012). *Standards of care for the health of transsexual, transgender, and gender-conforming people* (Version 7). https://www.wpath.org/publications/soc

Worthington, R. L., Dillon, F. R., & Becker-Schutte, A. M. (2005). Development, reliability, and validity of the Lesbian, Gay, and Bisexual Knowledge and Attitudes Scale for Heterosexuals (LGB-KASH). *Journal of Counseling Psychology, 52*(1), 104–118. https://doi.org/10.1037/0022-0167.52.1.104

Worthington, R. L., Navarro, R. L., Savoy, H. B., & Hampton, D. (2008). Development, reliability, and validity of the Measure of Sexual Identity Exploration and Commitment (MOSIEC). *Developmental Psychology, 44*(1), 22–33. https://doi.org/10.1037/0012-1649.44.1.22

IV

AFFIRMATIVE APPROACHES: ADVOCACY AND INTERNATIONAL ISSUES

9

REVIEW OF U.S. PUBLIC POLICY, LEGISLATIVE, AND JUDICIAL WORK ON CONVERSION EFFORTS

MELISSA J. GREY, SAM BRINTON, AND DOUGLAS C. HALDEMAN

Efforts to change sexual orientation or gender are inextricably linked with discrimination and sociocultural contexts that stigmatize sexual and gender minorities (SGM). Advocacy to end such conversion attempts is part of larger nondiscrimination and equality movements and is subject to unique challenges and opportunities. In this chapter, we use "conversion" or "conversion efforts" to include any attempts by professionals, authority figures, or others to change a person's sexual orientation or gender to be in alignment with heterosexual and cisgender norms. Conversion efforts have been referred to by many names, including conversion therapy, reparative therapy, reorientation therapy, and reintegrative therapy. However, decades of science demonstrate harm associated with conversion attempts, fails to support conversion proponents' claims of change or conversion, and shows sexual orientation and gender diversity (SOGD) are part of healthy human variation rather than being an illness or maladaptive behavior. Although lesbian, gay, bisexual, transgender, and questioning or queer (LGBTQ) advocates have sometimes reclaimed the term "conversion therapy," we chose to use the term "conversion efforts" to emphasize that these are not "therapy."

https://doi.org/10.1037/0000266-010
The Case Against Conversion "Therapy": Evidence, Ethics, and Alternatives,
D. C. Haldeman (Editor)

Public policy to prevent conversion is an important component of LGBTQ equality and liberation movements. Such public policy is vital to the efforts to end anti-LGBTQ stigma and the damage that stigma inflicts, and it is essential to bear witness to those who have survived "conversion therapy." Sam Brinton uses policy advocacy and their experience to ground us in the personal and particular ways conversion threatens wellness, justice, and freedom. As Brinton (2018a) wrote:

> In the early 2000s, when I was a middle schooler in Florida, I was subjected to a trauma that was meant to erase my existence as a newly out bisexual. My parents were Southern Baptist missionaries who believed that the dangerous and discredited practice of conversion therapy could "cure" my sexuality.
>
> For over two years, I sat on a couch and endured emotionally painful sessions with a counselor. I was told that my faith community rejected my sexuality; that I was the abomination we had heard about in Sunday school; that I was the only gay person in the world; that it was inevitable I would get H.I.V. and AIDS.
>
> But it didn't stop with these hurtful talk-therapy sessions. The therapist ordered me bound to a table to have ice, heat, and electricity applied to my body. I was forced to watch clips on a television of gay men holding hands, hugging, and having sex. I was supposed to associate those images with the pain I was feeling to once and for all turn into a straight boy. In the end it didn't work. I would say that it did, just to make the pain go away.
>
> I have begun to repair the damage that conversion therapy caused me and my family. But the failed promise of change has very likely caused a permanent tear in our relationship . . .
>
> Today I am proudly bisexual and gender fluid, and I serve as the head of advocacy and government affairs for The Trevor Project, the world's largest suicide prevention and crisis intervention organization for L.G.B.T.Q. youth. We constantly hear from survivors of conversion therapy who have been so hurt that they are contemplating suicide. So, we know the severity of the problem. (paras. 1–5)

Brinton's experience is one of many survivors' that is important to keep in focus as we work to understand the multiple influences on conversion efforts, which ultimately affect vulnerable, private domains of personal lives. In this chapter, we first contextualize conversion efforts in a brief history of U.S. policies that have impacted LGBTQ individuals and communities, and we then discuss the movement to end conversion as part of LGBTQ equality movements more broadly. Recognizing the movement to end conversion as an LGBTQ liberation or equality issue invites us to acknowledge the "messy" politics and social power dynamics that surround conversion efforts and that are often culturally distinct from the ostensible neatness of scientific and healthcare practice progress. With these historical and sociopolitical contexts in the backdrop, we review recent trends in regional, state, and federal legislation and professional regulations that prohibit conversion efforts, as well as judicial challenges to some of these. Given advocates' experiences in these arenas, we then provide practical information about strategies to end conversion efforts. Finally, we conclude with promising trends in the movement to end conversion. For the reader's reference, Table 9.1 presents a timeline of both policy and sociopolitical events related to conversion efforts.

NONLINEAR PROGRESS IS THE HISTORICAL CONTEXT OF CONVERSION

In the United States, public policy has often been used to protect privilege and advance the interests of dominant-culture groups while subjugating marginalized groups (see Zinn, 2003). The LGBTQ rights movement of the middle 20th century was a diverse and vibrant advancement toward freedom and was often disproportionately influenced by affluent, White, cisgender gay men, in a parallel reiteration of the control exerted by affluent White men over social policy in dominant culture. LGBTQ equality movement groups today are motivated to undermine the ineffectiveness and injustice of recapitulating oppressive dynamics, and they work to replace these dynamics by critiquing their own structures and strategies, taking intersectional perspectives, and centering marginalized voices (e.g., Butterworth, 2017; Collins & Bilge, 2016; Spade, 2015). LGBTQ equality movement groups have been growing stronger (Bronski, 2012; Stryker, 2017), and now many of us are visible; in many places, we are protected; public opinion is more often on our side; and many SGM enjoy freedoms that our foreparents could not even consider.

Prior to the LGBTQ equality movements in the 1950s, the daily life of SGM in the United States was marked by a lack of legal recognition, criminalization, and police harassment. Shifts in LGBTQ public policy, legislation, and judicial activity were driven by an LGBTQ activist movement and fueled by work in psychology, which began to dismantle the illness model it had once created. Psychological science shaped and followed public opinion. Ten years after Evelyn Hooker's (1957) research established that gay men were indistinguishable from a nonclinical sample of heterosexual men, the Stonewall rebellion ignited the official start of the modern LGBTQ rights movement, and 4 years after that, homosexuality was removed from the *Diagnostic and Statistical Manual of Mental Disorders (DSM)* and gender identity disorder emerged (Drescher, 2010; Minton, 2002).

There is rarely social change without backlash, and LGBTQ people who made significant gains for equality and respect through the 1970s learned quickly that such progress could provoke deep-seated bigotry and hatred (Bronski, 2012). Polarizing religious leaders and institutions targeted SGM, stoking fear

TABLE 9.1. Hallmark Policy and Sociopolitical Events Related to Conversion Efforts

Hallmark conversion event		Other LGBTQ related hallmarks
	1950	Mattachine Society established
Freud's letter to a mother of a gay man published in *The American Journal of Psychiatry*	1951	
The first *DSM* lists homosexuality as a disorder	1952	McCarran-Walter Act allows deportation of LGBTQ and other "subversive" immigrants
	1953	Executive Order 10450 prohibits gay federal workers in private contracts
	1955	Daughters of Bilitis established
	1957	Hooker's first study on gay men published
	1966	Compton Cafeteria Rebellion
	1969	Stonewall Rebellion
Homosexuality removed from the *DSM* (replaced with sexual orientation disturbance)	1973	
Love in Action established		
	1974	Kathy Kozachenko is the first openly gay elected public official
Exodus International established	1976	
Focus on the Family established	1977	*Richards v. US Tennis Association* decision finds Renee Richards can compete as an openly transgender woman
DSM-III lists Gender Identity Disorder and ego-dystonic homosexuality	1980	
	1981	Recognized beginning of the HIV/AIDS epidemic in the United States
	1986	*Bowers v. Hardwick* decision upheld Georgia's law criminalizing LGBTQ people
DSM-III-R removes ego-dystonic homosexuality	1987	
	1991	Joanne Conte is first openly transgender elected public official
National Association for Research and Therapy of Homosexuality established	1992	
American Academy of Pediatrics is first professional statement that conversion is "contraindicated"	1993	"Don't Ask Don't Tell"—U.S. military policy enacted

TABLE 9.1. Hallmark Policy and Sociopolitical Events Related to Conversion Efforts (Continued)

Hallmark conversion event		Other LGBTQ related hallmarks
	1996	*Romer v. Evans*
		Defense of Marriage Act (ends 2013)
		Boy Scouts of America v. Dale found the organization could refuse readmittance of a scout leader on the basis of his sexual orientation
Robert Spitzer's report claims sexual orientation change is possible	2003	*Lawrence v. Texas*
	2004	Massachusetts first state to enact marriage equality; 12 states amend state constitutions to ban marriage equality
	2008	California's Proposition 8 passes; Arizona and Florida ban marriage equality
	2009	The Matthew Shepard Act is passed
Robert Spitzer apologizes and retracts his 2003 report	2012	
California's SB1172 is first state law to prohibit conversion efforts		
Exodus International closes	2013	*Hollingsworth v. Perry* overturns Proposition 8; *United States v. Windsor* overturns DOMA
Gender Identity Disorder replaced with Gender Dysphoria in *DSM-5*		
Pickup v. Brown (and *Welch v. Brown*) decision upholds SB1172		
King v. Christie		
SAMHSA report on ending conversion therapy	2015	*Obergefell v. Hodges* brings marriage equality to all states
Ferguson v. JONAH		
Gender Identity Clinic at Ontario's Centre for Addiction and Mental Health closed		
First U.S. federal conversion prohibition proposed		
United Nations Human Rights Council report on conversion efforts	2020	*Bostock v. Clayton County* establishes LGBTQ workplace nondiscrimination protections

Note. This timeline is not exhaustive of all important events. It includes referenced events from the chapter in a linear timeline along with other lesbian, gay, bisexual, transgender, and questioning or queer (LGBTQ)-related public policies and sociopolitical events related to conversion efforts. *DSM* = Diagnostic and Statistical Manual of Mental Disorders; DOMA = Defense of Marriage Act; SAMHSA = Substance Abuse and Mental Health Services Administration.

and gathering supporters. At the same time, forces in psychoanalysis, in particular, were slow to relinquish pathologizing models of same-gender attraction and behavior, which were instrumental in promoting conversion efforts (Drescher, 2015). In fact, many of these psychoanalysts responded to the elimination of homosexuality from the *DSM* by doubling down on unsubstantiated theories of homosexuality resulting from parent–child or family dynamics (e.g., distant father, identification with different-gender parent; Bieber et al., 1962; Nicolosi, 1991; Socarides, 1978). Over time and with mounting disconfirming evidence, support for these theories among mainstream mental health practitioners diminished substantially (Drescher, 2015).

With mounting scientific evidence in support of SOGD and removing stigma from LGBTQ individuals, select religious and psychoanalytic leaders found common cause. In this way, the so-called "conversion therapy" project was born (Mattachine Society of Washington, DC, 2018). In 1973, Love in Action was formed as a religious ministry that used mental health frameworks to "treat" SGM. In 1977, religious fundamentalist and psychologist James Dobson founded Focus on the Family, an anti-LGBTQ religious organization dedicated to enshrining heteronormativity and anti-LGBTQ bigotry under the pretext of conservative values. Focus on the Family created an organization called Love Won Out, dedicated to promoting anti-LGBTQ ideals, hosting anti-LGBTQ conferences, and promoting "treatments" that claimed to rid people of "unwanted homosexual attractions." This organization was eventually subsumed by a similar group, Exodus International, which became the prime sponsor of conversion programs. In addition to advocating for several anti-LGBTQ laws, at its largest Exodus International supported conversion efforts in 17 countries through more than 400 ministries (see Chapter 10, this volume; Merritt, 2015).

Identifying LGBTQ people as part of the "social ills" of society garnered newfound conservative supporters, bolstered the backlash against feminists and antiwar activists, and built on preexisting racist ideology. Around this time, explicit racist rhetoric was falling out of favor in conservative politics for more subtle racism under the guise of opposition to big government overreach (Balmer, 2014). This subtle racism was combined with opposing the sexual revolution and abortion, for example, to politicize the religious right (Griffith, 2017). Racism relies on stereotypes of Black, Indigenous, and other People of Color's (BIPOC's) sexuality being viewed as animalistic and *heterosexually* promiscuous, for example. In order to rationalize such stereotypes, racist ideology rules out the possibility of Black sexual and gender diversity (Collins, 2005). Being BIPOC and LGBTQ was impossible inside this racist ideology, and so one function of rejecting BIPOC gender and sexual diversity is to reinforce racism and the political forces that benefit from racism.

The systems of racism, heterosexism, and cissexism are intertwined (Collins, 2005) in a politically expedient way. Although there were BIPOC participants in well-known conversion programs like Love in Action, BIPOC's race and ethnicity were often hidden, and so too have been the variety of other forms that conversion efforts have taken in Black communities (Hipp et al., 2019). The anti-LGBTQ focus of conservative politics built on previously useful oppressive ideology and garnered more opposition to social progress.

Although conversion efforts groups remained active for decades, and remain active today, public support for anti-LGBTQ discrimination decreased in the 1990s and through the 2000s (Flores, 2014). Several professional associations made statements opposing conversion efforts, including the American Academy of Pediatrics (1993), American Psychiatric Association (2000), and American Counseling Association (2013). The American Psychological Association (APA) adopted a policy cautioning practitioners about conversion efforts and addressing the "Appropriate Therapeutic Responses to Sexual Orientation" (APA, 1997), primarily using an ethical framework. However, this policy did not address antitransgender practices, nor did it state that psychologists should not attempt conversion efforts, owing in large part to the practice community's reluctance to prohibit any kind of "therapy" or limit psychologists' autonomy.

The patterns of progress and backlash persisted in public life, as psychological science worked toward clarifying the nature of conversion efforts. In 1996, in *Romer v. Evans*, the Supreme Court of the United States (SCOTUS) held that Amendment 2 to the Colorado State Constitution was unconstitutional, in that it was a violation of the Fourteenth Amendment equal protection rights to prohibit the extension of protections to LGB persons in housing, employment, and public accommodation in that there was no legitimate government interest to do so. Justice Anthony Kennedy, writing for the majority, stated, "The intent of the law is to single out one group and make it a stranger to the constitution's protections, and this the state of Colorado cannot do." With this landmark ruling, all other anti-LGB discrimination ordinances across the country fell immediately, and more jurisdictions passed legislation protective of LGB persons.

In 2004, Massachusetts was the first state to legalize marriage equality. The backlash was swift and predictable, and, as part of plans for divisive "wedge" politics, the party in power saw an opportunity to play on people's fears of the destruction of the institution of marriage by proposing ballot initiatives to ban same-sex marriage in 12 states. All of the ballot initiatives passed. As a sociopolitical attempt to maintain a heteronormative hold on the institution of marriage, this strategy worked, at least temporarily. LGBTQ equality activists would have to work another 9 years for redress.

The SCOTUS decision to strike down sodomy laws was a demonstration of the instrumental role of psychological science in the fight for SOGD civil rights. In 1986, SCOTUS had upheld the rights of states to enact sodomy prohibitions in *Bowers v. Hardwick*. The decision had a lasting and damaging effect on others seeking protection or relief from the law, including lesbian and gay parents who were stripped of their custodial rights because they exposed their children to criminal behavior by engaging in a same-gender relationship (Hegarty, 2018). Even with evidence from psychological science showing that the children of same-gender parents were healthy or similar to those with heterosexual parents, the courts still regarded same-gender relationships as criminal. Similar to the decision in *Romer*, however, *Bowers* was overturned in 2003, in the case of *Lawrence v. Texas*. According to Justice Kennedy, who wrote the decision in this case too, the Texas statute at issue served no legitimate state interest in criminalizing private behavior by one group when it such behavior was not criminal when done by another. It was clear that the law contained anti-LGB animus and there was harm in codifying this stigma against LGB people (Diamond & Rosky, 2016; Hegarty, 2018). An APA amicus brief opposing the Texas law applied psychological research showing that LGB people are "normal" and that sodomy statutes reinforce prejudice (Herek, 2008). Highlighting the problem of sexual prejudice and stigma helped to pave several paths through LGBTQ movements.

The toxicity of such discriminatory policies and public debates was traced onto the health of LGBTQ people during this period of advances and backlash. Early work by Russell (2000) during the Amendment 2 campaign in Colorado suggested that discriminatory policies actually made people sick: More depressive and anxiety symptoms were reported in persons living in areas where their civil rights were on the ballot. This research was replicated many times and found that those LGBTQ persons living in jurisdictions where marriage equality was on the ballot reported significantly greater symptoms of depression and anxiety than those living in more LGBT-supportive areas (Hatzenbuehler et al., 2010; Rostosky et al., 2009). Researchers in the 21st century made clearer that discriminatory treatment and legislation constitute minority stress (Meyer, 2003).

After the watershed ruling in *Lawrence*, LGBTQ activists saw openings and marshaled efforts for several advancements, including for marriage equality. During the tumult of the 1990s, President Clinton had signed the Defense of Marriage Act (DOMA), which denied federal benefits to same-gender couples even if their state passed marriage equality legislation; in 2003, the Bush administration made a failed attempt to strengthen federal opposition to marriage equality by defining marriage as only between one man and one woman. The next year, Massachusetts became the first state to legalize marriage equality. Marriage equality became a primary domain in which sociopolitical groups debated the lives of LGBTQ people, and between 2004 and 2012, voters in 27 states denied equality to their fellow residents by passing marriage equality bans. Most famously, Proposition 8 passed in California in 2008, overturning the state's marriage equality law. Arizona and Florida also passed bans that year, bringing the total to 40 states in which marriage equality was unlawful (McKinley & Goodstein, 2008). With this trend also came backlash legislation against access to other family structures, such as the 2008 legislation in Arkansas, which restricted adoption to married couples only (McKinley & Goodstein, 2008). The contentious context and codification of prejudice took significant tolls on LGBTQ people and rallied progressive activism (Herek, 2011; Maisel & Fingerhut, 2011). As tangible representation of couples as a battleground, 1,700 marriages that had been performed in California before the Proposition 8 ban were left hanging in limbo.

After several years of work lobbying the judiciary, California's Proposition 8 law was declared unconstitutional by a California district court in *Hollingsworth v. Perry* (2013). Although SCOTUS held there was no jurisdiction in that case, at nearly the same time, SCOTUS overturned DOMA in *United States v. Windsor* (2013). In the decision, the Court held that same-gender couples were qualified for equal protection status, and the law was interpreted as imposing a "disadvantage, a separate status, and so a stigma" on same-gender couples and their families. In fact, the court decided that DOMA "humiliates tens of thousands of children now being raised by same-sex couples" (*United States v. Windsor*, 2013). As in other marriage equality cases, DOMA was struck down with the help of psychological and other social science research highlighting the damage of its discriminatory nature. Analysts highlight this SCOTUS decision as a turning point in the legal construal of LGB lives: The courts had previously held that children needed protection *from* LGB people. *Windsor* now established that discrimination, including marriage inequality, was not only inimical to state interest but also harmful to children of same-gender couples (Diamond & Rosky, 2016). As DOMA fell, another case was advancing with the aim to open marriage equality throughout the United States. In *Obergefell v. Hodges* (2015), the SCOTUS again heard testimony from psychological scientists and distinguished between credible scientific evidence about marriage, relationships, and the nature of sexual orientation and claims that were "not credible"—for example, Mark Regnerus's claims that same-gender marriage led to poor outcomes for children (Regnerus, 2012). In 2015, the SCOTUS decided the right to same-gender marriage is constitutionally protected, citing due process and equal protection protections of the Fourteenth Amendment. All existing state bans fell and marriage equality became legal throughout the United States.

It was against the backdrop of events such as California Proposition 8 being struck down by SCOTUS, that the APA first revisited its 1997 policy on Appropriate Therapeutic Responses to Sexual Orientation. In the face of opposition and an email campaign from conservative Christian groups, the APA convened a task force to critically examine the extant literature on so-called "conversion therapy" and update its policy. This task force featured some of the top experts in the area, along with a content-naïve research methodology specialist who concluded that there was no empirical basis for supporting efforts to change sexual orientation. As of 2019, every major professional mental health association had made official statements against conversion efforts (see Chapter 8, this volume).

PROTECTIONS FROM CONVERSION EFFORTS ARE PART OF LGBTQ EQUALITY MOVEMENTS, AND MOVEMENTS ARE MESSY

When the first law attempting to protect minors from conversion efforts was signed in 2012, LGBTQ equality movements were in full swing. That year, the Equal Opportunity Commission ruled that the Civil Rights Act protects transgender people from illegal sex discrimination, three states legalized marriage equality by popular vote (Mayeski, 2012), and Robert Spitzer (2012) apologized for and retracted his past claims that supported conversion efforts. Although not without contention or setbacks, the trend was consistent with a general trajectory supporting LGBTQ-related awareness and justice.

Like other nondiscrimination initiatives, Youth Mental Health Protection Acts (YMHPAs) or legislation prohibiting the use of conversion efforts by licensed mental health professionals (LMHPs) are often moved by both political and professional/empirical dynamics. Fundamental psychological facts have supported much LGBTQ policy progress (e.g., YouGov, 2014), and these also support YMHPAs. Specifically,

(1) SOGD are natural, healthy human variations, and SGM show the same capacities as others do to lead healthy lives, work hard, raise families, and serve the community, which means the nature of SOGD does not provide a rationale for discrimination or preferring one form or expression of SOGD over another;

(2) there is a great deal of evidence in the United States of social and cultural stigma and prejudices of heterosexism, monosexism, and cissexism, from which discrimination and conversion efforts cannot be separated;

(3) inequality is bad for health; and

(4) like other expressions of stigma and prejudice, conversion efforts are harmful. (American Psychiatric Association, 2000; APA, 2009, 2021a, 2021b)

Analysts have highlighted that, although immutability of SOGD has been helpful in supporting steps in LGBTQ movements, immutability is no longer a clear pattern in SOGD and is an unnecessary rationale for rights won so far (Diamond & Rosky, 2016). Anti-LGBTQ advocates maintain a well of doubt about these well-supported SOGD-affirming facts, which fosters unnecessary fears in cautious legislators and other decision makers.

Attempts to promote conversion efforts are often coupled with research and practice distortions (Shidlo & Gonsiorek, 2017), and calls for more rigorous research to test the extraordinary claims of conversion proponents (e.g., APA, 2009) have not been met (APA, 2021a, 2021b; see also Chapter 1, this volume). Instead of meeting scientific critiques with stronger scientific methods, proponents of conversion efforts often misappropriate sexuality and gender research (Shidlo & Gonsiorek, 2017) and misrepresent facts. For example, in contrast to the assertions in a *Letter From Expert LGBTI Researchers* (2016), a transgender identity is not pathological, and gender affirming transition-related health care is an effective and safe option (APA, 2015). Other conversion proponents attempt to avoid scrutiny as health care professions (e.g., Substance Abuse and Mental Health Services Administration [SAMHSA], 2015) issue stronger warnings against conversion efforts; its proponents regroup with "newer" conversion efforts that maintain inaccurate and prejudicial tenets and stigmatizing practices while taking on the appearance of acceptance.

The contentious sociopolitical dynamics surrounding YMHPAs can make it difficult to discern that there is sometimes significant and widespread support for equality. As more individuals have relationships and connections to LGBTQ individuals, public support for nondiscrimination has also grown (Pew Research Center, 2016). When asked about conversion efforts specifically, most people in the United States do not support them, nor do they believe them to be effective (Merritt, 2015; YouGov, 2014). Within mental health professions, too, there have been notable shifts toward affirming diversity, particularly in light of scientific facts to support it, and shifts toward supporting the potential for individuals to synthesize ostensibly incompatible aspects of self, such as religiosity, gender, and sexuality.

RECENT TRAJECTORIES OF CONVERSION EFFORT POLICIES

As public policies to protect individuals from conversion efforts developed, Alan Chambers (leader of Exodus, the largest conversion efforts organization) disavowed the effectiveness of conversion efforts, apologized for the hurt they caused, and closed the organization (Payne, 2013). This was followed by the U.S. SAMHSA's (2015) experts' declaration of a consensus to end "conversion therapy." In the same year, following a YMHPA in Ontario, the Gender Identity Clinic at Ontario's Centre for Addiction and Mental Health closed. Many paths seemed to be converging to end conversion efforts.

Laws prohibiting conversion efforts have largely been active on the state level and debated in the courts. California SB 1172 ("Lieu. Sexual orientation conversion efforts," 2011–2012) was the first such YMHPA to be proposed, and it required that mental health providers who use conversion efforts with youth be disciplined by the provider's licensing board. During its legislative development, SB 1172 evolved to make clearer that it specifically prohibits only conversion efforts and does not prohibit legitimate forms of therapy (California Psychological Association, 2012). The law, enacted in September 2012, has been challenged several times on claims that it limits providers' free speech and freedom of religious expression. In each instance (*Pickup v. Brown*, 2012; *Welch v. Brown*, 2014), the law has been upheld. YMHPAs have been introduced in 40 states, with at least 20 adopting them as of this writing. As these laws have been adopted, they typically include in the definition of "change efforts" as attempts to change sexual orientation, gender identity, and gender expression. Most legislation prohibits conversion efforts with minors (notably, Washington, DC, also protects vulnerable adults), and they typically apply only to LMHPs.

Professional boards have the power to reasonably regulate their licensees and registrants, in order to protect clients, patients, or consumers of services; in fact, it is a professional board's duty to do so. As the trend in YMHPAs grew, calls for professional boards to strengthen their knowledge and regulations about conversion efforts also grew (Drescher et al., 2016); Ohio was the first state to make such progress. The Ohio mental health counseling, social work, and psychology boards issued advisory statements to licensed professionals stating that those regulated professionals who use conversion efforts with youth risk losing their license (Ohio Board of Psychology, 2016). Where attempts to pass YMHPAs have been repeatedly stalled in legislatures, as they were in Ohio, the health profession boards can make significant impacts to limit conversion efforts. After two attempts to pass YMHPAs stalled in Virginia, lawmakers raised the possibility of licensing boards regulating the issue directly. Taking that as their cue, Virginia's seven professional licensing boards took active steps to develop regulations prohibiting conversion efforts and clarifying that a complaint of a licensed professional practicing conversion efforts could result in a finding of misconduct, thus declaring conversion efforts to be formally regarded as a "violation of standard practices" (McNeill, 2019).

Professional board regulatory changes do not always require action from state legislators and may escape some of the political challenges to YMHPAs. At the same time, changing professional regulations is often a multistep process—in Virginia, for example, it included development of regulatory and guideline language; a public review process; a vote from the professional board; and official approval, including from the governor, attorney general, and the secretary of health and human services (Fischer, 2019). The workgroup of Virginia health profession boards developed guidance similar to YMHPAs, with essentially identical definitions of conversion efforts, application exclusively to practice on minors, and possible professional sanctions (see Virginia Board of Psychology, 2019). In March 2020, Virginia then passed a legislative YMHPA (Garcia, 2020). This process of developing professional regulations is fraught with potential for negative outcomes, including widely divergent regulations between different professions or defeat at any of the many votes or decision points along the way.

Conversion efforts regulations may represent movement toward legislation, or they may represent an effective substitute for legislation. After a failed attempt to pass statewide legislation, Utah developed professional licensing board regulations that reflect the same language found in YMHPAs. The regulations were ordered by a Republican governor and have the support not only of professional communities but also the Church of Jesus Christ of Latter-day Saints (Zaveri, 2020). Local ordinances, too, are a strategy to achieve the elimination of conversion efforts. At least 80 local ordinances have been passed in counties and cities, including in cities in considerably conservative areas in Kansas, Kentucky, and Alaska. Local ordinances and licensing regulations may use grassroots momentum to move state and finally federal legislation.

Several hallmark judicial decisions have supported the right of states to protect individuals, particularly youth, from the potential harms of conversion efforts. In *King v. Christie* (2013), a New Jersey state court case, conversion efforts legislation was upheld, with Judge Freda Wolfson concluding that the state law "restricts neither speech nor religious expression," and that the practitioners' challenge to the law "runs counter to the longstanding principle that a state generally may enact laws rationally regulating professionals, including those providing medicine and mental health services."

Opponents of conversion efforts have also sought to limit the practice on the theory that it constitutes an unfair business practice or commercial fraud. The court in *Ferguson v. JONAH* (2014) established a precedent for prosecuting practitioners under a state's existing consumer fraud protections. The court held that Jews Offering New Alternatives to Homosexuality (JONAH, a conversion efforts organization) violated the New Jersey Consumer Fraud Act by claiming that its services could change an individual's sexual orientation and that the failure of these claims resulted in substantial harm to the litigants. JONAH agreed to permanently cease operations as part of a settlement following a multimillion-dollar judgment. The JONAH case and others reflect both the damage done to many who have experienced conversion efforts and the power of the growing expert consensus that conversion efforts do not represent appropriate or effective treatment.

Beginning in 2015, members of Congress introduced the Therapeutic Fraud Prevention Act, which had more than 20 cosponsors. In the states, Illinois's legislation prohibiting conversion efforts directly amended the state's Consumer Fraud and Deceptive Business Practices Act; other states, including California, have introduced bills to do likewise. Proponents of conversion efforts assert that individuals have the freedom to select conversion efforts as a treatment and that LMHPs have the right to say what they want if it is religiously grounded. However, these claims have failed, especially when applied to minors, because of the well-established precedent that government may reasonably regulate and license the practice of medicine and professional conduct. It is not whether individuals have a right to their preferred "therapy" approach; it is that SGM have a right to be protected from dangerous and discredited practices masked as "help."

Although First Amendment claims have been rejected by two federal circuit courts of appeal (*King v. Christie*, 2013; *Pickup v. Brown*, 2012), interpretations of the scope of free speech protections are not static. Observers (Ford, 2018; Showalter, 2018) of the Clarence Thomas majority opinion upholding the right of pregnancy counseling centers to omit information from their speech to clients noted Thomas's connection to *Pickup*: "This Court has not recognized 'professional speech' as a separate category of speech. Speech is not unprotected merely because it is uttered by 'professionals'" (*National Institute of Family & Life Advocates v. Becerra*, 2018). At the same time, however, Thomas's opinion did reaffirm the power of states to regulate professional conduct, even when that conduct incidentally involves speech. Although proponents of conversion cling to Thomas's skepticism of the professional speech doctrine, advocates working to end conversion efforts continue to introduce and pass legislation secure in the state's ability to regulate activities that have no proven benefit and abundant evidence of harm as part of the government's duty to protect the health, safety, and well-being of residents.

Policy and judicial work in the United States has been happening in an international context of increasing recognition that conversion efforts are human rights violations. At the same time, it is becoming clearer that conversion efforts appear to be virtually ubiquitous (Bishop, 2019). In 2020, the Independent Expert on Protection Against Violence and Discrimination Based on Sexual Orientation and Gender Identity submitted to the United Nations Human Rights Council (UNHRC) a comprehensive investigation into conversion efforts. Around the world, conversion efforts are tied to pathologizing and unjustly stigmatizing views of SOGD and have been employed by a variety of persons, including health professionals, religious clergy, and clandestine groups. The UNHRC Investigator disavowed a religious basis for conversion and instead highlighted models of religious inclusivity. International communities are increasingly recognizing the lack of scientific basis for conversion efforts as well as physical and psychological injuries from conversion attempts (Bishop, 2019; UNHRC, 2020).

Citing the United Nations' (2013) consideration of conversion as consistent with torture, the 2020 report reinforces this classification when it is coercive or forced:

> Practices of "conversion therapy," based on the incorrect and harmful notion that sexual and gender diversity are disorders to be corrected, are discriminatory in nature. Furthermore, actions to subject lesbian, gay, bisexual, trans or gender-diverse persons to *practices of "conversion therapy" are by their very nature degrading, inhuman and cruel* and create a significant risk of torture. (UNHRC, 2020, p. 16, emphasis added)

Based on the recognition of the harm and stigma inherent in conversion efforts, international organizations call for reducing and preventing conversion efforts, including legislative bans and promotion of affirmative treatment and affirmative cultural norms for all SOGD (Bishop, 2019; UNHRC, 2020).

ADVOCACY STRATEGIES TO END CONVERSION EFFORTS

Some of the challenges and opportunities in the movement to end conversion efforts reflect the state of the larger political system, including difficulty gaining consistent bipartisan support for many initiatives. Other challenges might reflect the limits of respective fields. For example, social science and mental health often integrate a great deal of nuance in understanding gender and sexual orientation in contexts of faith, culture, and community; in contrast, the law can be a relatively blunt instrument. Some of the greatest challenges to the movement to end conversion efforts may be the breadth needed in advocacy approaches: support those in the margins of our communities to gain acceptance for all parts of ourselves, increase family and community acceptance, correct distortions in science, and prevent mental health professionals and others from exposing individuals to conversion efforts.

Although, by the time they are 18 years old, an estimated 57,000 youth will be exposed to conversion efforts by religious or spiritual practitioners who are not regulated by professional boards or laws that prohibit "conversion therapy," the first wave of YMHPAs, including in nine states and the District of Columbia, were estimated to help prevent conversion efforts being delivered to approximately 6,000 youth who live in those states with enacted protections (Mallory et al., 2018). In fact, due to efforts by national and state advocates against conversion efforts, 1,000 additional youth are estimated to have been protected against receiving "conversion therapy" from a licensed medical professional in 2018 alone (Brinton, 2018b). In 2019, the estimated number of protected youth in the 18 states with YMHPAs rose to 10,000 (Mallory et al., 2019). The passage of YMHPAs is a vital strategy for the movement to end conversion therapies.

Lessons in SOGD equality include a call to center the experiences and needs of those who are most affected by intersecting oppressive forces. There are increasing indications that the toll on marginalized youth is heavy; for example, in one survey, 57% of transgender and nonbinary youth who have experienced conversion attempts report a suicide attempt in the last year (Green et al., 2020). However, more research and community outreach are needed to connect resources for conversion efforts protections with those who are most affected by systemic inequalities, including transgender and gender nonconforming BIPOC youth and immigrant youth. Specifically, the link between family rejection and conversion efforts (e.g., Ryan et al., 2009, 2020) has downstream consequences on health, housing, and employment, particularly for gender minorities of color (James et al., 2016). Conversion attempts can magnify the impact of multiple stigmas and inequalities.

Research has begun to uncover manifestations and impacts of conversion efforts that might not be well-represented by mainstream portrayals of conversion. For example, transgender individuals in Southern Black communities might experience conversion efforts that include gate-keeping, violence, and church hurt (Hipp et al., 2019). These are not always framed as conversion efforts, even though they share common goals and stigma. LGBTQ youth with lower family incomes, from the South, whose parents use religion to say negative things about being LGBTQ, who are Hispanic/Latinx, and who are transgender or nonbinary have been overrepresented in reports of conversion efforts (Green et al., 2020). These data highlight that young people who report undergoing conversion efforts represent diverse backgrounds, and advocacy must confront the many ways conversion is experienced.

To begin to understand the impact of YMHPAs, more data collection is also needed. Whether BIPOC transgender, and gender nonbinary youth are being protected by developing protection acts is unknown. Rates of family acceptance for multiple marginalized youth in states with YMHPAs compared with those without them are also unknown. Intersectional policy analysis and research initiatives are needed to further understand this issue. At the same time, YMHPA advocates will need to address ongoing opposition, including by finding common ground and addressing conversion proponents' flawed claims, empirical and legal, that stall YMHPAs.

Like any other time when the political arena centers a debate on science, a significant challenge to ending conversion efforts is correcting the distortions of scientific literature, which can buoy antiequality efforts more broadly. Given pervasive distortions in this regard, it is worth clarifying that the traditional scientific method works by attempting to disconfirm a proposition, and regardless of one's philosophy of science, it is the conversion efforts proponents' burden of proof to demonstrate that their methods work and are safe. Having failed to do so, it is not the burden of proof of those targeted by conversion efforts to show that they were harmed and the methods are *not* effective; even so, evidence of harm has been gathered (e.g., Ryan et al., 2020; Shidlo & Schroeder, 2002). Research indicates that conversion efforts reinforce stigma (Davison, 1976; Tozer & Hayes, 2004), are an unfair burden on SGM, and are directly associated with harm. These harmful outcomes are important for making strong rationales to protect SGM, as reflected in other areas, where LGBTQ efforts have resulted in judicial and legislative progress.

Without credible evidence supporting conversion efforts, proponents may distort research discovering the nature of fluidity as though it lends credibility to conversion claims. Sexual fluidity describes the context-dependent nature of sexual responsiveness, regardless of sexual orientation. Diamond (2008) first described women's sexual fluidity in these terms:

> Though women—like men—appear to be born with distinct sexual orientations, these orientations do not provide the last word on their sexual attractions and experiences. Instead, women of all orientations may experience variation in their erotic and affectional feelings as they encounter different situations, relationships, and life stages. (p. 3)

Sexual fluidity does not equate to claims that external forces—packaged as therapeutic or otherwise—can manufacture such change. Similar claims about "persistence" rates among transgender and gender nonconforming youth can mistake fluidity for claims that intervention can alter the trajectory of gender identity.

Conversion efforts proponents sometimes use a false nature/nurture dichotomy in explanations for SOGD and emphasize the flaw in biological reductionist models of sexual orientation in particular. This reductionist model includes the false notion that if a human feature is not entirely biologically based, then it is a matter of "choice" or otherwise manipulatable. However, this is a straw person fallacy, a distortion of researchers' and advocates' claims about SOGD. Advocates working to end conversion attempts do not need biological essentialism to explain how conversion attempts are harmful, fail to show that they produce change, and are ethically and scientifically flawed (Diamond & Rosky, 2016). Regardless of what science discovers about how sexual orientation and gender develop, everyone deserves safe, affirming treatment.

Advocacy to end conversion efforts supports other equality goals and relies on making clear the direct and indirect negative consequences of conversion efforts. Direct harm includes exposure to stigma and discrimination in the conversion context (e.g., Shidlo & Schroeder, 2002). Indirect costs include the potential for conversion messages to bolster false ideas, for example, that SOGD is a matter of "choice," which is associated with prodiscrimination positions. Indeed, some of the value of YMHPAs may be in their expressive functions rather than prescriptive ones (George, 2017). Advocates against conversion efforts are fostering anticonversion and LGBTQ-affirming norms that may spread to religious practitioners and others who are not subject to regulation, potentially curbing the practice through culture change. More LGBTQ-affirming norms may also foster more supportive attitudes about other LGBTQ policy needs, such as nondiscrimination in employment and public accommodations (George, 2017). It is also important to distinguish what conversion efforts are not, including "free speech." False and harmful statements made by LMHPs in therapy are not acceptable; such statements are unethical (see Chapter 8, this volume), and when part of cultural stigma, they are also discriminatory.

Advocacy to end conversion efforts means people living longer, more satisfying, and more authentic lives, such that a step toward equality is a step toward health and wellness for individuals and communities. Advocates can connect to the movement to end conversion in many ways. The largest national campaign, *50 Bills 50 States*, which is run by The Trevor Project, the nation's crisis intervention and suicide prevention program for LGBTQ youth, helps to connect individuals to efforts to introduce protection acts in their states. As bills have developed through various state legislatures, sample legislation that utilizes these developments is available from advocacy organizations that provide consultation on developing policy strategies. Although each state and each locale has unique circumstances, several sections from bills are commonly included: legislative findings for historical context, definitions to provide legal recourse, and simple violation and enforcement mechanisms to protect minors.

Legislative findings include acknowledgment that same-gender attraction and behavior, as well as gender diversity, are normative variations of human expression and experience. In this area of legislation, it is it often important to establish that every major mental health association cautions against or opposes practices defined in the legislation as "conversion therapy," including the APA (2009, 2021a, 2021b), the American Psychiatric Association (2000), the American Academy of Pediatrics (1993), the American Medical Association (2017), the National Association of Social Workers (2015), the American Counseling Association (2013), the American School Counselor Association (Kull et al., 2018), the American Psychoanalytic Association (2012), the American Academy of Child and Adolescent Psychiatry (Adelson, 2012), the American Association of Sexuality Educators, Counselors, and Therapists (2017), the Pan American Health Organization (2012), and the American College of Physicians (Daniel et al., 2015).

A sample legislative definition of "conversion therapy" generally describes it as "any practices or treatments that seek to change an individual's sexual orientation or gender identity, including efforts to change behaviors or gender expressions or to eliminate or reduce sexual or romantic attractions or feelings toward individuals of the same gender." Although referring to these efforts as "therapy" is inaccurate, as described above, the term "conversion therapy" has retained practical utility in legislation and advocacy. The term also acknowledges the common context of these conversion efforts, and it communicates effectively by being carefully defined. It is important to also describe what "conversion therapy" is not in order to belay any fears of legislative overreach or to limit the therapeutically legitimate exploration and development of sexual orientation and gender identity. Other examples of what is not included in "conversion therapy" include affirmative counseling and support of gender-affirming transition.

Following the definition of "conversion therapy," legislation tends to then specify the violation and the subsequent enforcement mechanism, defining what will happen to a licensed medical professional who performs "conversion therapy" on a minor. The traditional violation simply states that no licensed provider shall engage in "conversion therapy" with a person under 18 years of age. The licensed medical professional in violation thereof is considered to have practiced "unprofessional conduct" and would be subjected to an investigation by and potential discipline from the practitioner's relevant professional licensing entity.

PROMISING TRENDS IN THE MOVEMENT TO END CONVERSION EFFORTS

Several promising trends characterize the ongoing work to end conversion efforts. Initial indications are that enacted laws are, in fact, protecting thousands of youth in several states (Brinton, 2018b; Mallory et al., 2018). Many YMHPAs are introduced in a variety of jurisdictions each legislative session; each time creates opportunities to provide more accurate information about SOGD and to lay the groundwork for a range of equality legislation. As of September 2020, 40 states across the country had submitted YMHPAs, with 20 states having passed such legislation or regulations. There are multiple signs of growing public support too, with more than 20,000 individuals joining *50 Bills 50 States* in 2018, and polls showing that 71% of Floridians and 80% of North Carolinians support protecting youth from conversion attempts (Kaplan, 2017; Nichols & Polaski, 2019).

Patterns in legislative behaviors also show promising levels of support. According to The Trevor Project, as of December 2018, over 2,136 legislators had voted for or sponsored legislation to protect minors from "conversion therapy" since the submission of the first bill in California in 2012. These votes continue to be bipartisan, with over 500 Republican lawmakers and six Republican governors supporting these efforts. In fact, rural cities across the country and traditionally conservative states, such as Kentucky, Idaho, and West Virginia, continue to be at the forefront of this conversation with strong bipartisan political support. Since the YMHPA was submitted in Utah for the first time in February 2019, the lack of opposition by the Church of Jesus Christ of Latter-day Saints and the sponsorship of the legislation by Republicans reminded the country that protecting youth from the harms of conversion efforts knows no political or religious bounds.

It is this important reminder of collaborative success that fuels the movement to pass legislation in every state across the country to protect LGBTQ youth from the harms of "conversion therapy." The number of states working to pass this legislation quadrupled in a matter of years. This movement has progressed faster than any other comparable LGBTQ movement, in large part thanks to groundwork having been laid for decades by mental health professionals recognizing the inherent dignity and mental health of LGBTQ people. From the halls of Congress to the courtroom to the movie screen, the legislative, litigative, and educative efforts of anticonversion therapy activists are bearing fruit.

Survivors of conversion efforts are stepping forward to perform survivor-based advocacy. As their stories are told and leaders in the faith and mental health community speak out against future harms, there will be even more legislative successes. And these successes will culminate in even more non-discrimination and equality movement successes as the reduction of sexuality and gender identity to a choice is removed, and the nation is reminded of a survivor's rallying call: "You can't change what I never chose."

REFERENCES

Adelson, S. L., & the American Academy of Child and Adolescent Psychiatry (AACAP) Committee on Quality Issues (CQI). (2012). Practice parameter on gay, lesbian, or bisexual sexual orientation, gender nonconformity, and gender discordance in children and adolescents. *Journal of the American Academy of Child & Adolescent Psychiatry, 51*(9), 957–974. https://doi.org/10.1016/j.jaac.2012.07.004

American Academy of Pediatrics, Committee on Adolescence. (1993). Homosexuality and adolescence. *Pediatrics, 92*(4), 631–634.

American Association of Sexuality Educators, Counselors, and Therapists. (2017). *Position on reparative therapy.* https://www.aasect.org/position-reparative-therapy

American Counseling Association. (2013). *Ethical issues related to conversion or reparative therapy.* https://www.counseling.org/news/updates/2013/01/16/ethical-issues-related-to-conversion-or-reparative-therapy

American Medical Association, Council on Scientific Affairs. (2017). *Health care needs of lesbian, gay, bisexual, transgender, and queer populations, H-160.991.* https://policysearch.ama-assn.org/policyfinder/detail/Health%20Care%20Needs%20of%20Lesbian,%20Gay,%20Bisexual%20and%20Transgender%20Populations%20H-160.991?uri=%2FAMADoc%2FHOD.xml-0-805.xml

American Psychiatric Association. (2000). Position statement on therapies focused on attempts to change sexual orientation (reparative or conversion therapies). *American Journal of Psychiatry, 157*(10), 1719–1721.

American Psychoanalytic Association. (2012). *Position statement on attempts to change sexual orientation, gender identity, or gender expression.* http://www.apsa.org/content/2012-position-statement-attempts-change-sexual-orientation-gender-identity-or-gender

American Psychological Association. (1997). Resolution on appropriate therapeutic responses to sexual orientation. *American Psychologist, 53*(8), 934–935.

American Psychological Association. (2009). Appropriate affirmative responses to sexual orientation distress and conversion efforts. *American Psychologist, 65*(5), 385–475. https://doi.org/10.1037/a0019553

American Psychological Association. (2014). *Amicus brief filed in* Obergefell v. Hodges. https://www.apa.org/about/offices/ogc/amicus/obergefell

American Psychological Association. (2015). Guidelines for psychological practice with transgender and gender nonconforming people. *American Psychologist, 70*(9), 832–864. https://doi.org/10.1037/a0039906

American Psychological Association. (2021a). *Resolution on gender identity change efforts.* https://www.apa.org/about/policy/resolution-gender-identity-change-efforts.pdf

American Psychological Association. (2021b). *Resolution on sexual orientation change efforts.* https://www.apa.org/about/policy/resolution-sexual-orientation-change-efforts.pdf

Balmer, R. (2014, May 27). The real origins of the religious right: They'll tell you it was abortion. Sorry, the historical record's clear: It was segregation. *Politico Magazine.* https://www.politico.com/magazine/story/2014/05/religious-right-real-origins-107133

Bieber, I., Dain, H. J., Dince, P. R., Drellich, M. G., Grand, H. G., Gundlach, R. H., Kremer, M. W., Rifkin, A. H., Wilbur, C. B., & Bieber, T. B. (1962). *Homosexuality: A psychoanalytic study.* Basic Books. https://doi.org/10.1037/11179-000

Bishop, A. (2019). *Harmful treatment: The global reach of so-called conversion therapy.* OutRight International Action. https://outrightinternational.org/reports/global-reach-so-called-conversion-therapy

Boy Scouts v. Dale, 706 A.2d 270 (N.J. Super. Ct. 1998), aff'd, 160 N.J. 562 (N.J. 1999), *rev'd and remanded,* 530 U.S. 640 (2000).

Brinton, S. (2018a, January 2). I was tortured in gay conversion therapy. And it's still legal in 41 states. *The New York Times.* https://www.nytimes.com/2018/01/24/opinion/gay-conversion-therapy-torture.html

Brinton, S. (2018b, December 27). I survived conversion therapy as a child. Now, I'm part of the movement to ban it for good. *USA Today.* https://www.usatoday.com/story/opinion/voices/2018/12/27/gay-conversion-therapy-lgbtq-law-harm-column/2413310002/

Bronski, M. (2012). *A queer history of the United States.* Beacon Press.

Butterworth, L. (2017). *Black Lives Matter co-founder Patrisse Cullors on intersectionality in activism: BUST interview by Bust Magazine.* https://bust.com/feminism/19122-the-making-of-a-movement-q-a-with-patrisse-cullors-of-blm.html

California Psychological Association. (2012, August 17). *California Psychological Association voices support for SB 1172 "(Lieu) Banning the use of sexual orientation conversion efforts (SOCE) with minors."* https://www.cpapsych.org/page/393

California S. B. 1172. Sexual orientation change efforts, 2011–2012 (2012). https://leginfo.legislature.ca.gov/faces/billTextClient.xhtml?bill_id=201120120SB1172

Collins, P. H. (2005). *Black sexual politics: African Americans, gender, and the new racism.* Routledge.

Collins, P. H., & Bilge, S. (2016). *Intersectionality.* Polity Press.

Daniel, H., Butkus, R., & the Health and Public Policy Committee of American College of Physicians. (2015). Lesbian, gay, bisexual, and transgender health Disparities: Executive summary of a policy position paper from the American College of Physicians. *Annals of Internal Medicine, 163*(2), 135–137. https://doi.org/10.7326/M14-2482

Davison, G. C. (1976). Homosexuality: The ethical challenge. *Journal of Consulting and Clinical Psychology, 44*(2), 157–162. https://doi.org/10.1037/0022-006X.44.2.157

Diamond, L. M. (2008). *Sexual fluidity: Understanding women's love and desire.* Harvard University Press.

Diamond, L. M., & Rosky, C. J. (2016). Scrutinizing immutability: Research on sexual orientation and U.S. legal advocacy for sexual minorities. *Journal of Sex Research, 53*(4–5), 363–391. https://doi.org/10.1080/00224499.2016.1139665

Drescher, J. (2010). Queer diagnoses: Parallels and contrasts in the history of homosexuality, gender variance, and the *Diagnostic and Statistical Manual. Archives of Sexual Behavior, 39*(2), 427–460. https://doi.org/10.1007/s10508-009-9531-5

Drescher, J. (2015). Out of *DSM*: Depathologizing homosexuality. *Behavioral Sciences, 5*(4), 565–575. https://doi.org/10.3390/bs5040565

Drescher, J., Schwartz, A., Casoy, F., McIntosh, C. A., Hurley, B., Ashley, K., Barber, M., Goldenberg, D., Herbert, S. E., Lothwell, L. E., Mattson, M. R., McAfee, S. G., Pula, J., Rosario, V., & Tompkins, D. A. (2016). The growing regulation of conversion therapy. *Journal of Medical Regulation, 102*(2), 7–12. https://doi.org/10.30770/2572-1852-102.2.7

Ferguson v. JONAH, 445 N.J. Super. 129 (N.J. Super. Ct. Law Div. 2014).

Fischer, J. (2019). *Virginia Board of Psychology votes to ban gay conversion therapy for minors.* https://www.wusa9.com/article/news/local/virginia/virginia-board-of-psychology-votes-to-ban-gay-conversion-therapy-for-minors/65-f832cb51-5612-44d9-bb6c-4f241e641d2b

Flores, A. R. (2014). *National trends in public opinion on LGBT rights in the United States.* Williams Institute. https://williamsinstitute.law.ucla.edu/wp-content/uploads/POP-natl-trends-nov-2014.pdf

Ford, Z. (2018). Is the Supreme Court poised to side with ex-gay conversion therapy? *Think Progress.* https://thinkprogress.org/supreme-court-ex-gay-therapy-78d7c1b00ac1/

Garcia, S. (2020). Virginia is first southern state to ban conversion therapy for minors. *The New York Times.* https://www.nytimes.com/2020/03/03/us/va-conversion-therapy-ban.html

George, M. A. (2017). Expressive ends: Understanding conversion therapy bans. *Alabama Law Review, 68*(3), 793–853.

Green, A. E., Price-Feeney, M., Dorison, S. H., & Pick, C. J. (2020). Self-reported conversion efforts and suicidality among US LGBTQ youths and young adults, 2018. *American Journal of Public Health, 110*(8), 1221–1227. https://doi.org/10.2105/AJPH.2020.305701

Griffith, R. M. (2017). *Moral combat: How sex divided American Christians and fractured American politics.* Basic Books.

Hatzenbuehler, M. L., McLaughlin, K. A., Keyes, K. M., & Hasin, D. S. (2010). The impact of institutional discrimination on psychiatric disorders in lesbian, gay, and bisexual populations: A prospective study. *American Journal of Public Health, 100*(3), 452–459. https://doi.org/10.2105/AJPH.2009.168815

Hegarty, P. (2018). *A recent history of lesbian and gay psychology: From homophobia to LGBT.* Taylor & Francis.

Herek, G. M. (2008). *Five years ago today: Reflections on* Lawrence v. Texas. https://herek.net/blog/five-years-ago-today-reflections-on-lawrence-v-texas/

Herek, G. M. (2011). Anti-equality marriage amendments and sexual stigma. *Journal of Social Issues, 67*(2), 413–426. https://doi.org/10.1111/j.1540-4560.2011.01705.x

Hipp, T. N., Gore, K. R., Toumayan, A. C., Anderson, M. B., & Thurston, I. B. (2019). From conversion toward affirmation: Psychology, civil rights, and experiences of gender-diverse communities in Memphis. *American Psychologist, 74*(8), 882–897. https://doi.org/10.1037/amp0000558

Hollingsworth v. Perry, 570 U.S. 693 (2013).

Hooker, E. (1957). The adjustment of the male overt homosexual. *Journal of Projective Techniques, 21*(1), 18–31. https://doi.org/10.1080/08853126.1957.10380742

James, S. E., Herman, J. L., Rankin, S., Keisling, M., Mottet, L., & Anafi, M. (2016). *The report of the 2015 U.S. Transgender Survey.* National Center for Transgender Equality.

Kaplan, D. (2017, April 13). Political climate forecast for Florida in 2018 looks positive for John Morgan, negative for gay conversion therapy, and uncertain on the future of American involvement in Syria. *Orlando Political Observer.* http://orlando-politics.com/2017/04/13/political-climate-forecast-for-florida-in-2018-looks-positive-for-john-morgan-negative-for-gay-conversion-therapy-and-uncertain-on-the-future-of-american-involvement-in-syria/

King v. Christie, 981 F. Supp. 2d 296 (D. N.J. 2013), *aff'd,* 767 F.3d 216 (3d Cir. 2014), *cert. denied,* 135 S. Ct. 2048 (2015).

Kull, R. M., Kosciw, J. G., & Greytak, E. A. (2018). Preparing school counselors to support LGBT youth: The roles of graduate education and professional development. *Professional School Counseling, 20*(1a). https://doi.org/10.5330/1096-2409-20.1a.13

Letter From Expert LGBTI Researchers. (2016, May 22). https://www.vumc.org/lgbti/files/lgbti/publication_files/ExpertLGBTIConcensusLetter.pdf

Maisel, N. C., & Fingerhut, A. W. (2011). California's ban on same-sex marriage: The campaign and its effects on gay, lesbian, and bisexual individuals. *Journal of Social Issues, 67*(2), 242–263. https://doi.org/10.1111/j.1540-4560.2011.01696.x

Mallory, C., Brown, T. N. T., & Conron, K. J. (2018). *Conversion therapy and LGBT youth.* The Williams Institute. https://williamsinstitute.law.ucla.edu/wp-content/uploads/Conversion-Therapy-Jan-2018.pdf

Mallory, C., Brown, T. N. T., & Conron, K. J. (2019). *Conversion therapy and LGBT youth: An update.* The Williams Institute. https://williamsinstitute.law.ucla.edu/wp-content/uploads/Conversion-Therapy-Update-Jun-2019.pdf

Mattachine Society of Washington. D.C. (2018). *The pernicious myth of conversion therapy: How love in action perpetrated a fraud on America.* http://www.nclrights.org/wp-content/uploads/2018/11/Mattachine-Society-Conversion-Therapy-White-Paper-Redacted.pdf

Mayeski, S. (2012, December 31). *Top ten events of 2012 in politics.* https://ivn.us/2012/12/31/top-ten-events-of-2012-in-politics/

McKinley, J., & Goodstein, L. (2008, November 5). Bans in 3 states on gay marriage. *The New York Times.* https://www.nytimes.com/2008/11/06/us/politics/06marriage.html

McNeill, J. M. (2019, April 5). State health officials take steps to ban conversion therapy. *AP News.* https://www.apnews.com/e34301d8e689497d8296ad67b56d205c

Merritt, J. (2015, October 6). The downfall of the ex-gay movement: What went wrong with the conversion ministry, according to Alan Chambers, who once led its largest organization. *The Atlantic.* https://www.theatlantic.com/politics/archive/2015/10/the-man-who-dismantled-the-ex-gay-ministry/408970/

Meyer, I. H. (2003). Prejudice, social stress, and mental health in lesbian, gay, and bisexual populations: Conceptual issues and research evidence. *Psychological Bulletin, 129*(5), 674–697. https://doi.org/10.1037/0033-2909.129.5.674

Minton, H. L. (2002). *Departing from deviance: A history of homosexual rights and emancipatory science in America.* University of Chicago Press.

National Association of Social Workers. (2015, May 1). *Sexual orientation conversion efforts (SOCE) and conversion therapy with lesbians, gay men, bisexuals, and transgender persons.* https://www.socialworkers.org/LinkClick.aspx?fileticket=IQYALknHU6s%3D&portalid=0

National Institute of Family & Life Advocates v. Becerra, 138 S. Ct. 2361 (2018).

Nichols, J. M., & Polaski, A. (2019). *Supermajority of NC Republicans and Democrats support protecting LGBTQ youth From "conversion therapy."* Protect Our Youth NC. https://bornperfectnc.org/bipartisanpolling.html

Nicolosi, J. (1991). *Reparative therapy of male homosexuality: A new clinical approach.* Jason Aronson.

Obergefell v. Hodges, 135 S. Ct. 2071 (2015).

Ohio Board of Psychology. (2016). *Advisory statement on sexual orientation change efforts.* https://psychology.ohio.gov/Portals/0/MISC%20PDFs/CONVERSION%20 THERAPY%20ADVISORY%20FINAL%204.14.16.pdf

Pan American Health Organization. (2012). *"Cures" for an illness that does not exist: Purported therapies aimed at changing sexual orientation lack medical justification and are ethically unacceptable.* https://www.paho.org/hq/dmdocuments/2012/ Conversion-Therapies-EN.pdf

Payne, E. (2013). Group apologizes to gay community, shuts down "cure" ministry. *CNN.* https://www-m.cnn.com/2013/06/20/us/exodus-international-shutdown/ index.html

Pew Research Center. (2016, September 28). *Vast majority of Americans know someone who is gay, fewer know someone who is transgender.* http://www.pewforum. org/2016/09/28/5-vast-majority-of-americans-know-someone-who-is-gay-fewer-know-someone-who-is-transgender/

Pickup v. Brown, 42 F. Supp. 3d 1347 (E.D. Cal. 2012, *aff'd,* 728 F.3d 1042 (9th Cir. 2013), *cert. denied,* 573 U.S. 945 (2014).

Regnerus, M. (2012). *New families structure study.* Inter-University Consortium for Political and Social Research. https://doi.org/10.3886/ICPSR34392.v1

Richards v. United States Tennis Ass'n, 93 Misc. 2d 713 (Sup. Ct., NY County, 1977).

Romer v. Evans, 517 U.S. 620 (1996).

Rostosky, S. S., Riggle, E. D. B., Horne, S. G., & Miller, A. D. (2009). Marriage amendments and psychological distress in lesbian, gay, and bisexual (LGB) adults. *Journal of Counseling Psychology, 56*(1), 56–66. https://doi.org/10.1037/a0013609

Russell, G. M. (2000). *Voted out: The psychological consequences of anti-gay politics.* New York University Press.

Ryan, C., Huebner, D., Diaz, R. M., & Sanchez, J. (2009). Family rejection as a predictor of negative health outcomes in White and Latino lesbian, gay, and bisexual young adults. *Pediatrics, 123*(1), 346–352. https://doi.org/10.1542/peds.2007-3524

Ryan, C., Toomey, R. B., Diaz, R. M., & Russell, S. T. (2020). Parent-initiated sexual orientation change efforts with LGBT adolescents: Implications for young adult mental health and adjustment. *Journal of Homosexuality, 67*(2), 159–173. https:// doi.org/10.1080/00918369.2018.1538407

Shidlo, A., & Gonsiorek, J. C. (2017). Psychotherapy with clients who have been through sexual orientation change interventions or request to change their sexual orientation. In K. A. DeBord, A. R. Fischer, K. J. Bieschke, & R. M. Perez (Eds.), *Handbook of sexual orientation and gender diversity in counseling and psychotherapy* (pp. 291–312). American Psychological Association. https://doi.org/10.1037/ 15959-012

Shidlo, A., & Schroeder, M. (2002). Changing sexual orientation: A consumer's report. *Professional Psychology, Research and Practice, 33*(3), 249–259. https:// doi.org/10.1037/0735-7028.33.3.249

Showalter, B. (2018). Supreme Court ruling protecting pregnancy centers dismantles "conversion therapy" bans, lawyer says. *The Christian Post.* https://www.christianpost. com/news/supreme-court-ruling-protecting-pregnancy-centers-dismantles-conversion-therapy-bans-lawyer-225555/

Socarides, C. W. (1978). The sexual deviations and the *Diagnostic Manual*. *American Journal of Psychotherapy, 32*(3), 414–426. https://doi.org/10.1176/appi.psychotherapy.1978.32.3.414

Spade, D. (2015). *Normal life: Administrative violence, critical trans politics, and the limits of law*. South End Press.

Spitzer, R. L. (2012). Spitzer reassesses his 2003 study of reparative therapy of homosexuality [Letter to the Editor]. *Archives of Sexual Behavior, 41*(4), 757. https://doi.org/10.1007/s10508-012-9966-y

Stryker, S. (2017). *Transgender history: The roots of today's revolution*. Seal Press.

Substance Abuse and Mental Health Services Administration. (2015). *Ending conversion therapy: Supporting and affirming LGBTQ youth* (HHS Publication No. 15-4928).

Tozer, E. E., & Hayes, J. A. (2004). Why do individuals seek conversion therapy? The role of religiosity, internalized homonegativity, and identity development. *The Counseling Psychologist, 32*(5), 716–740. https://doi.org/10.1177/0011000004267563

United Nations Human Rights Council. (February 2013). *Report of the Special Rapporteur on torture and other cruel, inhuman or degrading treatment or punishment* (A/HRC/22/53). https://www.ohchr.org/documents/hrbodies/hrcouncil/regularsession/session22/a.hrc.22.53_english.pdf

United Nations Human Rights Council. (May 2020). *Practices of so-called "conversion therapy": Report of the Independent Expert on protection against violence and discrimination based on sexual orientation and gender identity (A/HRC/44/53)*. https://www.ohchr.org/EN/Issues/SexualOrientationGender/Pages/ReportOnConversiontherapy.aspx

United States v. Windsor, 570 U.S. 744 (2013).

Virginia Board of Psychology. (2019). 125-9 Guidance document on the practice of conversion therapy, effective May 2, 2019. https://www.dhp.virginia.gov/psychology/psychology_guidelines.htm

Welch v. Brown, 58 F. Supp. 3d 1079 (E.D. Cal. 2014), aff'd, 834 F.3d 1041 (9th Cir. 2016).

YouGov. (2014). Brief for American Psychological Association et al., as amici curiae supporting plaintiff–appellee and in support of affirmance, *Windsor v. United States of America* (2012). View of LGBT people. http://cdn.yougov.com/cumulus_uploads/document/vvdwu87s7k/tabs_OPI_conversion_therapy_20140612.pdf

Zaveri, M. (2020). Utah is latest state to ban conversion therapy for children. *The New York Times*. https://www.nytimes.com/2020/01/22/us/utah-conversion-therapy-ban.html

Zinn, H. (2003). *A people's history of the United States: 1492–present*. Harper Collins.

10

SEXUAL ORIENTATION CHANGE EFFORTS AND GENDER IDENTITY CHANGE EFFORTS IN INTERNATIONAL CONTEXTS

Global Exports, Local Commodities

SHARON G. HORNE AND MALLAIGH McGINLEY

Sexual orientation change efforts (SOCE) and gender identity change efforts (GICE) occur in all regions of the world and have been documented in at least 68 countries (OutRight Action International, 2019; United Nations Human Rights Council, 2020). In a national survey of lesbian, gay, bisexual, and transgender (LGBT) participants in the United Kingdom, over 2,640 individuals (approximately 2% of the sample) reported undergoing conversion or reparative therapy and reported physical abuse, forced pregnancy, kidnapping, and other abuses (United Kingdom Government Equalities Office, 2019). Religious leaders and faith institutions appear to be primary perpetrators of SOCE/GICE in Africa, Latin America, and the Caribbean, but private and public mental health professionals are the most common perpetrators in Asia and many other regions of the world (OutRight Action International, 2019). SOCE/GICE by religious practitioners often involve exorcism or ritual cleanings via beatings or burnings during prayers, force-feeding, or food deprivation (Alempijevic et al., 2020). When SOCE/GICE are practiced by mental health professionals, these efforts typically take one of the following forms: psychotherapy; behavioral conditioning; electroconvulsive therapies

https://doi.org/10.1037/0000266-011
The Case Against Conversion "Therapy": Evidence, Ethics, and Alternatives,
D. C. Haldeman (Editor)

and aversive therapy treatments (e.g., electric shock to the hands or genitals and nausea-inducing drugs paired with homoerotic stimuli; medication, including antipsychotics, antidepressants, psychoactive drugs, and hormone injections; hypnosis, eye movement desensitization, or other trauma prevention therapies; hospitalization; Alempijevic et al., 2020).

This chapter explores the development and influence of SOCE/GICE in transnational contexts. First, we describe the historical development of transnational SOCE/GICE and the impact of religious teachings and colonization. Next, we explore SOCE/GICE in several areas of the world (i.e., India, Brazil, Russia, Hungary, and Uganda) and describe the particular challenges in each of these contexts. Finally, we cover international trends in SOCE/GICE and conclude with barriers and concerns related to SOCE/GICE, as well as strategies to combat global SOCE/GICE.

THE GLOBAL MOVEMENT TO END SOCE/GICE

Children and adolescents are most vulnerable to SOCE/GICE worldwide, due to pressures or coercion by family members, and these experiences may have lasting effects (OutRight Action International, 2019). Recalled exposure to GICE before age 10 has been found to be associated with increased odds of lifetime suicide attempts among transgender adults (Turban et al., 2020), and research has documented the negative impact of conversion therapy on mental health and psychological wellness, as well as its financial costs (e.g., Dehlin et al., 2015; Flentje et al., 2013).

The contemporary SOCE/GICE practices that use modern psychotherapy methods to attempt change efforts often require an infrastructure of mental health practice, typically formed from WEIRD (Western, Educated, Industrialized, Rich, and Democratic) constructions and institutions of psychology (Henrich et al., 2010). These WEIRD-informed psychologies have historically pathologized nonheteronormative sexualities and behaviors as well as gender nonconforming cisgender expressions and identities (Drescher, 2015). Historically, the United States has the highest number of reports of SOCE/GICE, as SOCE/GICE conversion practices took root at the same time as homosexuality was removed from the American Psychiatric Association's *Diagnostic and Statistical Manual of Mental Disorders (DSM)* in 1973. The Williams Institute estimates that 698,000 LGBT adults in the United States have received SOCE/GICE efforts at some point in their lives, including 350,000 LGBT adults who were exposed to efforts to reorient their sexual orientation and gender identity as minors (Mallory et al., 2019). In a large national nonprobability sample of 27,716 transgender individuals, 13.5% reported lifetime exposure to GICE, and approximately 5% reported exposure in the 5 years prior to the study (Turban et al., 2019).

Due to both greater awareness of the negative impact of these practices and the emergence of policies and guidelines issued by the major mental health organizations in the United States, SOCE/GICE appears to have declined, at least as practiced by licensed mental health professionals; and more than 20 states have passed laws to outlaw the use of SOCE/GICE with minors (see Chapter 9, this volume, for a full discussion).

Over the past decade, as efforts to discredit and deter SOCE and GICE have gained momentum in the United States, global attention to such concerns has also increased. Research indicates the emergence of international human rights norms pertaining to sexual orientation and gender identity (SOGI), which are reported to be steadily increasing (United Nations Human Rights Council, 2020). These norms include endorsement of human rights principles of universality, nondiscrimination, and equality pertaining to SOGI concerns; censure for the gravest human rights violations; prohibitions against violence and discrimination; and the obligation of the international community to respond to such violations (Baisley, 2016; Horne & Manalastas, 2020). Several international governing and advocacy groups have conducted official investigations into the prevalence and impact of SOCE and GICE across the globe, resulting in a series of formal reports condemning such practices. Following an investigation on protection against violence and discrimination based on sexual orientation and gender identity, in 2018, the United Nations Independent Expert presented such a report to the United Nations General Assembly of the Human Rights Council. The report stated that SOCE and GICE potentially constitute torture when state officials are involved, even if only by acquiescence, and it submitted a formal recommendation that nations ban all forms of SOCE and GICE.

The United Nations Independent Expert followed this exploration of SOGI violence and discrimination with a comprehensive and groundbreaking report of global practices of "so-called conversion therapy" (United Nations Human Rights Council, 2020). This report identified promoters and providers of SOCE/GICE, surveyed the scope of SOCE/GICE practices, and issued a series of recommendations to nation-states. The report condemned practices of conversion therapy as "discriminatory in nature" and recommended that nations ban practices of conversion therapy altogether. In addition, the report recommended defining prohibited conversion practices and banning the use of public funds to directly or indirectly support them, as well as any advertisements to promote them (United Nations Human Rights Council,

2020, p. 21). Additionally, the 2020 United Nations Human Rights Council report supported the creation of a system of sanctions for noncompliance with those SOCE/GICE bans; the supported sanctions would be commensurate with the severity of the violations, following the parameters for international human rights obligations on the "prohibition of torture and cruel, inhuman or degrading treatment or punishment" (p. 21). The report further recommended the establishment of mechanisms for support, as well as registration of complaints, to ensure that sexual and gender minorities with experiences of SOCE/GICE would be able to pursue reparations, rehabilitation, and legal support. It advocated for awareness campaigns regarding the ineffectiveness and lack of support for the use of SOCE/GICE, the development of affirmative mental health practices, the depathologization of SOGI diversity in health classifications and treatment, and the advancement of research on conversion therapy. Finally, the report called for the repeal of laws and policies that "enable, promote, or fuel practices" of conversion therapy and recommended the adoption of explicit antidiscrimination protections based on sexual orientation and gender identity (United Nations Human Rights Council, 2020, p. 22).

Both the 2018 and 2020 United Nations reports follow the United Nations High Commissioner for Human Rights (2015) report condemning conversion therapy as part of its mission to protect all persons—including lesbian, gay, bisexual, transgender, and intersex (LGBTI) individuals—from torture and other cruel, inhuman, or degrading treatment or punishment in custodial, medical, and other settings. The United Nations has reported that such therapies are unethical, unscientific, ineffective, and, in some instances, tantamount to torture. The 2015 report condemned a series of SOCE and GICE medical practices, including forced genital and anal examinations, forced and otherwise involuntary sterilization, and medically unnecessary surgery and treatment performed on or administered to intersex children (United Nations High Commissioner for Human Rights, 2015). A joint statement issued by 12 United Nations agencies, including the World Health Organization, cited SOCE practices as "unethical," "harmful," and a form of "abuse" (United Nations, 2015, p. 1).

In addition to the United Nations, other international organizations have declared SOCE and GICE practices unethical and ineffective. In 2011, the World Professional Association for Transgender Health released the *Standards of Care for the Health of Transsexual, Transgender, and Gender Nonconforming People*. The standards state that treatment efforts to change a person's gender identity and expression to become more congruent with sex assigned at birth are unethical. Further, in 2016, the World Psychiatric Association released a statement on SOCE/GICE indicating that such practices lack scientific evidence regarding efficacy and declaring SOCE/GICE unethical as purportedly treating something that is not a disorder.

Following a 2014 meeting of professional associations, regulators, and government departments, as well as both a decision by the National Health Service in England and campaigning groups in the United Kingdom (U.K.), a "Memorandum of Understanding on Conversion Therapy in the UK" (2017) was released; that document declared a shared commitment to protecting the public from the risks of conversion therapy. In the largest government survey to date, conducted in 2018, the U.K. government found that more than 2,000 LGBT people in a survey of 108,000 had reported receiving SOCE/GICE; the Prime Minister Teresa May vowed to end conversion therapy in the U.K. (LGBT Foundation, 2019). Although not finalized, the U.K. government has taken legislative steps toward a ban on the practice of conversion therapy (United Kingdom Government, 2021).

International empirical investigations have also found SOCE/GICE to be harmful. A 2012 report by the Pan American Health Organization found SOCE to lack medical indication and to represent a severe threat to the health and human rights of lesbian, gay, and bisexual individuals (Pan American Health Organization, 2012). The report asserted that such practices are unjustified and should be condemned, as well as subject to sanctions and penalties. The report included recommendations to government agencies, academic institutions, and professional associations regarding the depathologization of sexual diversity, as well as the need for interventions to prevent SOCE. Additionally, a consensus study by the Academy of Science of South Africa (2015), undertaken in collaboration with the Uganda National Academy of Sciences, reviewed the literature on the malleability of sexual orientation, the efficacy of SOCE, as well as the minority stress theory, and determined conversion therapy to be ineffective. They recommended the wide dissemination of these findings to health professionals across Africa and suggested that African health professionals and their associations should adopt affirmative stances toward LGBTI individuals, including psychosocial interventions to support the facilitation of adjustment to the stress, stigma, shame, and discrimination these individuals may face.

RELIGION-DRIVEN EFFORTS TO PERPETUATE SOCE/GICE

Despite such overwhelming global denouncement among governing bodies and professional mental health and medical organizations, the practice of SOCE/GICE is still common. Religion is the primary driving force that perpetuates SOCE/GICE.

Although Exodus International, which had been the largest ex-gay organization to endorse SOCE, was disbanded in 2013, Exodus Global Alliance, a separate but affiliated international coalition of ex-gay ministries, continues to operate with the mission of promoting conversion therapy practices globally through evangelical missionary work (Exodus Global Alliance, 2021a). Numerous other pro-SOCE and pro-GICE organizations have also formed: International Healing Foundation, Living Waters, Restored Hope Network, Hope for Wholeness Network, the Overcomers Network, Abiding Truth and Defending Family, Desert Streams, Global Mobilization Ministries, Teen Challenge, the Reintegrative Therapy Association, Family Watch International, Focus on the Family, and many others. In 2010, in Cape Town, 4,000 global evangelical leaders from 198 countries attended the "Third Lausanne Congress on World Evangelization," the largest gathering of global evangelical leaders in modern history (Queiroz et al., 2013). Exodus Global Alliance was a key leader in conference presentations, promoting the view that LGBT people need to be converted from "sinful" practices. *The Cape Town Commitment* (Lausanne Movement, 2011), which resulted from the Third Lausanne Congress gathering, was intended to serve as a road map for evangelical churches for the next decade (2011–2021); this call to action acknowledged that sexual identity and experience were "deep heart" issues, and that people who were drawn into "homosexual practice" should be treated with "love, compassion, and justice" (para. IIE, 2.A.4). However, it also clarified that "no person or situation is beyond the possibility of change and restoration," clarifying its stance on SOCE/GICE (Lausanne Movement, 2011, para. IIE, 2.A.5). Increasingly, conversion therapy practices have been rebranded as loving support for clients who struggle with same-sex attraction or gender identity, or folded into other treatment foci (e.g., substance use or family therapy; OutRight Action International, 2019).

A series of content and discourse analyses of "texts" from four of the leading ex-gay organizations—Exodus International, Exodus Global Alliance, the National Association of Research and Therapy of Homosexuality (NARTH), and Focus on the Family—explored the exportation of U.S. domestic ex-gay ministries into the global context (Robinson & Spivey, 2007, 2015; Spivey & Robinson, 2010). Such analyses have contributed to the understanding of international SOCE and GICE in relationship to evangelical Christianity missionary practices, which have grown steadily since the early 1970s, by increasingly investing resources in the political sphere and global expansion (Robinson & Spivey, 2007), and have led to WEIRD influences and neocolonization of many areas of the world, particularly the global South (Henrich et al., 2010). This transnational ex-gay movement is credited as the main purveyor of public antigay and lesbian rhetoric, contributing to the perpetuation of harmful SOCE/GICE practices and a conservative public policy agenda that promotes policies aimed at "genocide and the social death of LGBT people" (Robinson & Spivey, 2015; Spivey & Robinson, 2010, p. 70).

In the following sections, we share several examples of SOCE/GICE practices from regions around the globe. The examples illustrate a nation's stance toward its sexual and gender minorities, including LGBT people. The nation's attitude as to whether sexual and/or gender identities are alterable via SOCE/GICE is related to its developmental and cultural history (e.g., the role of colonization and organized religion), the particular sociocultural dimensions of how SOGI is stigmatized, and how mental health is construed and treatment given is provided (Horne, 2020). Although many factors have contributed to the stigmatization and marginalization of sexual and gender minority people, including political power expressed through authoritarianism, communism, neoliberal and colonizing practices; the influence of organized religions, such as Christianity and Islam; and indigenous communities that proscribed same-sex behaviors and gender nonconformity, the profound and disproportionate impact of Westernization, Christianity, and colonization on contemporary SOCE/GICE cannot be underestimated (Horne & Manalastas, 2020; OutRight Action International, 2019).

Although what follows is by no means a comprehensive review of the debate over so-called conversion therapies, our hope is that these cases portray a diverse perspective of global SOCE/GICE practices in the context of legislative action, the contributions of professional mental health organizations, and the global influence of conservative and evangelical Christianity.

India: The Lasting Impact of British Colonization

India, a country in South Asia, is the second most populous country in the world and the seventh largest in size. The constitutional republic is populated primarily by people who practice the religions of Hinduism and Islam. Although it is debated, precolonial India same-sex sexuality appears to not have been criminalized, or deemed sinful, and the concept of a third gender has long been part of Indian society. Since 2014, transgender Indians have had the right to change their identification from gender assigned at birth to their gender (but requires sex reassignment surgery), and/or identify as Third Gender as a social category. The legacy of British colonization and its imposition of criminality of same-sex sexuality through the adoption of Section 377 in 1861, however, has had deleterious effects on movement forward on LGBT rights in India.

In 2018, India made international headlines when its Supreme Court legalized same-sex sexuality. This overturned a 2013 judgment that had maintained the 157-year-old colonial-era law, Section 277, criminalizing "carnal intercourse against the order of nature with any man, woman, or animal," which was historically applied to same-sex sexuality and other "unnatural offenses" (BBC News, 2018). However, this decision was just one in a lengthy series of petitions and challenges to decisions both in disavowal and support of the law in the last 2 decades. A 2001 bid to repeal the law initiated was finally decided upon in 2009, when the Delhi High Court decided in favor of legalizing same-sex sexuality in the capital city (Timmons & Kumar, 2009). This decision was overturned in 2013 by the Indian Supreme Court, which reinstated the prohibition on certain sexual acts (Harris, 2013) and disproportionately affected those who were in same-sex relationships (BBC News, 2018).

Despite this 2018 decriminalization of same-sex sexuality, this result does not reduce the social and political pressures that reinscribe SOGI-related stigma in India and the rise of SOCE/GICE as a result. In the days following the 2009 decision overturning the prohibition on same-sex sexuality, a popular Hindu Guru, Swami "Baba" Ramdev, submitted a petition to India's Supreme Court claiming that homosexuality could be "cured" by yoga (Nelson, 2009). Then in 2013, just hours after the decision that upheld the criminalization of consensual sex between same-sex partners, he made a public offer to "cure homosexuals" at his ashram ("Ramdev offers," 2013). Ramdev had followers who were linked to senior Indian government ministers (Nelson, 2009), and *The New York Times* revealed, in a leaked 2015 announcement, that there were plans to initiate a state-sponsored program to assist young gay people to lead "a normal life" (Raj & Najar, 2015, para. 1). The Minister for Sports and Youth Affairs for the Indian state of Goa, Ramesh Tawadkar, announced a plan to set up "camps" to treat gay, bisexual, and transgender young people. Treatment would include counseling under Baba Ramdev's "expertise" in yoga instruction (Raj & Najar, 2015) and prescribed medicine to "make them normal" ("Minister Under Attack," 2015).

Although the minister's statement was summarily dismissed by State Chief Minister Laxmikant Parsekar, who condemned his cabinet colleague's "ignorance" and clarified that the government had no plans to set up such a program ("Minister Under Attack," 2015), the Goa State's antihomosexuality response and use of language was reminiscent of the historical teachings of the Christian missions of the 1540s, which categorized homosexuality as an "abomination" (Bhatia, 2015). The influence of Western Christianity in India is not merely a relic of the past. Exodus Global Alliance's online newsletter, *World News*, reports that, in 2010, Peter Lane stepped down from a 20-year tenure in his role as the director of Exodus South Pacific to launch a new ministry in India (Exodus Asia Pacific, 2021). Lane, under the guidance of Frank Worthen (then director of Love in Action) and Bob Davies (then the director of Exodus North America; Lane, 2021), were credited with building a platform for ex-gay ministries in Australia and New Zealand and ultimately forming a coalition under Exodus International (Exodus Global Alliance, 2021b).

Missionary work, such as Lane's, that aims to export Western ex-gay therapies continues to have implications both for the prevalence of SOCE practices in India and the political climate regarding legislative rights for LGBT people. SOCE practices have been offered by Catholic affiliate Indian organizations, such as Respect for Life India (n.d.), and lay doctors and "sexologists" throughout India (Sebastian & Vikram, 2015). A series of undercover videos released by *Mail Today*, a morning daily newspaper, revealed Delhi doctors offering to "cure" homosexuality with hormone therapy, seizure-inducing drugs, and even electric shocks (Mail Today, 2015a, 2015b; Sebastian & Vikram, 2015). The videos showed an essential lack of understanding regarding sexual orientation and gender identity among the doctors offering such practices. For example, one clinician promised to "cure" homosexuality with a hormone replacement therapy package and asserted that homosexuality in men is caused by higher levels of female hormones (Sebastian & Vikram, 2015). In 2018, a medical doctor was banned from medical practice by the Delhi Medical Council after it was discovered that he had been using electric shock and hormonal therapies with lesbian and gay patients (OutRight Action International, 2019). Such claims of cures demonstrate the lack of understanding of sexual orientation and gender identity, as practitioners offering such services often conflate the two. In a series of actions against conversion therapy, the Mumbai LGBTIQ organization, Humsafar Trust, engaged social media hashtags (e.g., #QueersAgainstQuacks, #Nothing2Cure) to create campaigns calling out false claims, promoting narratives of conversion harms, and challenging myths and misinformation (Baxter, 2016).

The fundamental assumption underlying SOCE, that homosexuality is a disease to be cured, has been used to argue for the continued prohibition of same-sex sexuality in India, as demonstrated in the most recent Supreme Court hearings regarding Section 377 (Withnall, 2018). During the final series of arguments in July 2018, two leaders of the evangelical community in India presented arguments opposing the legalization of same-sex sexuality, making Christianity the only faith represented in the opposition, as Hindu and Muslim religious groups had chosen not to oppose the decriminalization of Section 377 during the court hearings (Bhuyan, 2018).

The most recent ruling on Section 377 also demonstrated the importance of psychological professionals' contributions to the legislature's understanding of SOCE (Horne et al., 2019). In July 2018, just a month before the final hearings on Section 377, the Indian Psychiatric Society (IPS), the country's largest body of mental health professionals, released an announcement stating its official stance that homosexuality is not an illness (Pratap, 2018). We cannot know the full impact of this statement on the ultimate ruling to overturn Section 377, but it is noteworthy that one justice remarked in the ruling that homosexuality was "not an aberration, but a variation" just weeks after the IPS statement (Withnall, 2018). The process of legalizing same-sex sexuality in India highlighted the confluence of discourses emanating from Western and colonial historical influences—legal discourses surrounding the criminalization of homosexuality from the British colonial era that perpetuated the stigma and pathologization of SOGI; the assertion that SOCE/GICE could cure LGBT people through traditional methods (e.g., Ayurvedic treatment, homeopathy, yoga) and Western medical treatments (e.g., hormone replacement); and the disrupting discourses of the IPS, an institution similar in structure to Western psychiatry systems, which affirmed that homosexuality is a normal variation of sexuality (United Nations Human Rights Council, 2020).

China: The Persistent Pathologization of SOGI and SOCE/GICE in Mental Health Delivery

The People's Republic of China in East Asia is the most populous country in the world, with approximately 1.4 billion people. The majority of the population does not identify with an organized religion, and the government is a one-party socialist republic. Although there were many periods of history in which same-sex sexuality seems to have been common and not censured, during the founding of the People's Republic, particularly during the Cultural Revolution, homosexuality was persecuted (Hinsch, 1990; Wang et al., 2019). Same-sex sexuality was decriminalized in 1997, and transgender people have the right to change gender but only after sex reassignment surgery. Despite the 2001 declassification of homosexuality as a mental disorder by the Chinese Society of Psychiatry, pathologization of SOGI persists, and the National Health and Family Planning Commission has not updated its regulations to challenge (Human Rights Watch, 2017). As a result, conversion therapy is being practiced in many public and private hospitals throughout China (Glauert, 2019).

The current practice of SOCE/GICE in China reveals the limitations of statements by mental health organizations in determining policy. Although the Chinese Society of Psychiatry (CSP) released new guidelines in 2001 removing "homosexuality" from the Chinese Classification of Mental Disorders, a review by the Human Rights Watch of publicly available medical care regulations and guidelines of the National People's Congress and the National Health and Family Planning Commission indicated that there were no rules addressing conversion therapy (Human Rights Watch, 2017). Thus, clinics offering a "cure" for homosexuality remain a presence throughout China, as revealed by the undercover operations of a group of Chinese activists (Channel 4, 2015). Footage of these activists posing as patients seeking conversion therapy revealed the availability of aversion therapy, including electroshock treatments and prescription of nausea-inducing drugs, as techniques of SOCE/GICE. It has been reported that parents of recently "out" gay children are often the biggest proponents of conversion therapy (Channel 4, 2015; Human Rights Watch, 2017).

These anecdotal data were supported by a recently issued report from the Human Rights Watch, which presented findings from interviews conducted with 17 gay, lesbian, and transgender people who had undergone conversion therapy between 2009 and 2017 (Human Rights Watch, 2017). The interviews revealed that treatments were carried out in a variety of settings, including private psychiatric clinics and State-run hospitals. The influence of parents and families in the admissions process was nearly universal, and several cases involved parents or other family members physically and forcibly escorting the individuals to the treatment facilities. All interviewees said they were treated without their consent, and five were confined against their will at psychiatric hospitals or in the mental illness division of a hospital. Interviewees reported experiences likely to produce untold physical and psychological ramifications, including verbal harassment, forced administration of unidentified medication, and electroshock therapy. Investigations conducted by Queer Comrades, the Beijing LGBT Center, the United Nations Development Programme (UNDP), as well as OutRight Action International (2019) have all found reports of conversion therapy in China.

Such practices have resulted in two landmark civil suits in China. In 2014, a Beijing court awarded 3,500 yuan ($563) in compensation to Mr. Yang Teng, the plaintiff in a lawsuit against a psychiatric counseling center that administered hypnosis and electric shock treatments in an attempt to cure his homosexuality (Chin, 2014). However, although the court additionally ordered the clinic to post a public apology and to suspend any form of conversion therapy, as well as ordered an investigation into the clinic's license, the decision has not deterred the practice of conversion therapy at that clinic (Chin, 2014; Human Rights Watch, 2017). According to Human Rights Watch (2017), the clinic reopened within a few months with the same name, at the same location, and run by the same psychiatrist; as of 2017, it still offered conversion therapy services. The report by the Human Rights Watch also detailed a second lawsuit, brought by a former patient of a public hospital, for admitting the plaintiff against his will and forcing him to undergo conversion therapy. The ruling favored the plaintiff, finding that his rights were violated by his forced admission. Neither ruling, however, addressed the issue of conversion therapy itself, thus the rulings are unlikely to deter future perpetrators from engaging in SOCE. The Human Rights Watch has not been able to find any steps taken by the CSP in response to either ruling regarding conversion therapy.

The proliferation of SOCE in China did not occur in a vacuum. An anthropological investigation of Western influence on Asian LGBT rights advocacy reported that cultural perceptions of homosexuality in China are a direct exportation of Western values, as the Western scientific and medical perspective of homosexuality as pathological has engendered open hostility toward homosexuality in Chinese culture, as indicated by the rise of labor camps and electroshock practices (Laurent, 2005). This exportation has continued in the propagation of Western evangelical ex-gay ministries in East Asia, such as those under the direction of Exodus Global Alliance (Exodus East Asia, 2008). These practices continue despite the Chinese Psychological Society's explicit prohibition of sexual orientation discrimination and may be connected to the retention of "sexual orientation disorders" in the Chinese Classification of Mental Disorders (CCMD-3). In 2019, artists and activists launched a campaign against "conversion therapy" by emblazoning on the sides of trucks messages that questioned why these disorders were still retained (Taylor, 2019). To date, though, there have been no regulations or laws banning conversion therapy in China, and the financial incentives for hospitals, clinics, and psychiatric centers are enticing; therefore, SOCE/GICE treatment is widely available (Glauert, 2019).

Brazil: The Merging of Western Evangelical and Local Organized Religion on SOCE/GICE Efforts

The Federative Republic of Brazil is the largest country in South and Latin America, with approximately 211 million people. The primary religion in Brazil is Roman Catholic, and it is the only Portuguese-speaking country in the Americas. Brazil has been one of the most progressive countries for

SOGI rights, ushering in marriage rights in 2013, and rights to change one's legally listed gender have existed since 2009. It was also the first country to ban conversion therapy; however, SOCE/GICE continues through organized religious efforts.

The site of one of the world's largest annual gay pride parades, Brazil is often considered a leader in LGBT protections in Latin America. A world survey released by the International Lesbian, Gay, Bisexual, Trans, and Intersex Association reported that, as of 2017, Brazil was one of only three countries globally with provisions in place banning conversion therapy for licensed psychologists (Carroll & Mendos, 2017); passed in 1999, Resolution 1/99 was expanded in 2018 beyond sexual orientation to include gender identity and expression. However, recent years have seen a series of court decisions regarding the ban. Controversy followed a class-action suit brought by a group of psychologists, including one whose license was revoked in 2016 after she offered conversion therapies (Morais, 2017; Paletta & Goodwin, 2017). In September 2017, Federal Judge Waldemar de Carvalho overruled the 1999 decision by the Federal Council of Psychology (CFP) that forbade psychologists from offering treatments that claimed to "cure" gay people; instead, the court ruled in favor of Rozangela Justino, an evangelical Christian and practicing psychologist (Phillips, 2017). This injunction threatened to leave psychologists free to offer conversion therapy to "treat" homosexuality and prevented the CFP from prohibiting psychologists in Brazil from providing such treatments (Szpacenkopf & Guerra, 2017).

Facing a flood of international backlash (Morais, 2017), 3 months later, Judge Carvalho ultimately amended his decision and ruled that mental health professionals may provide care to people with "egodystonic sexual orientation" and can promote studies on the subject (Rodrigues & Morais, 2017, para. 2). The final ruling, however, eventually reinstated the power of the CFP to penalize psychologists who pathologize SOGI, and it reinstated the provisions of Resolution 1/99 (Rodrigues & Morais, 2017). Efforts to overturn Resolution 1/99 in favor of evangelical ex-gay practices are not a recent occurrence; in 2013, members of the evangelical caucus introduced a bill arguing that the resolution limits freedom of expression and psychologists' freedom of exercising their profession (Queiroz et al., 2013). Although it was later abandoned, this bill was initially approved by the Commission for Human Rights of Brazil's lower house of Congress (Carroll & Mendos, 2017), when the conservative, evangelical Social Christian Party secured the presidency, vice-presidency, and two thirds of the seats of the Human Rights and Minorities Commission of the House of Deputies that same year (Queiroz et al., 2013). Rev. Silmar Coelho, a Methodist minister, and his son, Filipe, who ran the Brazilian branch of Pat Robertson's American Center for Law and Justice, were linked to the development and support of the 2013 proposed legislation (Murphy, 2013).

In fact, the history of SOCE/GICE in Brazil is intimately tied to Western evangelical ex-gay ministries. According to an investigative report on SOCE in Latin America by the think tank Political Research Associates (PRA), Exodus Latin America, founded in 1994 and now based in Mexico, and its spinoff, Exodus Brasil, founded in 2002, remain under the umbrella of Exodus Global Alliance (Queiroz et al., 2013). Although there is a reported fundamental split between the two groups (Exodus Brasil states that the only way to be "healed" of homosexuality is through independently accepting Jesus, while Exodus Latin America promotes the efficacy of pastoral counseling services to the same end), both groups continue to actively promote SOCE/GICE in the region. In addition, the PRA report described the activities of Desert Stream/ Aguas Vivas, a network of ex-gay ministries operating in Latin America that was originally launched by the U.S.-based Desert Stream Ministries, whose practitioners are reportedly not trained mental health professionals. These perpetrators of SOCE/GICE continue to offer quasipsychological interpretations of injuries that supposedly produce homosexuality.

According to its website, Aguas Vivas remains networked with Exodus Latin America and NARTH (Desert Stream/Living Waters Ministries, 2021), and continues to export Western evangelical ideology regarding SOCE/GICE in the global context. The propagation of the belief that homosexuality can be "healed" is endorsed by Brazilian President Bolsonaro, who is reported to have said that he would rather have a dead son than a gay one, and that homosexuality was a result of a lack of beatings (Lopes, 2018). Lopes reported that Bolsonaro's remarks preceded a recent string of attacks on LGBT people by his supporters and heightened fears that homophobic violence has increased during his presidency. In recent developments, Jean Wyllys, a gay Brazilian lawmaker, resigned amid death threats, suggesting that the efforts to prevent a backsliding of LGBT rights, including the spread of SOCE/GICE, may be threatened (Biller, 2019).

Uganda: The Wholesale Western Exportation of SOCE/GICE

Uganda is a landlocked country located in East Africa with a population of approximately 43 million people. Christianity is practiced by the majority of the country, and the government is a presidential republic—President Museveni has been in office since 1986. Same-sex sexuality is illegal and can carry a penalty of life imprisonment; there are no rights for name change or other gender rights for transgender people. Western-style mental health services are limited in the country, but there are religious healing practices devoted to SOCE/GICE.

Perhaps the best-known example of the exportation of evangelical Christian policy agendas and influence on LGBT people is the case of Uganda. In 2009, several U.S.-based anti-LGBT advocates, including Scott Lively of Abiding Truth and Defend the Family, Don Schmierer of the former ex-gay group Exodus International, and Caleb Lee Brundidge, a representative of the International Healing Foundation, were invited by a Ugandan organization, the Family Life Network, to attend a workshop on the "Homosexuals Agenda," which contributed to the creation of the Ugandan Anti-Homosexuality Bill. This bill, dubbed the "Kill the Gays Bill" by LGBT activists, was signed into law in 2013; it widened criminalization of and violations for same-sex relations, including life imprisonment. It also penalized any abetting and aiding of same-sex sexual acts or relationships, including marriage. In 2014, the bill was declared unconstitutional. Lively, who had written a book that made the false claim that the Nazi party was led by gay men who were ultimately responsible for the Holocaust, made the case that LGBT people were intent on destroying the family and that abortion was a focus of the gay agenda. He emphasized Uganda's role as a last resort in stopping the progress of the LGBT movement. Lively also consulted with politicians and government workers, who would eventually support the drafted bill. The Parliament's Principal Research Officer, Charles Tuhaise, noted that Lively played an important role in influencing the Ugandan Parliament (Global Philanthropy Project, 2018).

With the passage of the bill, in 2014, a local newspaper printed photos of 200 LGBT people, outing many. Following Lively's visit and the proposed bill, David Kato, a Ugandan gay activist, was murdered after his name was listed in a similar local publication. Lively defended himself by stating that he recommended treatment, presumably in the form of SOCE/GICE, rather than imprisonment. The Ugandan example is a clear example of the neo-colonialist connection between Western-based religious extremism and nations with colonial pasts; several White U.S. religious leaders were provided access to the governing powers of a nation with the aim of furthering an anti-LGBT political agenda. They were assisted by the leader of a local Ugandan organization who had been responsible for the flow of developmental funds that had been earmarked for HIV funding in Uganda (Global Philanthropy Project, 2018).

Other countries in Africa that have strong anti-LGBT influences that are connected to U.S.-based movements and are reported to have significant SOCE/GICE, include Ghana, Nigeria, and Kenya, which are largely connected with U.S.-based Evangelical Protestant denominations, and Cameroon, which has a strong anti-LGBT stance influenced by Catholic faith organizations (Global Philanthropy Project, 2018). At the same time, other forms of SOCE/GICE are found in Sub-Saharan Africa, including acts of ritual cutting, forced fasting, beatings with brooms, and corrective rape (OutRight Action International, 2019). With the exception of South Africa, professional psychology is not established and rarely offers a counter to these practices of SOCE/GICE (Horne et al., 2019).

Russia: The Use of State-Sanctioned Homophobia/Transphobia for Political Aims

The Russian Federation is the largest country in the world, spanning the eastern side of Europe to the north of Asia, and it is home to approximately 146 million people. The primary religion is Russian Orthodox, and the government is considered a constitutional republic; however, President Putin has been in leadership since 1999, and he has extended his rights to the office until 2036. Although same-sex sexuality is not illegal and transgender people have the right to change their official gender following sex reassignment surgery, sexual and gender minority rights are limited and LGBT lives are restricted (Horne & White, 2019). Despite an established mental health system and a Russian Psychological Society ethics code that explicitly states that psychologists should respect individual and cultural differences, including sexual orientation and gender, and not to discriminate based on these personal characteristics, SOCE/GICE may continue due to persistent negative attitudes about LGBT people.

Russia presented a tremendous opportunity for the development of religious interests following the dissolution of the Soviet Union, which historically forbade organized religion. Along with the rise of the Russian Orthodox Church in Russia, there has been some influence from U.S.-based anti-LGBT advocates, which may have contributed to the passage of the damaging *2013 Propaganda Ban on Non-Traditional Sexual Relations,* which bans any representation of nontraditional sexual relations in the presence of minors in public and on social media. In 2006–2007, Lively held a speaking tour of 50 cities in Russia, espousing anti-LGBT rhetoric, connecting LGBT activism to Nazism and the destruction of the family, and constructing homosexuality as a personality disorder (Southern Poverty Law Center, 2021). At the conclusion of this speaking tour, Lively distributed a letter addressed to the Russian people advocating for anti-LGBT laws and measures; many of these cities later passed anti-LGBT legislation. Following the passage of the federal Propaganda Ban, Lively suggested he may have played a role and rejoiced in its passage. Since the Propaganda Ban, many LGBT organizations have shuttered, significant legal cases have been brought (e.g., against Deti-404, a website for LGBT and questioning youth), and hate crimes on the grounds of sexual orientation and gender identity have increased (Coalition of Civil Society Organizations, 2017). The most egregious example of what has occurred in Russia is the alleged torture and murder of gay men and lesbians from Chechnya, who were rounded up in police stings (Vasilyeva, 2019).

The role of U.S. evangelicals in Russian policy appears to be deep. Brian Brown, the president of the World Congress of Families and the National Organization of Marriage, visited Russia in 2016 to cultivate ties with members of the United Russia political party. He also sought funds from private donors to support these initiatives (Global Philanthropy Project, 2018). It is likely that these religious organizations, along with the teachings of the Russian Orthodox Church, are having an impact on mental health treatment for LGBT individuals in Russia; strong negative attitudes toward LGBT people in Russia continue (Horne et al., 2017). Although homosexuality was removed from official listing as a mental disorder in 1999, and the Russian Psychological Society has taken a firm position against SOCE/GICE, there have been many reports of SOCE/GICE and institutionalization of sexual and gender minority youth (Golubeva, 2017; Horne et al., 2009). In addition, the delivery of mental health treatment is unregulated in Russia, and there is no standard mechanism to censure therapists who engage in such treatments. Indeed, LGBT people have reported SOCE/GICE by mental health professionals that vary from subtle suggestions of change to aversion therapies and, in general, Russian psychologists are wary of treating LGBT minors for mental health issues due to the ban (Sabunaeva, personal communication, 2018).

Hungary: Copycat Laws and Anti-LGBT Political Football

Hungary is a moderate-size country in Eastern Europe with a population of about 10 million. The primary religion is Christianity, and it is part of the European Union. Hungary has a democratic parliamentary government; its leader, Prime Minister Victor Orban, has been in office since 2010. Same-sex sexuality is legal; however, marriage is prohibited for same-sex couples, and legal gender change was banned in 2020. Due to its far-right government, and anti-LGBT stance, sexual and gender minorities are exposed to SOCE/GICE efforts.

With Russia's legislative attack on LGBT people considered a success, Lively praised Vladimir Putin in an open letter in 2013 and then set his sights on Hungary. Lively wrote a letter to the Hungarian people suggesting that their leadership adopt the same type of antipropaganda law as was enacted in Russia. Hungary's right-wing government has been an oasis for anti-LGBT efforts, and, in 2017, President Orban welcomed the convention of the World

Congress of Families, which was designated a hate group by the Southern Poverty Law Center due to its anti-LGBT stance and its support for SOCE/ GICE (Tait, 2017). Recently, Hungarian State television aired interviews with a priest and two journalists who argued that homosexuality could be cured, and Hungary was selected as the site for a conference of a spinoff organization, the Reintegrative Therapy Association, formed following the death of NARTH's director in 2017 (Németh, personal communication, 2019). In May of 2020, during the COVID-19 pandemic, Orban ushered in legislation that ended the legal recognition of transgender persons, and redefined gender on the basis of sex at birth, as indicated by birth certificate, rendering transgender individuals vulnerable to discrimination, harm, and violence (Reynolds & Cotovio, 2020). Increasingly, U.S.-based and European anti-LGBT religious organizations are drawn to countries that are undergoing political or economic challenges and have been favorable to extreme-right positions (Kuhar & Paternotte, 2017; Sleptcov, 2018). Hungarian psychologists have been working to counter these efforts, although the fact that organized SOCE/GICE efforts are feeling welcome in Hungary is concerning, may increase SOCE/GICE.

FUTURE OF SOCE/GICE IN INTERNATIONAL CONTEXTS

A number of challenges remain in preventing the global spread of SOCE/GICE. First, international efforts to support affirming SOGI concerns are stymied; it is estimated that only .04% of official developmental support funds are allocated for sexual and gender minority concerns, and the vast majority of those funds have been prioritized for HIV/AIDS and human rights emphases. It is estimated that sexual and gender minorities make up a minimum of 4% of a population, suggesting that developmental dollars are at a minimum 100 times under the population's needs (UNDP, 2018). It is unknown how much developmental support religious congregations provide for SOCE/GICE, but that amount likely exceeds the developmental dollars specifically earmarked for mental health, including addressing SOCE/GICE.

Second, anti-LGBT concerns provide for a mechanism for coalition building among religious organizations that have not always historically seen eye to eye. Interreligious alliances involving Islamic, Protestant Evangelical, Mormon, and Catholic faiths have been formed around a common agenda: "U.S. politics seems to be the engine of the religious conservative activism working from the civil society in international scenarios, in a search for exporting local 'culture wars' to global arenas" (Global Philanthropy Project, 2018, p. 21; Kuhar & Paternotte, 2017). At global conventions and meetings, these coalitions are able to pool resources and coordinate actions to influence local and national priorities. In addition, LGBT refugee and asylum seekers will likely continue to be impacted by discrimination and marginalization in refugee camps; many resettlement organizations are faith-based and may be biased against or discriminatory toward LGBT asylum seekers and refugees (United Nations Commissioner for Human Rights, 2015).

Third, with the removal of homosexuality from the *DSM* and the *International Classification of Diseases, 11th Revision (ICD-11)*, and the removal of gender dysphoria from the mental health section of the *ICD-11* (although it remains in the sexual health section), the urgency around depathologization may be waning, at least in professional organizations and international bodies. In other words, there may be less of a need to defend against the pathologization of SOGI within mental health systems, and SOGI concerns may cease to be the purview of professional psychology and mental health organizations. Even many of the major ex-gay organizations have conceded that sexual orientation and gender identity are not alterable through therapeutic means. However, same-sex desire and gender nonconformity are being refashioned as moral and religious concerns, rather than psychological illnesses, and a celibacy movement has arisen in response (Freeman-Coppadge & Horne, 2019; OutRight Action International, 2019). In addition, struggles with one's sexual orientation are now treated as a symptom of treatment of addiction and trauma (e.g., in the new reintegrative therapy), so that SOCE/GICE may occur under the guise of substance use or PTSD treatment. Rather than emphasizing shame and pathology, new versions of SOCE/GICE in many areas of the world reflect a discourse of "choice," claiming that it is a client's right to be congruent with one's religious faith, even if that means abstinence or celibacy. It remains to be seen how this "kinder, gentler" version of "love the sinner, but hate the sin" will play out in places that have been hostile historically toward LGBT people. There are opportunities, however, for increasing supports for LGBT people who are struggling with conflict between SOGI and religion that do not involve SOCE/GICE. Many faiths have established affirming congregations, and all of the major religions have LGBT-affirmative organizations to support sexual and gender minorities; attending an affirming faith community has been found to be related to increased psychological wellness and greater spiritual well-being (Lease et al., 2005). Many of these faith communities have congregations and ministries that are global in scope, although they may not be as prevalent or widespread as evangelical ministries.

Although LGBT concerns have proved to be politically expedient in many places (e.g., Russia, Brazil, the United States), even in the most repressive countries and communities, LGBT activists are working toward justice and advocating for human rights (Horne & Manalastas, 2020; Horne et al., 2019).

These activists are increasingly aware of and informed about international standards and guidelines for LGBT concerns, and globalization has assisted with advancing and engendering transnational LGBT movements (Thoreson, 2014). In addition, mental health organizations are collaborating to take a stand on LGBT concerns and working towards inclusive SOGI ethics at the international level and focusing more specific efforts on transnational concerns (McGinley & Horne, 2020). For example, psychological organizations from more than 40 national and international organizations, including the Russian Psychological Society; all major psychology organizations in Brazil, Cameroun, South Africa, Bangladesh, Lebanon; the Hong Kong Psychological Society; and the Hungarian Psychological Society endorsed a shared statement in support of LGBT rights, and this statement proscribes SOCE/GICE (Horne et al., 2019; International Psychology Network for Lesbian, Gay, Bisexual, Transgender, and Intersex Concerns, 2018). It is now published in 10 languages, and recent endorsers, such as Polish psychological organizations, have used the statement to advocate for greater support and awareness of LGBT rights within professional psychology.

Finally, although there have been setbacks in legal and political rights in some countries, the explicit condemnation of conversion therapies by the U.N. Independent Expert on Sexual Orientation and Gender Identity, Victor Madrigal-Borloz, to the Human Rights Council is a major move forward on SOCE/GICE prevention and awareness. Moreover, the linkage of some SOCE/GICE practices with international resolutions on torture is an important reconceptualization and condemnation of these practices. As they attain more rights, sexual and gender minorities in different cultures and communities are constructing their own SOGI identities, norms, and supports. There is a great interest in reclaiming LGBT local history and communicating expectations for mental health within one's own cultural context. Recent LGBTI treatment guidelines crafted by the Psychological Society of South Africa (2017) and the nondiscrimination statement of the Psychological Association of the Philippines are exemplary cases in point (Manalastas & Torre, 2016). In addition, activist initiatives condemning conversion therapy, such as those described in China and India, are raising awareness of harmful practices more broadly.

Perhaps the greatest defense against SOCE/GICE will be sexual and gender minorities' freedom to define themselves and to openly express love and affection without interference from state and religious authorities. Globalization is having an impact on information flow and access to affirmative scientific literature, LGBT organizing, and transnational dialogue and support; and, over time, as in the recent case of India, justice often prevails. In the meantime, it is imperative that psychologists and other mental health professionals contest the fallacies and harms of SOCE/GICE and provide affirming mental health supports and policies for sexual and gender minorities throughout the world.

REFERENCES

Alempijevic, D., Beriashvili, R., Beynon, J., Birmanns, B., Brasholt, M., Cohen, J., Duque, M., Duterte, P., van Es, A., Fernando, R., Fincanci, S. K., Hamzeh, S., Hansen, S. H., Hardi, L., Heisler, M., Iacopino, V., Leth, P. M., Lin, J., Louahlia, S., . . . Viera, D. N. (2020). Statement on conversion therapy. *Journal of Forensic and Legal Medicine, 72*, 101930. https://doi.org/10.1016/j.jflm.2020.101930

Baisley, E. (2016). Reaching the tipping point? Emerging international human rights norms pertaining to sexual orientation and gender identity. *Human Rights Quarterly, 38*(1), 134–163. https://doi.org/10.1353/hrq.2016.0009

Baxter, R. M. (2016, May 17). #QueersAgainstQuacks: Gay community reminds Indian doctors that there is #NothingToCure. *Scroll.in.* https://scroll.in/article/808048/queersagainstquacks-gay-community-reminds-indian-doctors-that-there-is-nothingtocure

BBC News. (2018, September 6). *India court legalises gay sex in landmark ruling.* https://www.bbc.com/news/world-asia-india-45429664

Bhatia, K. (2015, January 16). *The imperial and religious roots of anti-homosexuality legislation in the Global South and Eastern Europe.* NATO Association of Canada. http://natoassociation.ca/the-imperial-and-religious-roots-of-anti-homosexuality-legislation-in-the-global-south-and-eastern-europe/

Bhuyan, A. (2018, July 18). At Supreme Court, all three religious groups backing Section 377 are Christian. *The Wire.* https://thewire.in/lgbtqia/at-supreme-court-all-three-religious-groups-backing-section-377-are-christian

Biller, D. (2019, January 24). *Gay Brazilian congressman resigns, citing death threats.* Bloomberg. https://www.bloomberg.com/news/articles/2019-01-24/gay-brazilian-congressman-resigns-his-seat-citing-death-threats

Carroll, A., & Mendos, L. A. (2017). *State-sponsored homophobia: A world survey of sexual orientation laws: Criminalisation, protection and recognition* (12th ed.). International Lesbian, Gay, Bisexual, Trans and Intersex Association (ILGA). https://ilga.org/downloads/2017/ILGA_State_Sponsored_Homophobia_2017_WEB.pdf

Channel 4 (Producer). (2015). China's gay shock therapy [Television series episode]. In *Unreported World.* https://www.channel4.com/programmes/unreported-world/on-demand/60446-009

Chin, J. (2014, December 19). Chinese court rules against clinic in country's first "gay conversion" case. *The Wall Street Journal.* https://blogs.wsj.com/chinarealtime/2014/12/19/chinese-court-rules-against-clinic-in-countrys-first-gay-conversion-case/

Coalition of Civil Society Organizations. (2017). *The situation of LGBT persons and men who have sex with men.* Submitted for the consideration of the 6th Periodic Report by the Russian Federation for the 62nd Session of the Committee on Economic, Social and Cultural Rights.

Dehlin, J. P., Galliher, R. V., Bradshaw, W. S., Hyde, D. C., & Crowell, K. A. (2015). Sexual orientation change efforts among current or former LDS church members. *Journal of Counseling Psychology, 62*(2), 95–105. https://doi.org/10.1037/cou0000011

Desert Stream/Living Waters Ministries. (2021). *Recommended friends.* https://desertstream.org/recommend-friends/

Drescher, J. (2015). Out of *DSM*: Depathologizing homosexuality. *Behavioral Sciences, 5*(4), 565–575. https://doi.org/10.3390/bs5040565

Exodus Asia Pacific. (2021). *Welcome to Exodus Asia Pacific.* https://www.exodusglobalalliance.org/exodusasiapacifics283.php

Exodus East Asia. (2008). A new region is formed. *World News.* Exodus Global Alliance.

Exodus Global Alliance. (2021a). *About Exodus.* https://www.exodusglobalalliance.org/aboutexoduss4.php

Exodus Global Alliance. (2021b). *How we began.* https://www.exodusglobalalliance.org/howwegotstartedc88.php

Flentje, A., Heck, N. C., & Cochran, B. N. (2013). Sexual reorientation therapy interventions: Perspectives of ex-ex-gay individuals. *Journal of Gay & Lesbian Mental Health, 17*(3), 256–277. https://doi.org/10.1080/19359705.2013.773268

Freeman-Coppadge, D., & Horne, S. G. (2019). "What happens if the cross falls and crushes me?" Psychological and spiritual promises and perils of lesbian and gay Christian celibacy. *Psychology of Sexual Orientation and Gender Diversity, 6*(4), 486–497. https://doi.org/10.1037/sgd0000341

Glauert, R. (2019, January 10). *In China, at least 130 places still offer LGBTI conversion therapy.* GayStarNews. https://www.gaystarnews.com/article/in-china-at-least-130-places-still-offer-lgbti-conversion-therapy/#gs.5svr8w

Global Philanthropy Project. (2018). *Religious conservatism on the global stage: Threats and challenges for LGBTI rights.* https://globalphilanthropyproject.org/2018/11/04/religious-conservatism-on-the-global-stage-threats-and-challenges-for-lgbti-rights/

Golubeva, A. (2017). *Hypnosis and holy water: Russian cures for gay people.* BBC News. https://www.bbc.com/news/world-europe-39777612

Harris, G. (2013, December 11). India's supreme court restores an 1861 law banning gay sex. *The New York Times.* https://www.nytimes.com/2013/12/12/world/asia/court-restores-indias-ban-on-gay-sex.html?module=inline

Henrich, J., Heine, S. J., & Norenzayan, A. (2010). The weirdest people in the world? *Behavioral and Brain Sciences, 33*(2–3), 61–83. https://doi.org/10.1017/S0140525X0999152X

Hinsch, B. (1990). *Passions of the Cut Sleeve: The male homosexual tradition in China.* University of California Press.

Horne, S. G. (2020). The challenges and promises of transnational LGBTQ psychology: Somewhere over and under the rainbow. *American Psychologist, 75*(9), 1358–1371. https://doi.org/10.1037/amp0000791

Horne, S. G., & Manalastas, E. J. (2020). Psychology and the global human rights agenda on sexual orientation and gender identity. In N. S. Rubin & R. L. Flores (Eds.), *The Cambridge handbook of psychology and human rights* (pp. 332–345). Cambridge University Press. https://doi.org/10.1017/9781108348607.023

Horne, S. G., Maroney, M. R., Nel, J. A., Chaparro, R. A., & Manalastas, E. J. (2019). Emergence of a transnational LGBTI psychology: Commonalities and challenges in advocacy and activism. *American Psychologist, 74*(8), 967–986. https://doi.org/10.1037/amp0000561

Horne, S. G., Maroney, M. R., Wheeler, E., & Peters, S. (2020). *The psychological development of LGBTQ activists* [Unpublished manuscript].

Horne, S. G., Maroney, M. R., Zagryazhskaya, E. A., & Koven, J. (2017). Attitudes toward gay and lesbian individuals in Russia: An exploration of the interpersonal contact hypothesis and personality factor. *Psychology in Russia, 10*(2), 21–34. https://doi.org/10.11621/pir.2017.0202

Horne, S. G., Ovrebo, E., Levitt, H. M., & Franeta, S. (2009). Leaving the herd: The lingering threat of difference for same-sex identities in postcommunist Russia. *Sexuality Research & Social Policy, 6*(2), 108–122. https://doi.org/10.1525/srsp.2009.6.2.88

Horne, S. G., & White, L. (2019). The return of repression: Mental health concerns of lesbian, gay, bisexual, and transgender people in Russia. In N. Nakamura & C. H. Logie (Eds.), *LGBTQ mental health: International perspectives and experiences* (pp. 75–88). American Psychological Association.

Human Rights Watch. (2017, November 14). *"Have you considered your parents' happiness?" Conversion therapy against LGBT people in China.* https://www.hrw.org/report/2017/11/15/have-you-considered-your-parents-happiness/conversion-therapy-against-lgbt-people

International Psychology Network for Lesbian, Gay, Bisexual, Transgender and Intersex Issues. (2018). *IPsyNet statement on LGBTQ concerns.* https://www.apa.org/ipsynet/advocacy/policy/statement-english.pdf

Kuhar, R., & Paternotte, D. (Eds.). (2017). *Anti-ge nder campaigns in Europe: Mobilizing against equality.* Rowman & Littlefield.

Lane, P. (2021). *God's call into ministry.* Exodus Global Alliance. https://www.exodusglobalalliance.org/godscallintoministryp15.php

Laurent, E. (2005). Sexuality and human rights: An Asian perspective. *Journal of Homosexuality, 48*(3–4), 163–225. https://doi.org/10.1300/J082v48n03_09

Lausanne Movement. (2011). *The Cape Town Commitment.* https://www.lausanne.org/content/ctc/ctcommitment

Lease, S., Horne, S. G., & Noffsinger-Frazier, N. (2005). Affirming faith experiences and psychological health for Caucasian lesbian, gay, and bisexual individuals. *Journal of Counseling Psychology, 52,* 378–388. https://doi-org.ezproxy.lib.umb.edu/10.1037/0022-0167.52.3.378

LGBT Foundation. (2019). *National LGBT survey: Summary report.* https://www.gov.uk/government/publications/national-lgbt-survey-summary-report/national-lgbt-survey-summary-report#the-results

Lopes, M. (2018, October 26). "More than fear": Brazil's LGBT community dreads looming Bolsonaro presidency. *The Washington Post.* https://www.washingtonpost.com/world/the_americas/more-than-fear-brazils-lgbt-community-dreads-looming-bolsonaro-presidency/2018/10/26/c9e7ac26-d890-11e8-a10f-b51546b10756_story.html

Mail Today. (2015a, May 27). Delhi doctors busted for trying to "cure" gays [Television series episode]. *India Today.* https://www.indiatoday.in/india/video/delhi-doctors-homosexuals-heterosexuals-gays-429797-2015-05-27

Mail Today. (2015b, May 27). Delhi doctors use hormone therapy, electric shock to treat homosexuality [Television series episode]. *India Today.* https://www.indiatoday.in/india/video/gay-cure-racket-delhi-doctors-homosexuality-lgbt-queers-429786-2015-05-27

Mallory, C., Brown, T. N. T., & Conron, K. J. (2019). *Conversion therapy and LGBT youth.* Williams Institute. https://williamsinstitute.law.ucla.edu/publications/conversion-therapy-and-lgbt-youth/

Manalastas, E. J., & Torre, B. A. (2016). LGBT psychology in the Philippines. *Psychology of Sexualities Review, 7*(1), 60–72.

McGinley, M., & Horne, S. G. (2020). An ethics of inclusion: Recommendations for LGBTI research, training, and practice. *Psychology in Russia, 13*(1), 54–69. https://doi.org/10.11621/pir.2020.0106

Memorandum of Understanding on Conversion Therapy in the UK, version 2. (2017). https://www.psychotherapy.org.uk/media/cptnc5qm/mou2-reva_0421_web.pdf

Mendos, L. R. (December, 2019). *State-sponsored homophobia 2019: Global legislation overview update.* International Lesbian, Gay, Bisexual, Trans, and Intersex Association (ILGA) World. https://ilga.org/state-sponsored-homophobia-report-2019-global-legislation-overview

Minister under attack for remarks on LGBT. (2015, January 13). In *Gulf Times.* https://www.gulf-times.com/story/423158/Minister-under-attack-for-remarks-on-LGBT

Morais, R. (2017, September 21). *"Cura gay": Juiz que proibiu punição a quem propõe tratamento nega ver homossexualidade como doença ["Gay cure": Judge who forbade punishment for those who propose treatment denies seeing homosexuality as a disease].* https://g1.globo.com/distrito-federal/noticia/cura-gay-juiz-que-proibiu-punicao-a-quem-propoe-tratamento-nega-ver-homossexuidade-como-doenca.ghtml

Murphy, T. (2013, June 28). *Brazilian evangelical lawmakers push gay conversion therapy bill* [Web log post]. Political Research Associates. https://www.politicalresearch.org/2013/06/28/brazilian-evangelical-lawmakers-push-gay-conversion-therapy-bill/

Nelson, D. (2009, July 8). Hindu guru claims homosexuality can be "cured" by yoga. *The Telegraph.* https://www.telegraph.co.uk/news/worldnews/asia/india/5780028/Hindu-guru-claims-homosexuality-can-be-cured-by-yoga.html

OutRight Action International. (2019). *Harmful treatment: The global reach of so-called conversion therapy.* https://outrightinternational.org/sites/default/files/ConversionFINAL_Web_0.pdf

Paletta, D., & Goodwin, L. (2017, September 19). *Brazil: Judge overturns ban on "conversion" therapy* [Web log post]. International Lesbian, Gay, Bisexual, Trans and Intersex Association (ILGA). https://ilga.org/lgbti-news-102-ilga-sep-2017

Pan American Health Organization. (2012). *"Cures" for an illness that does not exist: Purported therapies aimed at changing sexual orientation lack medical justification and are ethically unacceptable.* https://www.paho.org/hq/dmdocuments/2012/Conversion-Therapies-EN.pdf

Phillips, D. (2017, September 19). Brazilian judge approves "gay conversion therapy," sparking national outrage. *The Guardian.* https://www.theguardian.com/world/2017/sep/19/brazilian-judge-approves-gay-conversion-therapy

Pratap, A. (2018, June 6). Stop considering homosexuality as an illness: Psychiatric society to members. *Hindustan Times.* https://www.hindustantimes.com/india-news/stop-considering-homosexuality-as-an-illness-psychiatric-society-to-members/story-3ABklOaHu935ZmXuK1QxxL.html

Psychological Society of South Africa. (2017). *Practice guidelines for psychology professionals working with sexually and gender-diverse people.* https://www.psyssa.com/practice-guidelines-for-psychology-professionals-working-with-sexually-and-gender-diverse-people/

Queiroz, J., D'Elio, F., & Maas, D. (2013). *The ex-gay movement in Latin America: Therapy and ministry in the Exodus network.* Political Research Associates. https://

www.politicalresearch.org/sites/default/files/2018-10/Ex-Gay-Movement-in-Latin-America.pdf

Raj, S., & Najar, N. (2015, January 13). State in India plans to help gay youth "get over same-sex feelings." *The New York Times.* https://www.nytimes.com/2015/01/14/world/asia/indian-goa-program-counsel-gay-youths-to-become-straight.html

Ramdev offers to "cure homosexuals" at his Haridwar ashram. (2013, December 11). *Hindustan Times.* https://www.hindustantimes.com/india/ramdev-offers-to-cure-homosexuals-at-his-haridwar-ashram/story-UtnktIHM8qAdT5NKbG7QsO.html

Respect for Life India. (n.d.). *Our activities; Counselling.* http://respectforlifeindia.org/activities_co.html

Reynolds, E., & Cotovio, V. (2020, May 19). *Hungary bans people from legally changing gender.* CNN. https://www.cnn.com/2020/05/19/europe/hungary-trans-legal-recognition-intl/index.html

Robinson, C. M., & Spivey, S. E. (2007). The politics of masculinity and the ex-gay movement. *Gender and Society, 21*(5), 650–675. https://www.jstor.org/stable/27641004

Robinson, C. M., & Spivey, S. E. (2015). Putting lesbians in their place: Deconstructing ex-gay discourses of female homosexuality in a global context. *Social Sciences, 4*(3), 879–908. https://doi.org/10.3390/socsci4030879

Rodrigues, M., & Morais, R. (2017, December 15). *Juiz federal do DF altera decisão que liberou "cura gay" e reafirma normas do Conselho de Psicologia* [*Judge of the Federal District changes the decision that released "gay cure" and reaffirms norms of the Council of Psychology*]. https://g1.globo.com/df/distrito-federal/noticia/juiz-federal-do-df-altera-decisao-que-liberou-cura-gay-e-restabelece-normas-do-conselho-de-psicologia.ghtml

Sebastian, S., & Vikram, K. (2015, May 27). Mail Today exclusive: Delhi doctors use electric shock to treat homosexuality. *India Today.* https://www.indiatoday.in/mail-today/story/homosexuality-cure-delhi-doctors-exposed-conversion-therapy-254849-2015-05-27

Sleptcov, N. (2018). Political homophobia as a state strategy in Russia. *Journal of Global Initiatives: Policy, Pedagogy, Perspective, 12*(1), 140–161.

Southern Poverty Law Center. (2021). *Extremist files: Scott Lively.* https://www.splcenter.org/fighting-hate/extremist-files/individual/scott-lively

Spivey, S. E., & Robinson, C. M. (2010). Genocidal intentions: Social death and the ex-gay movement. *Genocide Studies and Prevention, 5*(1), 68–88. https://doi.org/10.3138/gsp.5.1.68

Szpacenkopf, M., & Guerra, R. (2017, September 18). *Justice allows psychologists to treat homosexuality as a disease.* O Globo: Sociedade. https://oglobo.globo.com/sociedade/justica-permite-que-psicologos-tratem-homossexualidade-como-doenca-21838339#ixzz4tAN6b2od

Tait, R. (2017, May 26). *Hungary's prime minister welcomes U.S. anti-LGBT hate group.* The Guardian. https://www.theguardian.com/world/2017/may/26/hungary-lgbt-world-congress-families-viktor-orban

Taylor, J. (2019, January 18). *Artist and policeman launch "three billboards" campaign against conversion therapy in China.* Newnownext.com. http://www.newnownext.com/china-conversion-therapy-protest/01/2019/

Thoreson, R. R. (2014). *Transnational LGBT activism: Working for sexual rights worldwide.* University of Minnesota Press. https://doi.org/10.5749/minnesota/9780816692712.001.0001

Timmons, H., & Kumar, H. (2009, July 2). Indian court overturns gay sex ban. *The New York Times*. https://www.nytimes.com/2009/07/03/world/asia/03india.html?module=inline

Turban, J. L., Beckwith, N., Reisner, S. L., & Keuroghlian, A. S. (2020). Association between recalled exposure to gender identity conversion efforts and psychological distress and suicide attempts among transgender adults. *JAMA Psychiatry*, *77*(1), 68–76. https://doi.org/10.1001/jamapsychiatry.2019.2285

Turban, J. L., King, D., Reisner, S. L., & Keuroghlian, A. S. (2019). Psychological attempts to change a person's gender identity from transgender to cisgender: Estimated prevalence across US states, 2015. *American Journal of Public Health*, *109*(10), 1452–1454. https://doi.org/10.2105/ajph.2019.305237

United Kingdom Government. (2021, May 21). *Government sets out plan to ban conversion therapy*. https://www.gov.uk/government/news/government-sets-out-plan-to-ban-conversion-therapy

United Kingdom Government Equalities Office. (2019, February 7). *National LGBT survey: Summary report*. https://www.gov.uk/government/publications/national-lgbt-survey-summary-report/national-lgbt-survey-summary-report

United Nations. (2015). *Ending violence and discrimination against lesbian, gay, bisexual, transgender and intersex people*. https://www.ohchr.org/Documents/Issues/Discrimination/Joint_LGBTI_Statement_ENG.PDF

United Nations. (2018). *Report of the Independent Expert on protection against violence and discrimination based on sexual orientation and gender identity*. Human Rights Council Thirty-eighth session (Report A/HRC/38/43). https://www.ohchr.org/Documents/Issues/SexualOrientation/ConversionTherapyReport.pdf

United Nations Development Programme. (2018, December 18). *The sustainable development goals: Sexual and gender minorities*. http://www.undp.org/content/undp/en/home/librarypage/hiv-aids/sexual-and-gender-minorities.html

United Nations High Commissioner for Human Rights. (2015). *Discrimination and violence against individuals based on their sexual orientation and gender identity* (Report A/HRC/29/23). http://www.un.org/en/ga/search/view_doc.asp?symbol=A/HRC/29/23&referer=/english/&Lang=E

United Nations Human Rights Council. (2020). *Practices of so-called "conversion therapy."* (Report A/HRC/44/53). https://daccess-ods.un.org/access.nsf/Get?Open&DS=A/HRC/44/53&Lang=E

Vasilyeva, N. (2019, January 11). *Reports: Several gay men and women detained in Chechnya*. Associated Press. https://apnews.com/article/88929f353d494b3a87843002d02ad155

Wang, Y., Hu, Z., Peng, K., Xin, Y., Yang, Y., Drescher, J., & Chen, R. (2019). Discrimination against LGBT populations in China. *Lancet Public Health*, *4*(9), e440–e441.

Withnall, A. (2018, July 14). India on brink of biggest gay rights victory as Supreme Court prepares to rule on gay sex ban. *The Independent*. https://www.independent.co.uk/news/world/asia/india-gay-rights-lgbt-homosexuality-supreme-court-decision-section-377-a8447361.html

World Professional Association for Transgender Health. (2011). *Standards of care for the health of transsexual, transgender, and gender nonconforming people*. https://www.wpath.org/media/cms/Documents/Web%20Transfer/SOC/Standards%20of%20Care%20V7%20-%202011%20WPATH.pdf

EPILOGUE

DOUGLAS C. HALDEMAN

What does it mean for a mental health provider or pastoral counselor to attempt to change someone's sexual orientation or gender identity, and what are the possible outcomes of such attempts? In this book, we have seen that both sexual orientation change efforts (SOCE) and gender identity change efforts (GICE) stem from a socially constructed devaluation of same-sex attraction and behavior and gender nonconformity rooted in a heterocentric, cisgender paradigm. SOCE and GICE bypass a thoughtful exploration of why a person might wish—or why parents might wish for their child—to conform to a social standard that bears little relevance to the individual's experience. That process—with a practitioner-determined agenda, aided and abetted by a client who is likely suffering from internalized shame—is not how therapy is intended to work. Additionally, there is ample evidence to suggest that SOCE and GICE can contravene professional ethics by harming people.

Clearly, as long as the heterocentric and cisgender values enshrined by some political perspectives and organized religions continue, these dangerous and discredited practices will continue. SOCE residential camps have proliferated over the course of the past decade, and evidence suggests that the aversive methods of old have not disappeared but have simply gone

https://doi.org/10.1037/0000266-012
The Case Against Conversion "Therapy": Evidence, Ethics, and Alternatives,
D. C. Haldeman (Editor)

underground. The situation with GICE may be even more dire, as noted by Glassgold and Ryan in Chapter 4 of this volume, indicating that those youth obliged to undergo efforts to change their gender identities are at a significantly greater risk of attempting suicide. Despite these warnings, much remains unchanged about the mindset of those who conduct SOCE and GICE in their misguided efforts to create a straight, cisgender society. So where do we go now?

Although much remains the same (albeit sometimes in careful repackaging) with the SOCE and GICE industries, much has changed. A recent study by the Williams Institute indicates that 56% of adults now oppose the use of SOCE with minors (Mallory et al., 2019). This finding suggests that the significant amount of visibility and public criticisms of these potentially dangerous practices has raised public awareness and shifted public opinion. Thus, continued efforts to educate the public—through the dissemination of new research findings and strengthened social policy based on such research—are more important than ever.

Perhaps no area of this national discussion is more critical than the experiences of transgender, genderfluid, and nonconforming individuals— particularly persons of color. "Trans-panic"-style legislation attempting to force transgender and gender nonconforming (TGNC) persons into using the bathrooms designated for their natal sex, an executive order prohibiting TGNC persons from military service, trans persons being murdered on a near-weekly basis, and other examples have emerged as signs of the severity of this problem. TGNC youth are at significantly elevated risk for suicide attempt and completion. TGNC youth are put at significant risk for adverse health effects by attempting to force them into presenting and behaving in ways that are inconsistent with their feelings. We know we should not be using GICE, so what should we be doing for TGNC youth and/or their parents instead?

For children, the most ethical and effective therapeutic solution—at least given what we know now—may be to do nothing. Research indicates that the vast majority of gender nonconforming children will not go on to endorse a transgender identity. Allowing them the freedom to simply explore and be themselves—critical developmental tasks in childhood—minimizes the risk of doing harm while allowing parents and health care providers to provide social and emotional support. In addition, TGNC kids who choose to socially transition often benefit from an "environmental scan" to determine the relative safety of the social context that enables parents, school personnel, and health care providers to advocate systemically on their behalf. Counseling should be supportive and nondirective. Other models of counseling, including the facilitation of social transition at a very early age and the use of prepubertal hormone blockers, show promise from initial research. One study shows a significant inverse relationship between the use of hormone blockers and suicidality in TGNC kids (Turban et al., 2020). Other studies indicate that hormone blockers are safe and reversible; in any case, more research is needed in this area. For TGNC adults, supportive, nondirective counseling is also best. A host of complexities relative to transition (and the degree thereof), housing and employment, family and support system, and physical well-being may be profitably addressed in treatment.

SOCE are also dangerous for youth and should never be used (American Psychological Association, 2021). But how should we address the needs of adults who are attracted to the same sex and who believe that "gay is just not me"? As noted in the 2009 American Psychological Association report, a variety of methods to explore internal conflict between sexual orientation and personal belief systems do not involve SOCE. One important method employs classic person-centered psychotherapy along with psychoeducation about options for integrating sexual orientation with more compatible belief systems or religious affiliations. A corollary recommendation involves conducting a thoughtful inquiry into the person's motivations behind seeking SOCE. Invariably, those factors (e.g., choice of religious identification) are far easier to change than is sexual orientation.

Research efforts in this area have been notoriously difficult for two reasons. First, it is difficult to base meaningful conclusions on research that uses convenience samples. This concern is diminishing, however, as more population-based studies with robust data are published. We are beginning to see population-based studies of those who have undergone SOCE (Blosnich et al., 2020; Green et al., 2020). These studies indicate that SOCE are indeed as harmful as we have thought, given the adverse mental health effects reported by SOCE participants. Second, continued support for research on issues related to sexuality and gender are crucial. Nonetheless, it is incumbent on those conducting research in this area to stop supporting the continued use of SOCE based on the argument that it has yet to be "proven" harmful. Instead, they should attempt to prove that it isn't; or better yet, stop research on the benefits of SOCE altogether.

Finally, the legislative, regulatory, and judicial arenas are those in which SOCE and GICE are likely to see the most activity in coming years. As noted in this book, scientific evidence, public opinion, and social policy have created seismic changes since California adopted the first SOCE ban in 2012. As of this writing, 20 states plus the District of Columbia have prohibited licensed mental health professionals from conducting SOCE (and, in some places, GICE). The Trevor Project's (2021) 50 Bills 50 States campaign has been instrumental in this regard. However, most of the jurisdictions that have adopted this ban are politically in the "deep blue" category, which means that the climb toward 50 at this point swings sharply uphill. To bypass the recalcitrance of conservative lawmakers in banning SOCE/GICE, advocacy and professional groups in many (more conservative) places are turning to regulatory agencies, such as state boards of psychology, psychiatry, and counseling, for amendments to their states' licensing laws.

To date, courts have dismissed legal challenges to anti-SOCE/anti-GICE legislation. In one case, SOCE was found to be a form of consumer fraud. This judgment not only earned the complainants compensation for pain and suffering but also put the SOCE organization in question out of business. This judgment served as the basis for a recent effort in the California legislature to label all SOCE as a form of consumer fraud.

But despite the major gains that the courts have delivered to the lesbian, gay, bisexual, transgender, and questioning or queer (LGBTQ) community over the past years, we cannot take the judiciary's support as a given. The case of *Masterpiece Cakeshop, Ltd. v. Colorado Civil Rights Commission* (2018) demonstrated that the Supreme Court's recent tack to the right may jeopardize any and all of the hard-fought gains toward LGBTQ equality. Despite passage by both houses of the California state legislature and virtual assurance of the governor's signature, the SOCE Consumer Fraud Act was pulled before it become law—by the bill's own sponsor. Apparently, this lawmaker had learned that not only this (new) legislation but all other pro-LGBTQ legislation was threatened by renewed appeals from far-right legal organizations that hope to benefit from a newly conservative U.S. Supreme Court.

In 1975, Begelman observed, "[Conversion therapies] by their very existence constitute a significant causal element in reinforcing the social doctrine that homosexuality is bad; therapists . . . further strengthen the prejudice that homosexuality is a 'problem behavior,' since treatment may be offered for it" (p. 180). Forty-five years later, the SOCE and GICE industries are alive and well. The Williams Institute (2018) estimates that every year some 20,000 youth will undergo a form of SOCE/GICE with a licensed mental health provider before the age of 18 and that an additional 57,000 will receive such interventions from a pastoral counselor or clergy person.

SOCE and GICE are maintained by social and cultural stigma that devalues same-sex attraction and nonbinary gender identities. In 1994, I wrote,

> Psychology cannot free people from stigma by continuing to support or tacitly endorse conversion therapy. Psychology can only combat stigma with a vigorous avowal of empirical truth. The appropriate focus of the profession is what reverses prejudice, not what reverses sexual orientation. (Haldeman, 1994, p. 226)

We hope that this book will serve to inform the ongoing battle to protect our LGBTQ community and its future generations. In these days of straight and cisgender supremacy, combating the stigma that serves as the foundation for SOCE and GICE is more than a goal to which health care professionals should aspire—it is also an ethical mandate.

The LGBT community has gained increased visibility since I wrote those words so many years ago, and we have seen a concomitant positive shift in public opinion. At one time, lesbian and gay characters in film and television were a rarity; now, in many major media markets, same-sex couples are featured in advertisements for everything from car insurance to laundry detergent. We are also seeing a similar visibility of and support for TGNC persons. Trans characters, played by trans actors, are featured in movies and television. Numerous corporations promote trans-positive policies, and an increasing number of jurisdictions protect TGNC persons from discrimination in housing and employment.

However, none of this progress should lull us into a false sense of security that we can rest in our advocacy for competent treatment of LGBT individuals. The cultural backlash against progress in LGBT equality mirrors the larger national conversations about race and immigration, in which we see that the so-called culture wars in our polarized society are intensifying. With the rise of theocratic ideology that enshrines bigotry so long as it is justified in scriptural terms, and an increasingly conservative judiciary, it is our duty to remember that the best weapons we have in this fight are what we know best: evidence, effects, and alternatives.

REFERENCES

American Psychological Association. (2021). *Policy on sexual orientation change efforts*.

Begelman, D. A. (1975). Ethical and legal issues of behavior modification. In M. Hersen, R. Eisler, & P. M. Miller (Eds.), *Progress in behavior modification* (pp. 175–188). Academic Press.

Blosnich, J. R., Henderson, E. R., Coulter, R. W. S., Goldbach, J. T., & Meyer, I. H. (2020). Sexual orientation change efforts, adverse childhood experiences, and suicide ideation and attempt among sexual minority adults, United States, 2016–2018. *American Journal of Public Health, 110*(7), 1024–1030. https://doi.org/10.2105/AJPH.2020.305637

Green, A. E., Price-Feeney, M., Dorison, S. H., & Pick, C. J. (2020). Self-reported conversion efforts and suicidality among US LGBTQ youths and young adults, 2018. *American Journal of Public Health, 110*(8), 1221–1227. https://doi.org/10.2105/AJPH.2020.305701

Haldeman, D. C. (1994). The practice and ethics of sexual orientation conversion therapy. *Journal of Consulting and Clinical Psychology, 62*(2), 221–227. https://doi.org/10.1037/0022-006X.62.2.221

Mallory, C., Brown, T., & Conron, K. (2019). *Update: Conversion therapy and LGBT youth*. The Williams Institute. https://williamsinstitute.law.ucla.edu/demographics/conversion-therapy-and-lgbt-youth/

Masterpiece Cakeshop, Ltd. v. Colorado Civil Rights Commission, 584 U.S. __ (2018). https://www.supremecourt.gov/opinions/17pdf/16-111_j4el.pdf

The Trevor Project. (2021). *50 Bills 50 States*. https://www.thetrevorproject.org/get-involved/trevor-advocacy/50-bills-50-states/

Turban, J. L., King, D., Carswell, J. M., & Keuroghlian, A. S. (2020). Pubertal suppression for Transgender youth and risk of suicidal ideation. *Pediatrics, 145*(2), e20191725. https://doi.org/10.1542/peds.2019-1725

Williams Institute. (2018). *More than 20,000 teens will be subjected to conversion therapy*. https://williamsinstitute.law.ucla.edu/press/conversion-therapy-release/

Index

About the Editor

Douglas C. Haldeman, PhD, is chair of the doctoral program in clinical psychology at John F. Kennedy University in Pleasant Hill, California, where he is also a professor of assessment. He was in full-time independent practice for 30 years in Seattle, Washington, primarily working with the lesbian, gay, bisexual, and transgender (LGBT) communities. He has also worked extensively with the American Psychological Association on policy and guideline development, as well as having served on a number of APA boards and committees, the Council of Representatives, the Council Leadership Team, and the Board of Directors. Dr. Haldeman served as chair of the Board of the American Insurance Trust, is a member of the board of the American Psychological Foundation, and is a past president of the California Psychological Association. Since 1991, Dr. Haldeman has published numerous articles and book chapters critiquing so-called "conversion therapy" and has advocated in state legislatures for laws to prohibit these practices. He is currently developing mental health programs for LGBT asylum seekers who are fleeing countries where same-sex behavior is criminalized.